Health Informatics: A Systems Perspective

Health Informatics: A Systems Perspective

Editor: Patrick Garter

AMERICAN
MEDICAL PUBLISHERS
www.americanmedicalpublishers.com

AMERICAN
MEDICAL PUBLISHERS
www.americanmedicalpublishers.com

Cataloging-in-Publication Data

Health informatics : a systems perspective / edited by Patrick Garter.
p. cm.
Includes bibliographical references and index.
ISBN 978-1-63927-690-5
1. Medical informatics. 2. Medicine--Data processing.
3. Information storage and retrieval systems--Medicine.
4. Information storage and retrieval systems--Health.
I. Garter, Patrick.
R858 .H45 2023
610.285--dc23

American Medical Publishers,
41 Flatbush Avenue,
1st Floor, New York,
NY 11217, USA

ISBN 978-1-63927-690-5 (Hardback)

Contents

Preface

The purpose of the book is to provide a glimpse into the dynamics and to present opinions and studies of some of the scientists engaged in the development of new ideas in the field from very different standpoints. This book will prove useful to students and researchers owing to its high content quality.

Health informatics is the intersection of computer science, information science and health care. Its aim is to develop technologies and methods for processing, acquisition and study of patient data. This data is derived from various sources and modalities including medical scans, electronic health records and diagnostic test results. The healthcare sector faces multiple difficulties, which can be resolved or managed using computational techniques. Health informatics is a multidisciplinary field that involves the design and development of computational innovations for improving health care. It uses data, knowledge, and information for delivery and improvement of healthcare services, while enhancing the patient outcomes. Data analysis involves collecting, processing, and interpreting data, while informatics involves applying the information derived from analysis. The purpose of health informatics is to derive conclusions from healthcare information and support in decision-making. This book provides significant information to help develop a good understanding of health informatics. It presents researches and studies performed by experts across the globe. The extensive content of this book provides the readers with a systems perspective on the subject.

At the end, I would like to appreciate all the efforts made by the authors in completing their chapters professionally. I express my deepest gratitude to all of them for contributing to this book by sharing their valuable works. A special thanks to my family and friends for their constant support in this journey.

Editor

1

Analysis of Emergency Medical Vulnerability and Survival Rates Following Real-Time Traffic Information

Jeongbae Jeon [1], Solhee Kim [2], Gu Hyun Kang [3] and Kyo Suh [4,*]

1 Spatial Information Research Institute, Korea Land and Geospatial Informatix Corporation, Jeonju 54870, Korea; jbjeon@lx.or.kr
2 Interdisciplinary Program in Agricultural and Forest Meteorology, College of Agriculture and Life Sciences, Seoul National University, Seoul 08826, Korea; solhee1101@snu.ac.kr
3 Department of Emergency Medicine, KangNam Medical Center, College of Medicine, Hallym University, Seoul 07441, Korea; emkang@hallym.or.kr
4 Graduate School of International Agricultural Technology, Institute of Green Bio Science Technology, Seoul National University, Pyeongchang 25354, Korea
* Correspondence: kyosuh@snu.ac.kr

Abstract: Providing rapid access to emergency medical services (EMS) within the "golden time" for survival is important to improve the survival rate of emergency patients. This study analyzes the accessibility of EMS based on driving speed changes following real-time road traffic conditions by time to estimate vulnerable areas for EMS and survival rates of emergency patients. The key results of the network analysis based on real-time road speed and this evaluation of vulnerable areas by village level across South Korea reveal the different characteristics of urban and rural areas to access emergency medical facilities. In urban areas, road traffic congestion during rush hour delays the patients' access time to EMS. In contrast, in rural areas, the long geographical distance to an emergency medical facility is a hurdle for receiving care from an EMS during the "golden time" because emergency medical facilities are mostly located in urban areas. The existing standard to assess vulnerable areas of EMS accessibility is based on the speed limit of roads, but the time may be underestimated because the speed limit alone does not reflect the real road conditions. The study results show that an effective way to increase the survival rate is receiving immediate first aid treatment, which means that the government should continuously train the public to perform cardiopulmonary resuscitation (CPR) as well as install automated external defibrillators (AEDs) in populated places, and train the public to use them. Reducing assess time to emergency medical centers in urban areas and providing additional manpower to help with first aid in rural areas are reasonable ways to improve the survival rate of emergency patients.

Keywords: emergency medical service; accessibility; vulnerability; survival rate; golden time; real-time; network

1. Introduction

Rapid access to emergency medical facilities within the "golden time" as well as prompt and appropriate first aid are essential factors to improve the survival rate of emergency patients [1–4]. The emergency medical services (EMS) system enables manpower, facilities, and equipment to be organically operated to effectively and quickly provide medical care in emergencies [5]. The EMS system is divided into the pre-hospital and in-hospital phases depending on the place before and after receiving help from an EMS. In the pre-hospital phase, emergency responders provide appropriate first aid to patients onsite before promptly and safely transferring the patient to a hospital for treatment [6]. In the pre-hospital phase, accessibility to EMS is evaluated by the time and distance to arrive at the best EMS facility in a short time, mainly considering the available EMS resources and the transfer time [7]. The method used to evaluate accessibility to EMS considers service availability, population coverage, and time-based geographic delivery of emergency services.

Differences in the locational distribution of emergency medical facilities in urban and rural areas also need to be considered to improve accessibility to EMS in vulnerable areas [8–11]. Among Organization for Economic Cooperation and Development (OECD) countries, the accessibility and mobility of medical services in Korea are generally evaluated as excellent based on a statistical evaluation with a high rate of receiving medical service benefits per person [12]. However, medical facilities and manpower are concentrated in urban areas [13]. As of 2019, most medical centers (3699 medical facilities including general hospitals and clinics) were concentrated in cities (90.4% of general hospitals, 85.2% of common hospitals, and 88.8% of clinics), indicating that there is a broad gap in medical service quality between urban and rural areas [14]. Unlike cities, poor medical access in rural areas makes the transfer distance and time to emergency medical facilities longer.

Emergency situations occur more frequently among the elderly. For conditions such as cardiovascular diseases and respiratory diseases, rapid first aid significantly affects the survival rates of patients [15]. For the elderly in Korea, deaths from cardiovascular and cerebrovascular diseases that require immediate first aid have increased by about 63% in the last 10 years (from 15 thousands in 2006 to 24 thousands in 2016), and the ratio has increased annually by about 6% for the last 10 years [16]. The aging population rate of rural areas (23.1% as of 2019) is more than twice as high as that of urban areas (10.9%) [17]. The rapid pace of aging compared to urban areas also makes it more likely that emergencies with a high risk of death will occur in rural areas. Thus, poor medical facilities and aging in rural areas further widen the gap of preventable or amendable mortality between rural and urban areas [7,18].

New methods such as calculating the traffic flow speed and dispatch time of emergency medical technician-paramedics (EMT-P) in real time to determine the appropriate response time to an emergency situation are very effective in identifying vulnerable areas for EMS based on practical accessibility [19]. Korean government defines vulnerable areas for EMS as areas where the local EMS center cannot be reached within 30 min or residents cannot reach a regional emergency medical center within 60 min [20]. This standard was revised in 2017 to apply the concept of the golden time to accessible time based on the accessibility to emergency medical facilities for a population of less than 150,000 in a rural area. The time to reach an emergency medical facility is calculated as the time required from where patient's emergency occurred to a local/regional emergency medical center by mainly calculating the time based on the legal speed limit of the roads. Using this standard, 99 administrative districts (Si, Gun, and Gu) across the country in Korea (approximately 44%) could not receive EMS within the appropriate time [19]. However, the number of vulnerable areas for EMS increases if the real-time traffic conditions to reach the emergency medical facility are considered. In addition, the dispatch time by an emergency medical technician (e.g., the EMT-P or ambulance workers from the 119-safety center) who can provide first aid should also be considered. In particular, an evaluation of time-based accessibility is an essential requirement considering real-time road conditions by region, because the survival rate could vary significantly depending on whether or not rapid first aid is given in emergencies, such as an acute cardiac arrest.

Many studies on accessibility to medical or healthcare-related facilities have been conducted in various fields based on physical distance to identify vulnerable areas [21–25]. However, few related studies have used real-time traffic flow as well as driving speed data. Studies related to accessibility have mainly based the calculations on the physical distance, such as the Euclidean distance (linear distance), the estimated road distance using a circuity factor, and the actual road distance [26–34]. However, Kim [13] and Li [35] pointed out that the linear distance is more likely to result in excessive distortion compared to actual road distances because the linear distance does not reflect the geographical features such as the terrain or road geometry. Kim [13] suggested that calculating the estimated road distance by applying circuity factors to linear distance could be a substitute for the actual road distance for the vulnerability assessment of access to medical facilities. Studies on accessible vulnerability using physical distance have recently improved, and now estimate the accessible time using data about the shape of the road network and legal speed limit provided by the Korean government [36]. However, calculating accessibility using the speed limit of the road has limitations since it does not reflect the effects of slower vehicle speed during traffic jams or traffic signals.

The goal of this study is to analyze EMS accessibility using real-time road traffic conditions with driving speed changes by time of day and to estimate the vulnerable areas and survival rate of emergency patients. We also compare the results of urban areas and rural areas. For this purpose, we established a nationwide road network map across Korea to identify the current status of road use distribution following real road speed flow by time. In addition, we evaluated vulnerable areas for EMS by estimating the real-time access time via an optimal route from a village to an emergency medical facility using network analysis. We set up four cases according to the patient transfer process to an EMS facility, considering whether the patient receives first aid or not, and the dispatch time of an EMT-P. We also examined the changes in the survival probability for each case in urban areas compared to rural areas.

2. Data and Methods

2.1. Data

To analyze the access vulnerability to EMS by region in South Korea based on real-time road traffic flow speed, we established spatial big data including road and position information of relevant facilities (Figure 1). The facility information we established using spatial big data included community centers in urban and rural villages, emergency centers, 119-safety centers, community health centers, population and road network maps, as well as traffic speed flow data (Table 1).

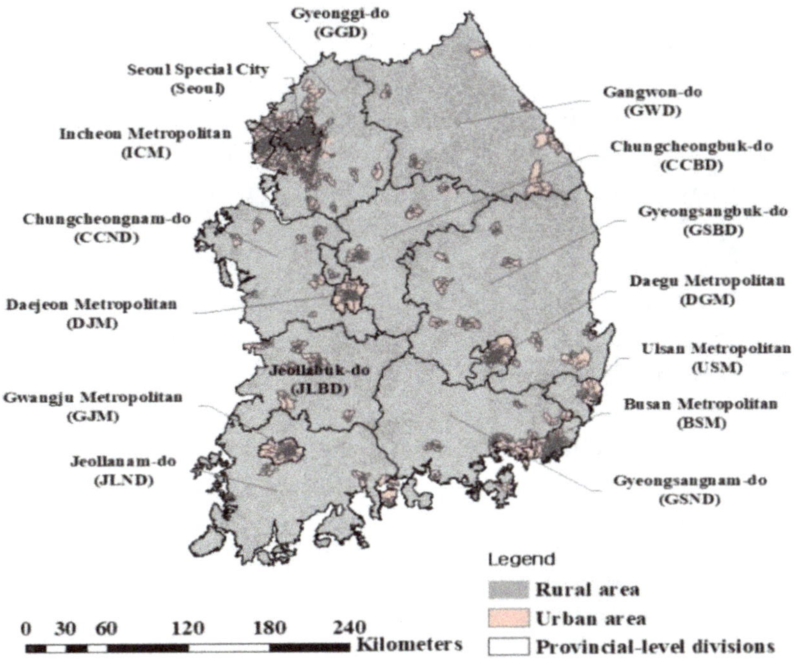

Figure 1. Location of provincial-level divisions in South Korea except for Jeju island. South Korea consists of 17 first-tier administrative divisions: 6 metropolitan cities, 1 special city, 1 special self-governing city, and 9 provinces. The gray and pink areas indicate rural and urban areas, organized sub-municipal level divisions (Dong (neighborhood in Urban) and Ri (Village in Rural).

Table 1. List of available data (facility, population, and traffic speed data) to analyze the vulnerable areas for emergency medical services (EMS). The facility data include data about community centers and medical centers. Each type of data includes a description of the data, the number of available statistics (urban and rural), and reasons for exceptions. The data were provided by the Korean government, and the source of each type of data is shown.

Category		Description	Number of Available Data			Source
			Urban	Rural	Exception [1]	
Facility data						
Community center		Coordinate information on community centers in urban and rural villages	3507	15,171	907	MIS [2]/RAISE [3]
Medical center	Emergency medical center	Coordinate information on emergency medical facilities including local emergency rooms and regional medical centers	397	112	14	NMC [4]
	119-safety centers	Coordinate information on 119-safety centers	709	1112	110	NFA [5]
	Community health center	Converting addresses to coordinate information of local community health centers	287	3195	321	MHW [6]
Traffic speed data						
Roadmap		Polyline information	531,843 links			ITS [7]
Traffic speed		Text information	358,143 links			MLIT [8]

[1] Each facility for assessing accessibility of emergency medical center in island and military zone excepts in this study; [2] Ministry of the Interior and Safety (MIS); [3] Rural Areas Information Service (RAISE); [4] National Medical Center (NMC); [5] National Fire Agency (NFA); [6] Ministry of Health and Welfare (MHW); [7] Intelligent Transport Systems (ITS); [8] Ministry of Land, Infrastructure and Transport (MLIT).

We used 17,771 addresses of community centers in urban and rural villages (as the facility point to represent the center of a village (3507 urban community centers and 14,264 rural community centers) as of 2019 [37]. Community centers, as landmarks of villages, are a space for culture, administration, and communication for village residents in the villages which are the sub-municipal level divisions (Dong and Ri) [38–40].

We also acquired data on the addresses of the medical facilities including emergency centers, community health centers, and 119-safety centers. Data were provided by various sources: data on emergency centers were provided by the National Medical Center (NMC) [41], community health centers were provided by the Ministry of Health and Welfare (MHW) [42], and 119-safety centers were provided by the National Fire Agency (NFA) [43]. The addresses were taken from the Open Application Programming Interface (Open API) and converted into coordinate data through a geocoding method.

We used traffic-related data such as road network maps and traffic speed information. The road network map was provided by the Intelligent Transport Systems (ITS) of the Ministry of Land, Infrastructure and Transport (MLIT) [44], and the traffic speed was provided by the Traffic and Road Information Service of MLIT [45]. The road network maps were based on 2019 data, and the traffic speed information was also acquired from the Open API of ITS from February to April in 2020.

2.2. Method

2.2.1. Accessibility Using Network Analysis

We used network analysis to evaluate vulnerable areas for EMS in urban and rural areas. The network analysis for calculating accessibility was performed using the Network Analyst extension of the Geographic Information System (ArcGIS™), which provides various techniques for network-based spatial analysis, such as optimal path analysis on a road network, identification of the nearest facility, analysis of service ranges, and other accessibility functions [46]. Among the various network analyst functions, we used the origin-destination cost matrix (O-D cost matrix) to create a matrix of the origins and destinations. The optimal path was extracted to determine the least time to arrive at the destinations. The transfer path for emergency patients was determined as the route from the community center (through 119-safety centers or community health center) to the nearest emergency center.

2.2.2. Emergency Medical Vulnerability and Survival Rates by Emergency Case

(1) Emergency situation cases

Since the golden time is very important for emergency patients, their survival rate can increase if prompt and appropriate first aid is administered. For example, with myocardial infarction, the survival rate may double when someone (e.g., the primary respondent around the patient) promptly performs cardiopulmonary resuscitation (CPR) and may triple when an automated external defibrillator (AED) is used [47]. Since the golden time is just 5 to 10 min for cardiac arrest, the survival rate of emergency patients depends not only on the real-time road traffic flow speed but also appropriate first aid administered before or during transportation [48–50].

We evaluated changes in vulnerable areas and survival rates of an emergency by setting up four emergency medical response cases considering the presence of first aid and dispatching of EMT-P (Table 2). Case 1 is when a patient moves to an emergency center in person without initial emergency treatment. This case simulates the same situation that has been used in previous assessments of vulnerable areas of EMS. Case 2 is when a person near the emergency patient performs first aid according to the first aid directions provided by a telephone operator (dispatcher) and then the EMT-P arrives on-site to transport the patient to an emergency center by ambulance. Case 3 is when an EMT-P arrives onsite, provides first aid, and then transports the patient to an emergency center by ambulance. Case 4 is when an EMT-P or a community health center healthcare provider who is nearest to the emergency patient arrives onsite and provides first aid first, and then the EMT-P transports the patient to an emergency center.

Table 2. Description of emergency cases considering first-aid and transfer systems.

Case	Description	Emergency First Aid
Case 1	A patient moves to the nearest emergency center using a personal means of transportation.	X
Case 2	An emergency medical technician-paramedic (EMT-P) is dispatched, but a person near the patient immediately provides first aid according to the first aid instructions given by a telephone operator (dispatcher). After arriving onsite, the EMT-P transfers the patient to the nearest emergency center.	O
Case 3	An EMT-P is dispatched. After arriving onsite, the EMT-P provides first aid, and then transfers the patient to the nearest emergency center.	O
Case 4	An EMT-P or an additional healthcare provider from a community health center is dispatched, provides first aid on-site, and then the EMT-P transfers the patient to the nearest emergency center.	O

(2) Vulnerable areas for emergency medical services (EMS)

Based on the relevant laws and regulations about vulnerable areas in Korea, the vulnerable area of EMS is defined as an area where an emergency medical center cannot be accessed within 30 min. Although data in previous studies on vulnerability to EMS within 30 min have been analyzed based on the road network and legal speed limit of the roads, these analyses do not reflect the real-time traffic flow speed. We evaluated the accessible time every five minutes according to the real traffic speed based on the traffic speed information provided by the Traffic and Road Information Service.

(3) Survival rates

The survival rate of patients with myocardial infarction decreased by 3–4% each minute the patient did not receive CPR, and by 8–10% each minute CPR was not performed [51,52]. Therefore, the survival rate was assumed to decrease by 3% for each minute first aid was not provided by a person near the emergency patient, an EMT-P, or a community health center worker, and by 10% each minute no first aid was provided.

3. Results and Discussion

3.1. *Vulnerable Areas for Emergency Medical Services (EMS)*

3.1.1. The Distribution State of EMS in Urban and Rural Areas

We examined the current states of medical facilities to identify whether the medical environment is balanced between rural and urban areas (Figure 2). The number of medical facilities includes 495 emergency medical centers (Figure 2a), 3161 community health centers (Figure 2b), and 1711 119-safety centers in Korea (Figure 2c). Of these facilities, 80.2% of the emergency medical centers (397 centers) are concentrated in urban areas. Since most emergency medical centers are concentrated in urban areas that are highly populated, emergency patients in rural areas are relatively vulnerable to health emergencies.

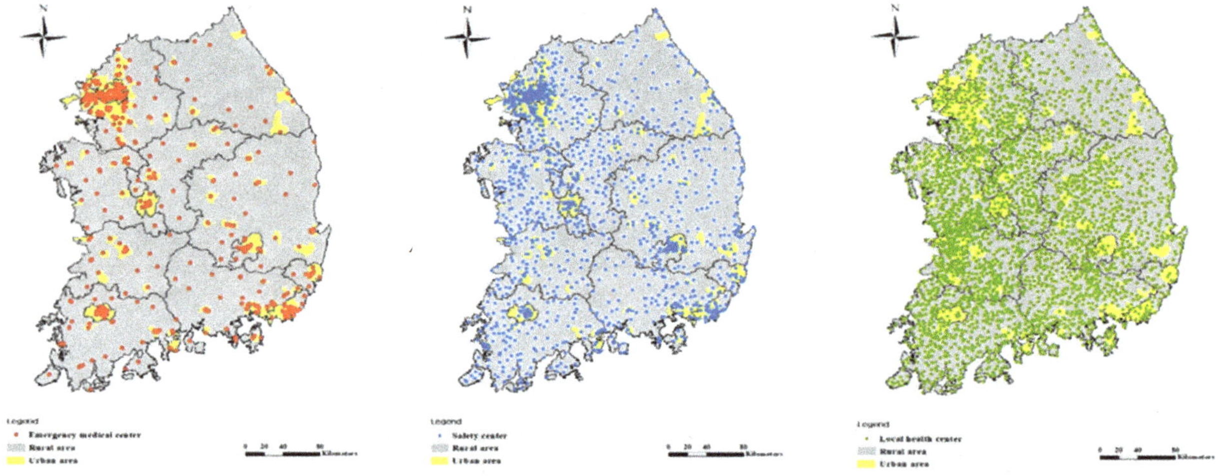

(**a**) Emergency medical center (**b**) 119-Safety center (**c**) Community health center

Figure 2. Distribution of medical facilities in Korea. The yellow and gray areas indicate urban and rural areas, respectively. The individual medical facilities are represented by dots. Red dots in (**a**) are emergency medical centers, blue dots in (**b**) are community health centers, and green dots in (**c**) are 119-safety centers. There are 495 emergency medical centers, 3161 community health centers, and 1711 safety centers.

Community health centers and 119-safety centers are also balanced between urban and rural areas because they are managed by the government to improve and promote residents' public health. They provide protective services for residents' health and property according to the Regional Public Health Act and the Framework Act on fire-fighting services [53]. Approximately 90.9% of community health centers seem to be concentrated in rural areas, but in fact one health center is located in each jurisdictional county in each urban and rural village. The distribution of 119-safety centers is relatively balanced between urban and rural areas with 41.4% (709 centers) in urban areas and 58.6% (1002 centers) in rural areas.

3.1.2. Comparison of Speed Limit and Real Speed of Traffic Flow

We established a road network map that can be used to analyze accessibility in 5-min units by combining a standard node link and traffic communication information. We compared the legal speed limit of each road to the real speed in the established road network.

Data on the speed range showed a descriptively statistical range within 5-min for 3 months. The speed of vehicles in urban areas is not as easily available as the speed limit, but in rural areas, the speed of vehicles can be sufficiently calculated at a speed corresponding to the speed limit of the road (Figure 3). In the capital city (Seoul), for example, the highest population density, on average, vehicles traveled 20–30 km/h on roads with a 60 km/h speed limit and 40–60 km/h on roads with an 80 km/h speed limit (Figure 3a). However, the vehicle speed decreased remarkably around the morning and evening rush hour (8 a.m. and 5 p.m.). By contrast, vehicles in Hongcheon, a typical rural area located in a mountainous region, on average, vehicles can travel at a similar speed to a speed limit of 60 km/h and 60–70 km/h on the road with an 80 km/h speed limit (Figure 3b).

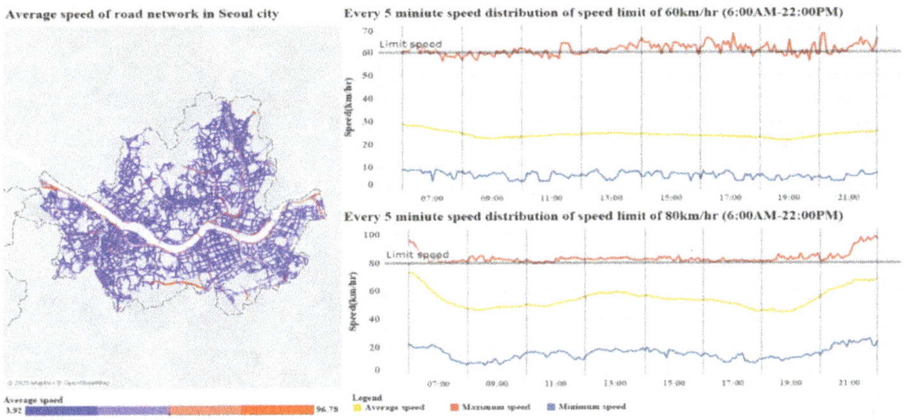

(**a**) Vehicle speeds in the road network measured at a 5-min unit by road type in Seoul (Urban)

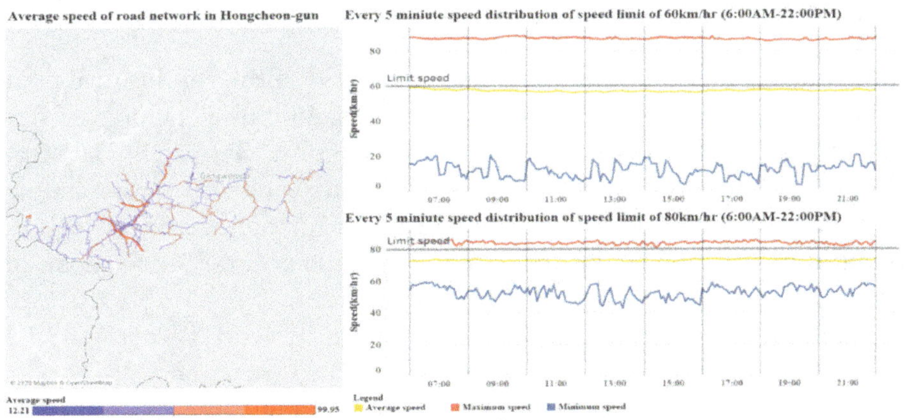

(**b**) Vehicle speeds in the road network measured at a 5-min unit by road type in Hongcheon-gun (Rural)

Figure 3. Vehicle speeds in the road network measured at a 5-min unit by road type in urban and rural areas. The average speed of roads is shown in blue to red on each road map. The distribution of the actual vehicle speed is indicated by road type (speed limit of 60 km/h and 80 km/h) on the right side in the line graph.

3.1.3. Vulnerable Areas for EMS

We evaluated and compared the vulnerable areas of EMS, which are defined as areas where a patient from a community center cannot reach the nearest emergency center within 30 min according to the speed limit, and the real speed (Figure 4). When a patient goes directly to the emergency medical center in an emergency situation as in Case 1, the speed limit-based assessment is underestimated using the current method of assessing emergency medical vulnerability compared to the real speed-based assessment. In particular, the number of vulnerable areas of EMS was 659 villages based on the speed limit (Figure 4a), but 3618 villages based on the real speed (Figure 4b). Rural areas had the most vulnerable areas that increased using the real speed.

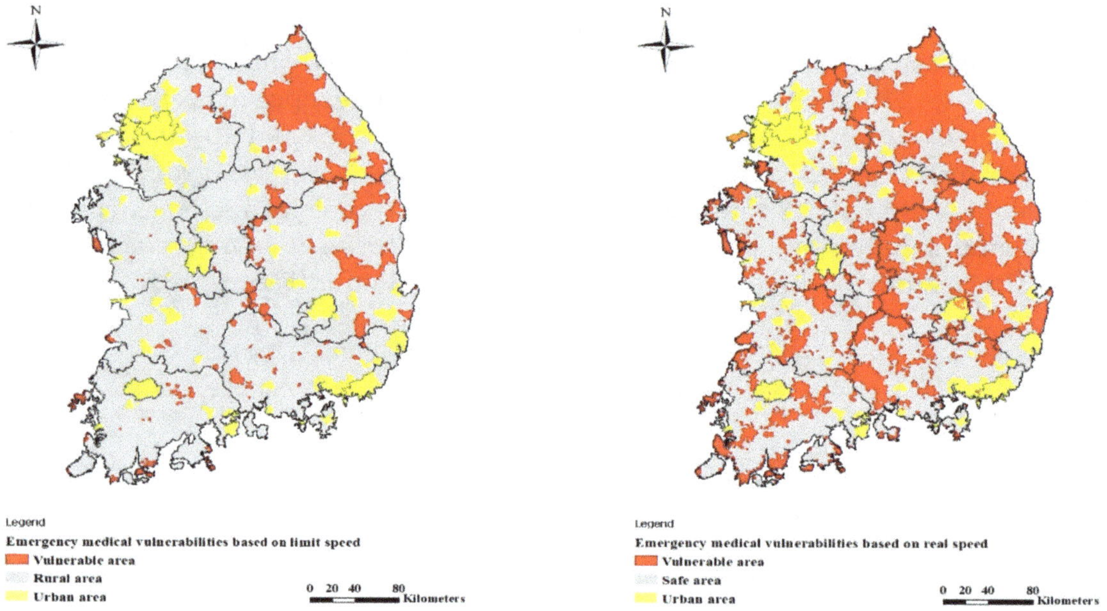

(**a**) Vulnerable areas based on speed limits of roads (**b**) Vulnerable areas based on real speed of roads

Figure 4. Vulnerable areas depending on the road traffic flow speed. The yellow and gray areas indicate urban and rural areas, respectively. The red areas indicate vulnerable areas of EMS, where an emergency patient could not arrive at an emergency medical center within 30 min. (**a**) shows 659 vulnerable areas (4 urban areas and 655 rural areas). (**b**) shows 3618 vulnerable areas (48 urban areas and 3570 rural areas).

An assessment using a 5-min unit based on the real speed of the road reveals that vulnerable areas occurred mostly during afternoon rush hour. In urban areas, 48 villages were considered vulnerable at 6:35 p.m. In rural areas, 3570 villages were vulnerable at 6:25 p.m. (Figure 5). The trend of real speed of the road by time shows that rural areas are relatively insensitive to traffic congestion during rush hour compared to urban areas, but the trend was still the highest during afternoon rush hour. We think that this tendency refers to locations around emergency medical centers. Since most emergency medical centers are located in cities (397 emergency medical centers, 80.2%), the real traffic flow of roads entering the city from rural areas slowed down when patients were transferred from a rural area to an urban emergency medical center, which ultimately led to increased vulnerability of villages in rural areas.

3.2. *Survival Rate of Patients by Emergency Case*

3.2.1. Survival Rate by Time Slot in Urban and Rural Areas

We estimated the survival rate of emergency patients by emergency case considering first aid status and dispatching EMT-paramedics (Figure 6). In Case 1 (Figure 6a), the average survival rate in urban areas was about 31.7% higher than those in rural areas: 36.6% in urban areas and 4.9% in rural areas. In Case 2 (Figure 6b), the average survival rate was 59.4% in urban areas and 22.2% in rural areas, which is about 22.9% higher for urban areas and 17.3% higher in rural areas than Case 1. As the survival rate in rural areas in Case 2 was about 4.5 times higher than those of Case 1, immediate CPR action can remarkably increase the survival rate of emergency patients in Case 2.

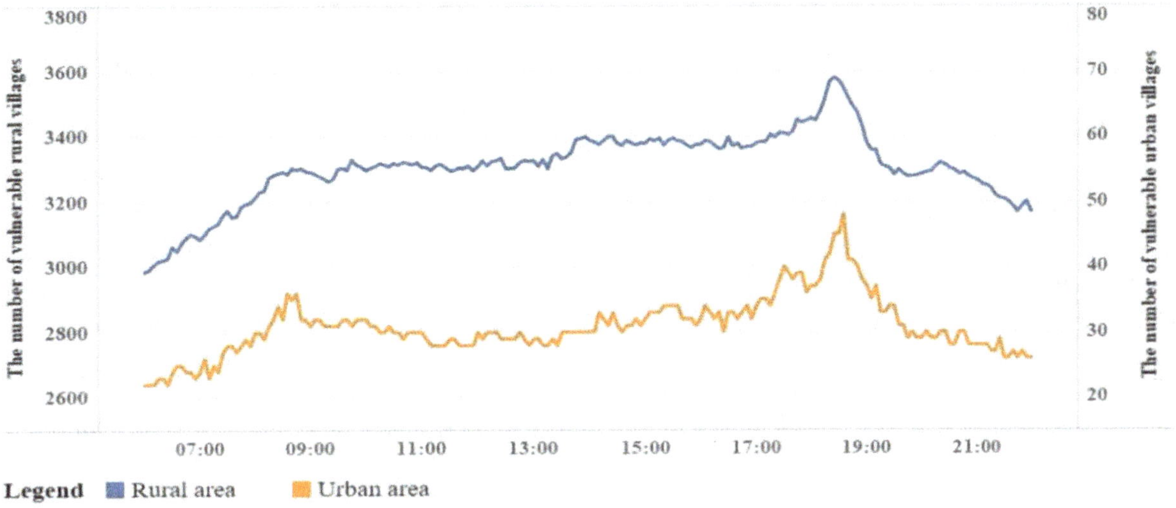

Figure 5. Number of vulnerable areas of EMS in urban and rural areas based on the real road traffic speed in five-minute units. The number of vulnerable areas is marked as an orange line for urban areas and as a blue line for rural areas. The time slots when the number of vulnerable areas reach a peak during afternoon rush hour (17:00–20:00). The highest is 6:35 p.m. (48 villages) in urban areas, and 6:25 p.m. (3570 villages) in rural areas.

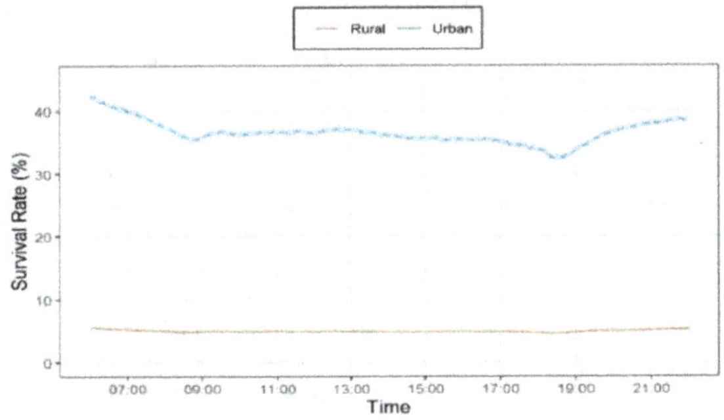

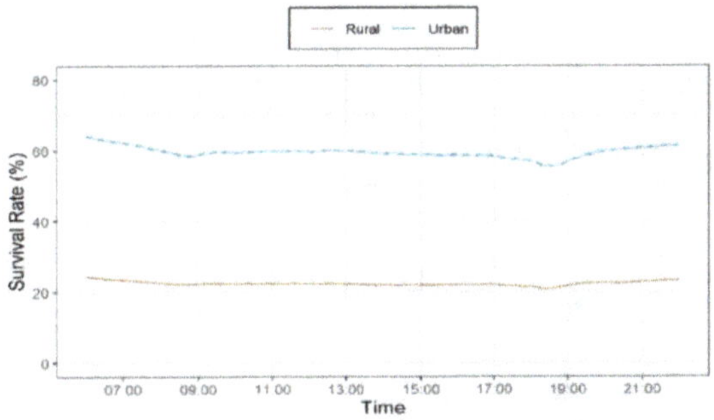

(**a**) Case 1 (Average rate; urban 36.6%, rural 4.9%) (**b**) Case 2 (Average rate; urban 59.4%, rural 22.2%)

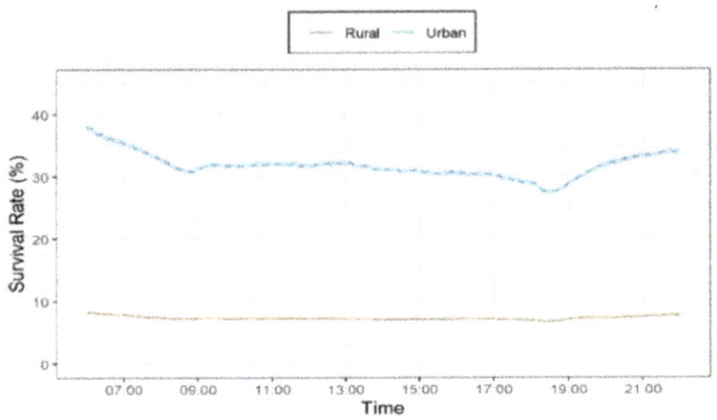

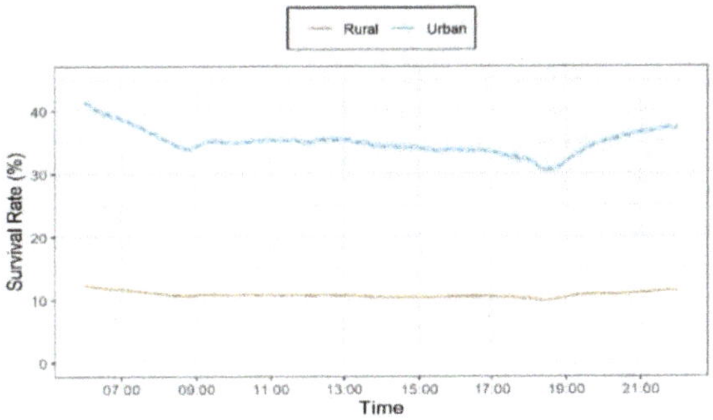

(**c**) Case 3 (Average rate; urban 31.8%, rural 7.3%) (**d**) Case 4 (Average rate; urban 35.0%, rural 10.8%)

Figure 6. Survival rates in urban and rural areas by emergency response case. The survival rates in different timeslots are shown according to the emergency response cases described in Table 2. Among the four cases, the highest survival rate is Case 2, which is when a patient receives cardiopulmonary resuscitation (CPR) by someone near the patient.

In Case 3 (Figure 6c), the survival rate was 31.8% in urban areas and 7.3% in rural areas. In Case 4 (Figure 6d), the survival rate was 35.0% in urban areas and 10.8% in rural areas. The survival rate in urban areas in Case 3 was about 5% lower than that in Case 1, indicating that the survival rate of patients decreases because of the delayed arrival time of an EMT-P to assist the patient and the longer transfer time to an emergency medical center due to low speed flow in urban areas. In contrast, the lower survival rate in rural areas was because of the long distance to an emergency medical facility. Despite these negative impact factors, dispatching an EMT-P can positively affect the overall survival rates of emergency patients.

In Case 4, the survival rate in urban areas also generally decreased to the same as Case 3, since the dispatch time of an EMT or healthcare provider has a negative effect on improving patient survival. In rural areas with Case 4, however, the survival rate was about two times as high as that in Case 1. Because rapid first aid can increase the survival rate of patients in rural areas, where there is a longer distance to a fire station or an emergency center, the survival rate could double when personnel at the nearest community health center are used. When personnel from a community health center are combined with first aid provided promptly by a person near the patient, the survival rate can increase by more than four times.

3.2.2. Survival Rates by Region Depending on Emergency Cases

We examined the survival rate by region (urban and rural areas) with different emergency situations (Case 2, Case 3, and Case 4) compared to Case 1 (Figure 7). In Case 2 when patients immediately receive CPR, the survival rate increased in 12,439 villages compared to Case 1 (Figure 7a). Case 2 seems to be an ideal situation because the survival rate increased in 70% of the villages throughout the country. This result supports the other studies [54–56] that first aid provided by a person near the patient before an EMT arrives is important in improving the survival rate. In Case 3 where first aid is provided after the EMT arrives onsite, the survival rate increased in 3440 villages, but decreased in 2627 villages in mainly Busan, Gwangju, and Gyeonggi compared to Case 1 (Figure 7b). However, the survival rate in Seoul with Case 3 increased in some areas and decreased in other areas.

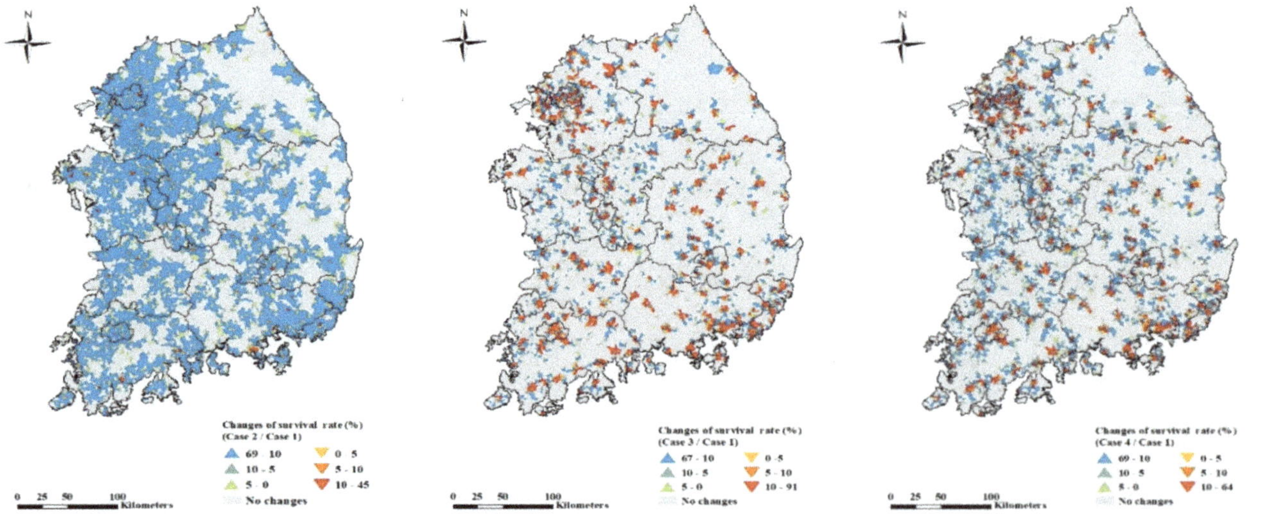

(**a**) Changes in the survival rate for Case 2 compared to Case 1

(**b**) Changes in the survival rate for Case 3 compared to the Case 1

(**c**) Changes in the survival rate for Case 4 compared to the Case 1

Figure 7. Survival rates in emergency response cases compared to Case 1. The blue areas represent the areas where the survival rate increases through expanded emergency responses by local individuals compared to Case 1. Red areas represent areas where the survival rate decreases. In both urban and rural areas, the emergency response in Case 2 was found to be the most effective in improving the survival rate.

In Case 4 where first aid is provided by a healthcare provider or an EMT-P nearest the patient, the survival rate increased in 5309 villages, but decreased in 2217 villages in urban areas such as Seoul,

Busan, Gwangju, Daegu, and Gyeonggi (Figure 7c). Case 4 does not seem to be applicable to urban areas as a policy because the time to receive help from a healthcare provider or an EMT-P increases and the time required to transfer the patient to an emergency medical facility increases. However, the survival rate in rural areas increased for 4060 villages in Case 4. This shows that establishing a system for medical staff in community health centers to provide first aid before an EMT-P arrives is an appropriate method to improve the survival rate. However, Case 4 is not a suitable method in Gangwon province, a representative mountainous region in Korea, because of the low road density and because the major medical facilities are concentrated in the central areas that are highly populated. Therefore, another alternative EMS is needed in this region to more effectively increase the survival rate of local residents.

4. Discussion

We suggest policy-based support to provide rapid first aid using local personnel. As the current major medical infrastructure is concentrated in urban areas, more emergency medical facilities should be established in rural areas to improve accessibility to EMS. However, it may be less efficient to build new emergency medical centers to cover all rural areas due to the personal and social expenditure needed. Instead, a more efficient method is to provide first aid to emergency patients to improve the survival rate. Based on our analysis, when first aid is provided by a primary respondent before an EMT-P arrives, the survival rate increased by 70% of the villages in rural areas. In addition, the survival rate increased in rural areas where an EMT-P or a healthcare provider provides first aid and then transfers the patient to an emergency medical facility. In urban areas, however, access by an EMT-P or a healthcare provider increased the time required for patient transfer and ultimately decreased the survival rate. Healthcare providers can also be used as additional personnel in rural areas to provide prompt and proper first aid. To further reduce the transfer time of emergency patients in urban areas, the government should consider introducing a traffic sign control system based on artificial intelligence on the road.

Based on some studies revealing the importance of reducing EMT-P dispatch time and implementing AED by the public [57–59], establishing an efficient response system that could increase patients' survival rate if they receive quick first aid could be through additional dissemination of AEDs to places with potential risks (e.g., with many acute cardiac arrest patients, highly populated, and largely transient populated places) as well as through continuous training for the public on how to use AEDs and CPR. Because the most effective way to increase the survival rate is immediate first aid treatment, the government should train the public to administer CPR as well as to install and educate AEDs in populated places. One effective way to offer faster first aid is to foster the human infrastructure, including police, general staff of community health centers, apartment or building managers, and village representatives (town chiefs), to increase opportunities to provide first aid. These approaches would also be reasonable ways to improve the survival rate of emergency patients considering both the access time to emergency medical centers in urban areas and more people who can help provide first aid in rural areas before an EMT-P arrives.

5. Conclusions

We explored the vulnerable accessibility to emergency medical services (EMS) by region and time considering the speed limit and real speed of roads. The main findings showed that urban and rural areas have different characteristics in terms of access to an emergency medical facility. In urban areas, the congested road traffic flow (particularly during rush hour) delays the access time. In contrast, in rural areas, the far physical distance to an emergency medical facility increases the travel time, because most emergency medical facilities are concentrated in urban areas. We also found that assessing vulnerable areas to EMS based on the speed limit of roads, as in the existing standard, underestimates the time to a medical facility because it does not reflect the real road conditions.

This study delivers significant meaning to the existing government's approach to define vulnerable areas for emergency care and shows the potential possibility of the underestimation to reflect real world through big data analysis using activity data (real-time road speed) and geographical data (spatial information). However, the study results can be improved with more data sources for the following: First, we assume that there is no delay time due to traffic signals as well as no extra time to prepare the EMT-P's dispatch in 119-safety center which would ultimately have affected the survival rate of emergency patients. Second, we supposed that all emergency patients will be transferred to the nearest emergency medical center although patients can be transferred to different emergency centers following the patient's choices or medical conditions of the center such as medical manpower and equipment. Third, the influence of epidemic conditions such as COVID-19 cannot be considered even though pandemic diseases potentially restrict the accessibility of emergency patients because of uncertain information and related laws to prevent the possibility of infection for medical personnel and other patients in the medical facilities.

We expect that future studies overcome current data availability issues for modeling precise cases including EMT-P's actual dispatch time and arrival time as well as the exact transferred emergency center location of emergency patients. Our ongoing studies will not only provide more accurate assessment of vulnerable areas for EMS but also suggest optimal transport systems for regional emergency medical services.

Author Contributions: Conceptualization, J.J., S.K., and K.S.; methodology, J.J.; software, J.J.; validation, G.H.K. and K.S.; formal analysis, J.J.; investigation, S.K. and K.S.; resources, J.J. and G.H.K.; data curation, J.J., G.H.K. and K.S.; writing—original draft preparation, J.J. and S.K.; writing—review and editing, J.J., S.K. and K.S.; visualization, J.J. and S.K.; supervision, K.S.; project administration, K.S.; funding acquisition, K.S. All authors have read and agreed to the published version of the manuscript.

References

1. Hoffman, E. Mortality and morbidity following road accidents. *Ann. R. Coll. Surg. Engl.* **1976**, *58*, 233. [PubMed]
2. Weber, E.J. Travel or Traffic: Either Way, Emergency Service May Be Delayed. *Ann. Emerg. Med.* **2009**, *2*, 270–271. [CrossRef] [PubMed]
3. Carr, B.G.; Branas, C.C.; Metlay, J.P.; Sullivan, A.F.; Camargo, C.A., Jr. Access to emergency care in the United States. *Ann. Emerg. Med.* **2009**, *54*, 261–269. [CrossRef] [PubMed]
4. Carr, B.G.; Caplan, J.M.; Pryor, J.P.; Branas, C.C. A meta-analysis of prehospital care times for trauma. *Prehosp. Emerg. Care* **2006**, *10*, 198–206. [CrossRef] [PubMed]
5. Eisenberg, M.S.; Cummins, R.O.; Damon, S.; Larsen, M.P.; Hearne, T.R. Survival rates from out-of-hospital cardiac arrest: Recommendations for uniform definitions and data to report. *Ann. Emerg. Med.* **1990**, *19*, 1249–1259. [CrossRef]
6. Noble-Mathews, P.M. *Pre-Hospital Care*; Elsevier Health Sciences: London, UK, 2005; pp. 61–69.
7. Bigdeli, M.; Khorasani-Zavareh, D.; Mohammadi, R. Pre-hospital care time intervals among victims of road traffic injuries in Iran. A cross-sectional study. *BMC Public Health* **2010**, *10*, 406. [CrossRef]
8. Lee, E. Designing service coverage and measuring accessibility and serviceability of rural and small urban ambulance systems. *Systems* **2014**, *2*, 34–53. [CrossRef]
9. Shin, K.; Lee, T. Improving the measurement of the Korean emergency medical System's spatial accessibility. *Appl. Geogr.* **2018**, *100*, 30–38. [CrossRef]
10. Grossman, D.C.; Kim, A.; Macdonald, S.C.; Klein, P.; Copass, M.K.; Maier, R.V. Urban-rural differences in prehospital care of major trauma. *J. Trauma Acute Care Surg.* **1997**, *42*, 723–729. [CrossRef]
11. Chng, C.L.; Collins, J.; Eaddy, S. A comparison of rural and urban emergency medical system (EMS) personnel: A Texas study. *Prehosp. Disaster Med.* **2001**, *16*, 159–165. [CrossRef]

12. OECD. *OECD Health Care Quality Review: Korea*; Organization for Economic Cooperation and Development Publishing: Paris, France, 2012.
13. Kim, S.; Kim, T.; Suh, K. Assessment of accessibility to medical facilities in rural areas using real road distance focusing on Pyeongchang-gun. *J. Korean Soc. Agric. Eng.* **2015**, *57*, 39–49. [CrossRef]
14. HIRAS. *Healthcare Bigdata Hub*; Health Insurance Review & Assessment Service: Wonju-si, Korea, 2020; Available online: https://opendata.hira.or.kr/home.do (accessed on 17 September 2020).
15. Lloyd-Jones, D.M.; Leip, E.P.; Larson, M.G.; d'Agostino, R.B.; Beiser, A.; Wilson, P.; Wolf, P.A.; Levy, D. Prediction of lifetime risk for cardiovascular disease by risk factor burden at 50 years of age. *Circulation* **2006**, *113*, 791–798. [CrossRef] [PubMed]
16. KOSIS. *2017 Causes of Death Statistics*; Korean Statistical Information Service, Statistics Korea: Daejeon, Korea, 2017.
17. KOSIS. *Population Ageing*; Korean Statistical Information Service, Statistics Korea: Daejeon, Korea, 2019.
18. Van den Heuvel, W.; Ghinescu, M.; Olaroiu, M. How to Prevent Preventable Death. *SM Prev. Med. Public Health* **2017**, *1*, 1004. [CrossRef]
19. Jeon, J.; Park, M.; Jang, D.; Lim, C.; Kim, E. Vulnerable Analysis of Emergency Medical Facilities based on Accessibility to Emergency Room and 119 Emergency Center. *J. Korean Soc. Rural Plan.* **2018**, *24*, 147–155. [CrossRef]
20. Health and Welfare. Public Health and Medical Services Act. In *Article 12 (Designation and Public Announcement of Areas Lacking Medical Services)*; Korea Legislative Research Institute: Bangok-dong, Korea, 2018.
21. Barbarisi, I.; Bruno, G.; Diglio, A.; Elizalde, J.; Piccolo, C. A spatial analysis to evaluate the impact of deregulation policies in the pharmacy sector: Evidence from the case of Navarre. *Health Policy* **2019**, *123*, 1108–1115. [CrossRef] [PubMed]
22. Ikram, S.Z.; Hu, Y.; Wang, F. Disparities in spatial accessibility of pharmacies in Baton Rouge, Louisiana. *Geogr. Rev.* **2015**, *105*, 492–510. [CrossRef]
23. Neutens, T. Accessibility, equity and health care: Review and research directions for transport geographers. *J. Transp. Geogr.* **2015**, *43*, 14–27. [CrossRef]
24. Pu, Q.; Yoo, E.-H.; Rothstein, D.H.; Cairo, S.; Malemo, L. Improving the spatial accessibility of healthcare in North Kivu, Democratic Republic of Congo. *Appl. Geogr.* **2020**, *121*, 102262. [CrossRef]
25. Wang, F. Measurement, optimization, and impact of health care accessibility: A methodological review. *Ann. Assoc. Am. Geogr.* **2012**, *102*, 1104–1112. [CrossRef]
26. Ehara, A. Accessibility of pediatric inpatient services in Japan. *PLoS ONE* **2018**, *13*, e0201443. [CrossRef]
27. Jin, M.; Liu, L.; Tong, D.; Gong, Y.; Liu, Y. Evaluating the spatial accessibility and distribution balance of multi-level medical service facilities. *Int. J. Environ. Res. Public Health* **2019**, *16*, 1150. [CrossRef] [PubMed]
28. Bruno, G.; Cavola, M.; Diglio, A.; Piccolo, C. Improving spatial accessibility to regional health systems through facility capacity management. *Socio-Econ. Plan. Sci.* **2020**, *71*, 100881. [CrossRef]
29. Wielebski, Ł.; Medyńska-Gulij, B. Graphically supported evaluation of mapping techniques used in presenting spatial accessibility. *Cartogr. Geogr. Inf. Sci.* **2019**, *46*, 311–333. [CrossRef]
30. Liu, S.; Qin, Y.; Xu, Y. Inequality and Influencing Factors of Spatial Accessibility of Medical Facilities in Rural Areas of China: A Case Study of Henan Province. *Int. J. Environ. Res. Public Health* **2019**, *16*, 1833. [CrossRef] [PubMed]
31. Dejen, A.; Soni, S.; Semaw, F. Spatial accessibility analysis of healthcare service centers in Gamo Gofa Zone, Ethiopia through Geospatial technique. *Remote Sens. Appl. Soc. Environ.* **2019**, *13*, 466–473. [CrossRef]
32. Kim, S.; Kim, T.; Suh, K. Analysis of the implication of accessibility to community facilities for land price in rural areas using a hedonic land price model. *J. Korean Soc. Rural Plan.* **2016**, *22*, 93–100. [CrossRef]
33. Jeon, J.; Kim, S.; Kwon, S.M. The Effects of Urban Containment Policies on Public Health. *Int. J. Environ. Res. Public Health* **2020**, *17*, 3275. [CrossRef]
34. Kim, S.; Jeon, J.; Suh, K. Evaluating Educational Fairness of Commuting Distances for Rural Villages following the Closing of Elementary Schools. *J. Korean Soc. Agric. Eng.* **2020**, *62*, 29–38. [CrossRef]
35. Li, L.; Du, Q.; Ren, F.; Ma, X. Assessing spatial accessibility to hierarchical urban parks by multi-types of travel distance in Shenzhen, China. *Int. J. Environ. Res. Public Health* **2019**, *16*, 1038. [CrossRef]
36. Jeon, J.; Kim, S.; Suh, K.; Yoon, S. Analysis of Village Safety Index using Accessibility to Public Facilities. *J. Korean Soc. Rural Plan.* **2016**, *22*, 121–129. [CrossRef]

37. Rural Areas Information Service (RAISE). Available online: https://www.raise.go.kr/raise/index.do (accessed on 16 September 2020).
38. Chin, H.S.; Park, M.J.; Yun, D.S. Evaluating Accessibilities to Village Community Centers via Rural Amenity Resources Information. *J. Korean Soc. Rural Plan.* **2014**, *20*, 57–69. [CrossRef]
39. Kim, S.; Kim, T.; Suh, K. Evaluation of Accessibility to Elementary and Secondary Educational Facilities on Village Level in Rural Areas. *J. Korean Soc. Rural Plan.* **2017**, *23*, 121–131. [CrossRef]
40. Wikipedia. Administrative Divisions of South Korea. Available online: https://en.wikipedia.org/wiki/Administrative_divisions_of_South_Korea (accessed on 16 September 2020).
41. National Medical Center (NMC). Available online: https://www.nmc.or.kr/main.asp (accessed on 16 September 2020).
42. Ministry of Health and Welfare (MHW). Available online: http://www.mohw.go.kr/react/index.jsp (accessed on 16 September 2020).
43. National Fire Agency (NFA). Available online: https://www.nfa.go.kr/nfa/ (accessed on 16 September 2020).
44. Intelligent Transport Systems (ITS). Available online: http://nodelink.its.go.kr/ (accessed on 16 September 2020).
45. Traffic and Road Information Service. Available online: http://openapi.its.go.kr/data/centerTraffic.do (accessed on 16 September 2020).
46. ESRI. What is the ArcGIS Network Analyst Extension? Available online: https://desktop.arcgis.com/en/arcmap/latest/extensions/network-analyst/what-is-network-analyst-.htm (accessed on 16 September 2020).
47. Eisenberg, M.S.; Cummins, R.O.; Larsen, M.P. Numerators, denominators, and survival rates: Reporting survival from out-of-hospital cardiac arrest. *Am. J. Emerg. Med.* **1991**, *9*, 544–546. [CrossRef]
48. Gottschalk, A.; Burmeister, M.-A.; Freitag, M.; Cavus, E.; Standl, T. Influence of early defibrillation on the survival rate and quality of life after CPR in prehospital emergency medical service in a German metropolitan area. *Resuscitation* **2002**, *53*, 15–20. [CrossRef]
49. May, S.; Zhang, L.; Foley, D.; Brennan, E.; O'Neil, B.; Bork, E.; Levy, P.; Dunne, R. Improvement in Non-Traumatic, Out-Of-Hospital Cardiac Arrest Survival in Detroit From 2014 to 2016. *J. Am. Heart Assoc.* **2018**, *7*, e009831. [CrossRef]
50. Eisenberg, M.S.; Horwood, B.T.; Cummins, R.O.; Reynolds-Haertle, R.; Hearne, T.R. Cardiac arrest and resuscitation: A tale of 29 cities. *Ann. Emerg. Med.* **1990**, *19*, 179–186. [CrossRef]
51. Larsen, M.P.; Eisenberg, M.S.; Cummins, R.O.; Hallstrom, A.P. Predicting survival from out-of-hospital cardiac arrest: A graphic model. *Ann. Emerg. Med.* **1993**, *22*, 1652–1658. [CrossRef]
52. European Resuscitation Council. Part 6: Advanced cardiovascular life support. Section 8: Postresuscitation care. European Resuscitation Council. *Resuscitation* **2000**, *46*, 195–201.
53. Health and Welfare. Regional Public Health Act. In *Article 3 of the Framework Act on Health and Medical Services*; Act No. 16262; Korea Legislative Research Institute: Bangok-dong, Korea, 2019.
54. Holmberg, M.J.; Vognsen, M.; Andersen, M.S.; Donnino, M.W.; Andersen, L.W. Bystander automated external defibrillator use and clinical outcomes after out-of-hospital cardiac arrest: A systematic review and meta-analysis. *Resuscitation* **2017**, *120*, 77–87. [CrossRef]
55. Hasselqvist-Ax, I.; Riva, G.; Herlitz, J.; Rosenqvist, M.; Hollenberg, J.; Nordberg, P.; Ringh, M.; Jonsson, M.; Axelsson, C.; Lindqvist, J. Early cardiopulmonary resuscitation in out-of-hospital cardiac arrest. *N. Engl. J. Med.* **2015**, *372*, 2307–2315. [CrossRef]
56. Park, Y.M.; Do Shin, S.; Lee, Y.J.; Song, K.J.; Ro, Y.S.; Ahn, K.O. Cardiopulmonary resuscitation by trained responders versus lay persons and outcomes of out-of-hospital cardiac arrest: A community observational study. *Resuscitation* **2017**, *118*, 55–62. [CrossRef] [PubMed]
57. Lee, S.Y.; Do, Y.K.; Do Shin, S.; Park, Y.J.; Ro, Y.S.; Lee, E.J.; Lee, K.W.; Lee, Y.J. Community socioeconomic status and public access defibrillators: A multilevel analysis. *Resuscitation* **2017**, *120*, 1–7. [CrossRef] [PubMed]

58. Hawkes, C.; Booth, S.; Ji, C.; Brace-McDonnell, S.J.; Whittington, A.; Mapstone, J.; Cooke, M.W.; Deakin, C.D.; Gale, C.P.; Fothergill, R. Epidemiology and outcomes from out-of-hospital cardiac arrests in England. *Resuscitation* **2017**, *110*, 133–140. [CrossRef] [PubMed]
59. Nishi, T.; Takei, Y.; Kamikura, T.; Ohta, K.; Hashimoto, M.; Inaba, H. Improper bystander-performed basic life support in cardiac arrests managed with public automated external defibrillators. *Am. J. Emerg. Med.* **2015**, *33*, 43–49. [CrossRef] [PubMed]

2

A Comparison of Deep Learning Methods for ICD Coding of Clinical Records

Elias Moons [1,*], Aditya Khanna [1,2], Abbas Akkasi [1] and Marie-Francine Moens [1]

1 Department of Computer Science, KU Leuven, 3000 Leuven, Belgium; adityakhanna@iitb.ac.in (A.K.); abbas.akkasi@kuleuven.be (A.A.); sien.moens@cs.kuleuven.be (M.-F.M.)
2 Department of Electrical Engineering, IIT Bombay, Maharashtra 400076, India
* Correspondence: elias.moons@cs.kuleuven.be

Abstract: In this survey, we discuss the task of automatically classifying medical documents into the taxonomy of the International Classification of Diseases (ICD), by the use of deep neural networks. The literature in this domain covers different techniques. We will assess and compare the performance of those techniques in various settings and investigate which combination leverages the best results. Furthermore, we introduce an hierarchical component that exploits the knowledge of the ICD taxonomy. All methods and their combinations are evaluated on two publicly available datasets that represent ICD-9 and ICD-10 coding, respectively. The evaluation leads to a discussion of the advantages and disadvantages of the models.

Keywords: ICD coding; hierarchical classification; electronic healthcare

1. Introduction

The International Classification of Diseases (ICD), which is endorsed by the World Health Organization, is the diagnostic classification standard for clinical and research purposes in the medical field. ICD defines the universe of diseases, disorders, injuries, and other related health conditions, listed in a comprehensive, hierarchical fashion. ICD coding allows for easy storage, retrieval, and analysis of health information for evidenced-based decision-making; sharing and comparing health information between hospitals, regions, settings, and countries; and data comparisons in the same location across different time periods (https://www.who.int/classifications/icd/en/) . ICD has been revised periodically to incorporate changes in the medical field. Today, there have been 11 revisions of the ICD taxonomy, where ICD-9 and ICD-10 are the most studied when it comes to their automated assignment to medical documents. In this paper, we compare state-of-the-art neural network approaches to classification of medical reports written in natural language (in this case English) according to ICD categories.

ICD coding of medical reports has been a research topic for many years [1]. Hospitals need to label their patient visits with ICD codes to be in accordance with the law and to gain subsidies from the government or refunds from insurance companies. When the documents are in free text format, this process is still done manually. Automating (a part of) this process would greatly reduce the administrative work.

In this paper, we compare the performance of several deep learning based approaches for ICD-9 and ICD-10 coding. The codes of ICD-9 consist of, at most, five numbers. The first three numbers represent a high level disease category, a fourth number narrows this down to specific diseases, and a fifth number differentiates between specific disease variants. This leads to a hierarchical taxonomy with four layers underneath a root node. The first layer ($L1$) consists of groups of 3-numbered categories, the next three layers ($L2$ through $L4$) correspond to the first 3, 4, or 5 numbers of the ICD code as is displayed in the upper part of Figure 1. In the lower part of this figure, a concrete example of the coding is shown.

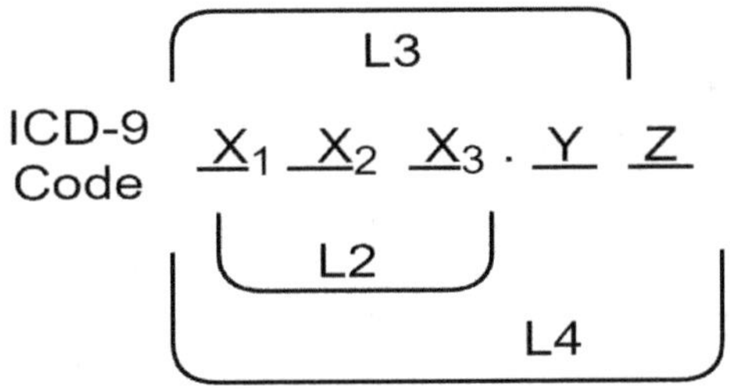

240-279: Endocrine, nutritional and metabolic diseases (L1)
250: Diabetes mellitus (L2)
250.2: Diabetes with hyperosmolarity (L3)
250.21: Diabetes with hyperosmolarity of type 1 (L4)

Figure 1. ICD-9 code structure with second through fourth layer representations and diabetes as an example.

In this paper, we survey state-of-the-art deep learning approaches for ICD-9 coding. We especially focus on the representation learning that the methods accomplish.

Experiments with ICD-9 are carried out on the MIMIC-III dataset [2]. This dataset consists of over 50,000 discharge summaries of patient visits in US hospitals. These summaries are in free textual format and labeled with corresponding ICD-9 codes, an example snippet is visible in Figure 2. Most discharge summaries are labeled with multiple categories, leading to a multiclass and multilabel setting for category prediction.

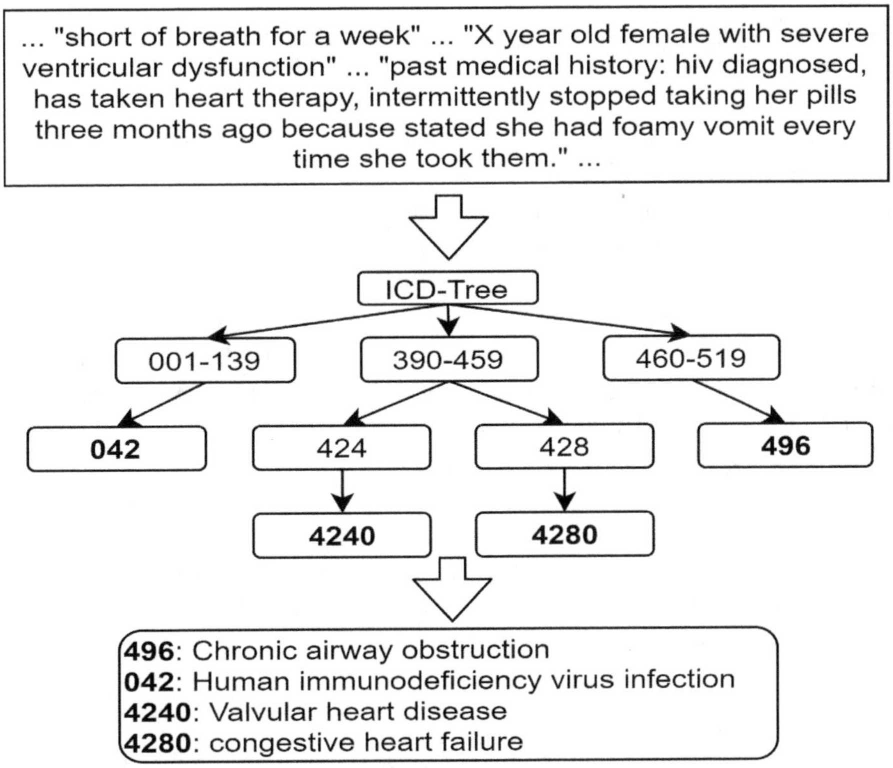

Figure 2. Example snippet of discharge summary from the MIMIC-III dataset with corresponding target International Classification of Diseases (ICD) codes.

Codes from the ICD-10 version are very similar to those of ICD-9. The main difference is that they consist of up to seven characters of which at least the first three are always present, the latter four are optional. The first character is an uppercase alphabetic letter, all other characters are numeric. The first three characters indicate the category of the diagnoses, and the following three characters indicate the etiology, anatomic site, severity, or other clinical details. A seventh character indicates an extension. An example of the ICD-10 structure is visible in Figure 3, it visualizes the same diagnosis as in Figure 1 but for ICD-10 instead of ICD-9.

Experiments with ICD-10 are conducted on the CodiEsp dataset, which is publicly available. This dataset consists of 1000 discharge summaries of patient visits in Spain. The documents are in free text format, which is automatically translated to English from Spanish, and they are manually labeled with ICD-10 codes by healthcare professionals.

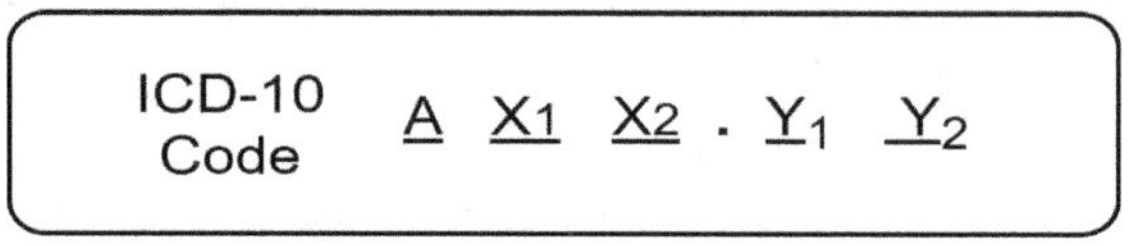

E:	Endocrine, nutritional and metabolic diseases	(L1)
E10:	Insulin dependent diabetes mellitus	(L2)
E10.6:	Diabetic arthropathy	(L3)
E10.69:	Diabetes with hyperosmolarity of type 1	(L4)

Figure 3. ICD-10 code structure with second through fourth layer representations and diabetes as an example.

The deep learning methods that we discuss in this paper encompass different neural network architectures including convolutional and recurrent neural networks. It is studied how they can be extended with suitable attention mechanisms and loss functions and how the hierarchical structure of the ICD taxonomy can be exploited. ICD-10 coding is especially challenging, as in the benchmark dataset that we use for our experiments the ICD coding model has to deal with very few manually labeled training data.

In our work we want to answer the following research questions. What are the current state-of-the-art neural network approaches for classifying discharge summaries? How do they compare to each other in terms of performance? What combination of techniques gives the best results on a public dataset? We hypothesize the following claims. (1) A combination of self-attention and convolutional layers yields the best classification results. (2) In a setting with less training samples per category, attention on description vectors of the target categories improves the results. (3) Using the hierarchical taxonomy explicitly in the model improves classification on a small dataset. The most important contribution of our work is an extensive evaluation and comparison of state-of-the-art deep learning models for ICD-9 and ICD-10 coding which currently does not exist in the literature.

The remainder of this paper is organized as follows. In Section 2, related work relevant for the conducted research will be discussed. Section 3 will elaborate on the datasets used in the experiments and how this data is preprocessed. The compared deep learning methods are described in Section 4. These methods are evaluated on the datasets in different settings and all findings are reported in Section 5. The most important findings will be discussed in Section 6. Finally, we conclude with some recommendations for future research.

2. Related Work

The most prominent and more recent advancements in categorizing medical reports with standard codes will be described in this section.

2.1. *Traditional Models for ICD Coding*

Larkey and Croft [3] are the first to apply machine learning techniques to ICD coding. Different techniques including a *k*-nearest neighbor classifier, relevance feedback, and a Bayesian classifier are applied to the texts of inpatient discharge summaries. The authors found that an ensemble of models yields the best results. At that time, and still later, one has experimented with rule-based pattern matching techniques, which are often expressed as regular expressions (see, e.g., in [4]). Farkas et al. [5] have proposed a hybrid system that partially relied on handcrafted rules and partially on machine learning. For the latter, the authors compare a decision tree learner with a multinomial logistic regression algorithm. The system is evaluated on the data from the CMC Challenge on Classifying Clinical Free Text Using Natural Language Processing, support vector machines (SVMs) were also a popular approach for assigning codes to clinical free text (see, e.g., in [6] who evaluate a SVM using *n*-gram word features on the MIMIC-II dataset). A systematic overview of earlier systems for automated clinical coding is found in [7]. The authors of [8] show that datasets of different sizes and different numbers of distinct codes demand different training mechanisms. For small datasets, it is important to select relevant features. The authors have evaluated ICD coding performance on a dataset consisting of more than 70,000 textual Electronic Medical Records (EMRs) from the University of Kentucky (UKY) Medical Center tagged with ICD-9 codes. Integrating feature selection on both structured and unstructured data is researched by the authors of [9] and has proven to aid the classification process. Two approaches are evaluated in this setting: early and late integration of structured and unstructured data, the latter yielding the better results. Documents are tagged with ICD-9 and ICD-10 medical codes.

2.2. *Deep Learning Models for ICD Coding*

More recently, and following a general trend in text classification, deep learning techniques have become popular for ICD coding. These methods learn relevant features from the raw data and thus skip the feature engineering step of traditional machine learning methods. Deep learning proved its value in computer vision tasks [10], and rapidly has conquered the field of text and language processing. Deep learning techniques also have been successfully applied to Electronic Health Records (EHR) [11]. In the 2019 CLEF eHealth evaluation lab, deep learning techniques had become mainstream models for ICD coding [12].

A deep learning model that encompasses an attention mechanism is tested by the authors of [13] on the MIMIC-III dataset. In this work, a Long Short-Term Memory network (LSTM) is used for both character and word level representations. A soft attention layer here helps in making predictions for the top 50 most frequent ICD codes in the dataset. Duarte et al. [14] propose bidirectional GRUs for ICD-10 coding of the free text of death certificates and associated autopsy reports. Xie et al. [15] have developed a tree-of-sequences LSTM architecture with an attention mechanism to simultaneously capture the hierarchical relationships among codes. The model is tested on the MIMIC-III dataset. Huang et al. [16] have shown that deep learning-based methods outperform other conventional machine learning methods such as a SVM for predicting the top 10 ICD-9 codes on the MIMIC-III dataset, a finding confirmed by Li et al. [17], who have confirmed that ICD-9 coding on the MIMIC-II and MIMIC-III datasets outperforms a classical hierarchy-based SVM and a flat SVM. This latter work also shows that convolutional neural networks (CNNs) are successful in text classification given their capability to learn global features that abstract larger stretches of content in the documents. Xu et al. [18] have implemented modality-specific machine learning models including unstructured text, semistructured text, and structured tabular data, and then have used an ensemble method to integrate all modality-specific models to generate the ICD codes. Unstructured and semistructured text is handled by a deep neural network, while tabular data are converted to binary features which are input as features in a decision tree learning algorithm [19]. The text classification problem can also be modeled as a joint label-word embedding problem [20]. An attention framework is proposed that measures the compatibility of embeddings between text sequences and labels. This technique is evaluated on both the MIMIC-II and MIMIC-III datasets but achieves inferior results to the neural models presented further in this paper. Zeng et al. [21] transfer MeSH domain knowledge to improve automatic ICD-9 coding but improvements compared to baselines are limited. Baumel et al. [22] have introduced the Hierarchical Attention bidirectional Gated Recurrent Unit model (HA-GRU). By identifying relevant sentences for each label, documents are tagged with corresponding ICD codes. Results are reported both on the MIMIC-II and MIMIC-III datasets. Mullenbach et al. [23] present the Convolutional Attention for Multilabel classification (CAML) model that combines the strengths of convolutional networks and attention mechanisms. They propose adding regularization on the long descriptions of the target ICD codes, especially to improve classification results on less represented categories in the dataset. This approach is further extended with the idea of multiple convolutional channels in [24] with max pooling across all channels. The authors also shift the attention from the last prediction layer, as in [23], to the attention layer. Mullenbach et al. [23,24] achieve state-of-the art results for ICD-9 coding on the MIMIC-III dataset. As an addition to these models, in this paper a hierarchical variant of each of them is constructed and evaluated.

Recently, language models have become popular in natural language processing. The use of Bidirectional Encoder Representations from Transformers (BERT) models, which uses a transformer architecture with multi-head attention, and especially BioBERT has improved the overall recall values at the expense of precision compared to CNN and LSTM models when applied in the ICD-10 coding task at CLEF eHealth in 2019 [25], a finding which we have confirmed in our experiments. Therefore, we do not report on experiments with this architecture in this survey.

Finally, Campbell et al. [26] survey the literature on the benefits, limitations, implementation, and impact of computer-assisted clinical coding on clinical coding professionals. They conclude that human coders could be greatly helped by current technologies and are likely to become clinical coding editors in an effort to raise the quality of the overall clinical coding process. Shickel et al. [11] review deep learning models for EHR systems by examining architectures, technical aspects, and clinical applications. Their paper discusses shortcomings of the current techniques and future research directions among which the authors cite ICD coding of free clinical text as one of the future challenges.

2.3. Hierarchical Models for Classification

In this paper, we foresee several mechanisms to exploit the hierarchical taxonomy of ICD codes in a deep learning setting, in other words we exploit the known dependencies between classes. Although this is a rather novel topic, hierarchical relationships between classes have been studied in traditional machine learning models. Deschacht et al. [27] have modeled first-order hierarchical dependencies between classes as features in a conditional random field and applied this model to text classification. Babbar et al. [28] study error generalization bounds of multiclass, hierarchical classifiers using the DMOZ hierarchy and the International Patent Classification by simplifying the taxonomy and selectively pruning some of its nodes with the help of a meta-classifier. The features retained in this meta-classifier are derived from the error generalization bounds. Furthermore, hierarchical loss functions have been used in non-deep learning approaches. Gopal et al. [29] exploit the hierarchical or graphical dependencies among class labels in large-margin classifiers, such as a SVM, and in logistic regression classifiers by adding a suitable regularization term to their hinge-loss and logistic loss function, respectively. This regularization enforces the parameters of a child classifier to be similar to the parameters of its parent using a Euclidean distance function, in other words, encouraging parameters which are nearby in the hierarchy to be similar to each other. This helps classes to leverage information from nearby classes while estimating model parameters. Cai and Hofmann [30] integrate knowledge of the class hierarchy into a structured SVM. Their method also considers the parent–child relationship as a feature. All parameters are learned jointly by optimizing a common objective function corresponding to a regularized upper bound on the empirical loss. During training it is enforced that the score of a training example with a correct labeling should be larger than or equal to the score of a training example of an incorrect labeling plus some loss or cost. It is assumed that assignment of confusing classes that are "nearby" in the taxonomy is less costly or severe than predicting a class that is "far away" from the correct class. This is realized by scaling the penalties for margin violation. A similar idea is modeled in a deep learning model for audio event detection [31]. These authors propose the hierarchy-aware loss function modeled as a triplet or quadruplet loss function that favors confusing classes that are close in the taxonomy, over ones that are far away from the correct class. In [32], an hierarchical SVM is shown to outperform that of a flat SVM. Results are reported on the MIMIC-II dataset. In a deep neural network setting, recent publications on hierarchical text classification outside the medical field make use of label distribution learning [18], an hierarchical softmax activation function [33], and hierarchical multilabel classification networks [34].

Recent research shows the value of hierarchical dependencies using hierarchical attention mechanisms [22] and hierarchical penalties [34], which are also integrated in the training of the models surveyed in this paper.

If the target output space of categories follows a hierarchy of labels—as is also the case in ICD coding—the trained models efficiently use this hierarchy for category assignment or prediction [32,35,36]. During categorization the models apply a top-down or a bottom-up approach at the classification stage. In a top-down approach parent, categories are assigned first and only children of assigned parents are considered as category candidates. In a bottom-up approach, only leaf nodes in the hierarchy are assigned which entail that parent nodes are assigned.

In the context of category occurrences in hierarchical target spaces, a power-law distribution is described in [37]. Later, the authors of [38] have addressed this phenomenon quantitatively deriving a relationship in terms of space complexity for those kind of distributions. They have proved that hierarchical classifiers have lower space complexity than their flat variants if the hierarchical target space satisfies certain conditions based on, e.g., maximum branching factor and the depth of the hierarchy. The hierarchical variants discussed in this survey are of different shape than those discussed in these works, layer-based instead of node-based, and do not suffice the necessary conditions for these relationships to apply.

2.4. Models Relevant for This Survey

The experiments reported in Section 5 are carried out starting with and expanding the models described in [23,24]. These models are evaluated against common baselines, partly inspired by other models e.g., the GRU form [22]. For all models, the state-of-the-art, and the baselines, a hierarchical version is constructed using the principles explained in [34]. This hierarchical version duplicates the original model for each layer in the corresponding ICD taxonomy (ICD-9 or ICD-10). These are then trained in parallel. Furthermore, the weights in these networks are influenced by the weights of neighboring layers via the addition of a hierarchical loss function. This loss function penalizes hierarchical inconsistencies that arise when training the model. This leads to a clear comparison between all tested models among themselves as well as with their hierarchical variants.

3. Materials

3.1. ICD-9 Datasets

The publicly available MIMIC-III dataset [2] is used for ICD-9 code predictions. MIMIC-III is an openly accessible clinical care database. For this research, following the trends of previous related work, the patient stay records from the database are used. Every hospital admission has a corresponding unique HADM-ID. In the MIMIC-III database, some patients have also an added Addendum to their stay. Based on earlier studies, records of only those patients who have discharge summaries linked are selected. The addendum is concatenated to the patient's discharge summary. Analogous to the work in [24], out of the the original database, three sub-datasets are extracted. These datasets are used for the experiments and allow for evaluation in different settings. The sub-datasets are the following.

- **Dis-50** consists of a selection of the discharge summaries from the MIMIC-III dataset (11,369 out of 52,726) for the classification of Top-50 ICD-9 codes. We use the publicly available split [23] for training (8066), testing (1729), and development (1574) of the models.
- **Dis** describes the full label setting where all Diagnostic (6918) and Procedural (2011) ICD-9 codes are used. This leads to a total of 8929 Unique codes on the 52,726 discharge summaries. We again use the publicly available split for training (47,723), testing (3372), and development (1631) of the models.
- **Full** extends the **Dis** dataset with other notes regarding the patient (radiology notes, nursing notes, etc.) in addition to the discharge summaries. This dataset, contains almost thrice the number of tokens for training. We use the same test, train, development split as used in the **Dis** dataset.

3.2. ICD-10 Dataset

The **CodiEsp** corpus [39] consists of 1000 clinical cases, tagged with various ICD-10 codes by health specialists. This dataset is released in the context of the CodiEsp track for CLEF ehealth 2020. The dataset corresponding to the subtask of classifying diagnostic ICD codes is used. The original text fragments are in Spanish but an automatically translated version in English is also provided by the organizers, this version is used in this research. The publicly available dataset contains a split of 500 training samples, 250 development samples, and 250 test samples. In total, the 1000 documents comprises of 16,504 sentences and 396,988 words, with an average of 396.2 words per clinical case. The biggest hurdle while training with this dataset is the size and consequently the small number of training examples for each category present. Figure 4 gives a sorted view of all categories present in the training dataset and the amount of examples tagged with that specific category.

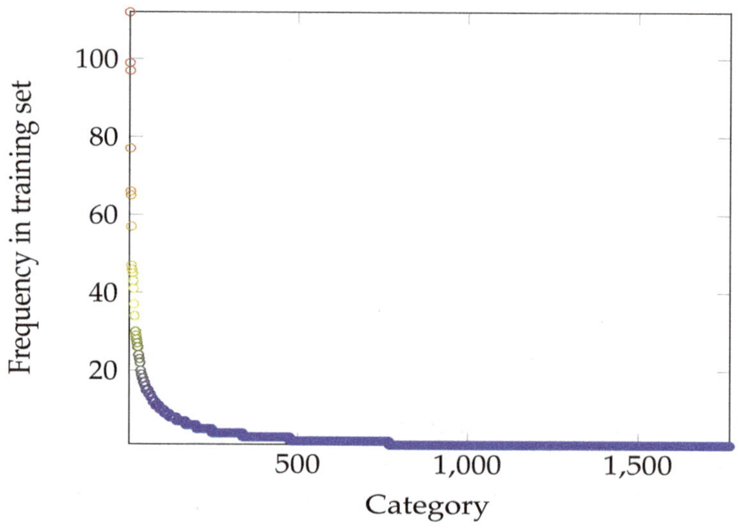

Figure 4. Category frequencies of CodiEsp training dataset.

There are in total 1767 different categories spread out over only 500 training documents. Every document is labeled with on average 11.3 different categories and each category is on average represented by 3.2 training examples. Even the top 50 most frequently occurring categories have only between 15 and 112 corresponding positive training documents. Therefore, tests for this dataset are conducted on these 50 categories. Table 1 gives an overview of statistics for all discussed training datasets. The specifics for the corresponding development and test sets are similar. Displayed statistics for the Dis and the Full dataset are the same since the only difference lies in larger text fragments, resulting in 72,891 unique tokens for the Full dataset compared to 51,917 for Dis. There are no differences concerning the labels.

Table 1. Dataset specifics overview.

Dataset	#Training Docs	#Labels	Avg. #Labels/Doc	Avg. #Training Docs/Label
Dis-50	8067	50	5.7	920
Dis	47,724	8922	15.9	85
Full	47,724	8922	15.9	85
CodiEsp	500	1767	11.3	3.2

3.3. Preprocessing

The preprocessing follows the standard procedure described in [23], i.e., tokens that contain no alphabetic characters are removed and all tokens are put to lowercase. Furthermore tokens that appear in fewer than three training documents are replaced with the "UNK" token. All documents are then truncated to a maximum length of 2500 tokens.

4. Methods

In this section, all tested models will be discussed in detail. First, a simple convolutional and a recurrent baseline commonly used in text classification are described. Then, two recent state-of-the-art models in the field of ICD coding are explained in detail. These models are implemented by the authors following the original papers and are called **DR-CAML** [23] and **MVC-(R)LDA** [24], respectively. We discuss in detail the attention mechanisms and loss functions of these models. Afterwards, as a way of handling the hierarchical dependencies of the ICD-codes, we propose various ways of their integration in all models. This is based on advancements in hierarchical classification as inspired by [34].

All discussed models have for each document i as input a sequence of word vectors x^i as their representation and as output a set of ICD-codes y^i.

4.1. Baselines

The performance of all models will be evaluated and compared against two simple common baselines used for handling sequential input data (text). These models are, respectively, based on convolutional and recurrent neural principles.

4.1.1. Convolutional

The baseline convolutional neural network model, or **CNN**, consists of a 1D temporal convolutional neural layer. This convolutional layer consists of different kernels, which are filters with a specific pattern that are tested against all sequences of the input data with the same length. This is followed by a (max-)pooling layer, to reduce the data size by only remembering the maximum value over a certain range. More formally, for an input x and a given 1D kernel f on element s of the input sequence, the convolutional and pooling operation can be defined as follows.

$$F_1(s) = (x \circledast f)(s) = \sum_{i=0}^{k-1} f(i) \cdot x_{s-i} \tag{1}$$

$$F_2(s) = max_{i=0}^{l-1} F_1(s-1) \tag{2}$$

The amount of filters k and l in the convolutional and pooling layer, respectively, as well as their sizes are optimizable parameters of this model. For both layers a stride length, i.e., the amount by which the filter shifts in the sequence, can be defined leading to a trade-off between output size and observability of detailed features.

4.1.2. Recurrent

As the recurrent neural network baseline, two common approaches are considered.

BiGRU

The **GRU**, or Gated Recurrent Unit, is a gating mechanism in recurrent neural networks. It is the mechanism of recurrent neural networks allowing the model to "learn to forget" less important fragments of the data and "learn to remember" the more important fragments with respect to the learning task. More formally, consider an input vector x_t, update gate vector z_t, reset gate vector r_t, and output vector h_t at time t. The respective values can be calculated as follows.

$$z_t = \sigma(W_z \cdot [h_{t-1}, x_t] + b_z) \tag{3}$$
$$r_t = \sigma(W_r \cdot [h_{t-1}, x_t] + b_r) \tag{4}$$
$$h_t^* = tanh(W_h \cdot [t_t \times h_{t-1}, x_t] + b_h) \tag{5}$$
$$h_t = (1 - z_t) \times h_{t-1} + z_t \times h_t^* \tag{6}$$

This leads to weight matrices W_z, W_r, and W_h to train as well as biases b_z, b_r, and b_h, σ stands for the sigmoid activation function. **BiGRU** is the bidirectional variant of such a model that processes the input data front-to-back and back-to-front in parallel.

BiLSTM

An **LSTM**, or Long Short-Term Memory neural network model, is very similar to a GRU but replaces the update gate with a forget gate and an additional output gate. This way it usually has more computational power than a regular GRU, but at the expense of more trainable parameters and more chance of overfitting when the amount of training data is limited [40–42]. Formally, consider again an input vector x_t and a hidden state vector h_t at time t. Activation vectors for the update gate, forget gate, and output gate are, respectively, represented by z_t, f_t, and o_t. These states relate to each other like follows.

$$z_t = \sigma(W_z \cdot [h_{t-1}, x_t] + b_z) \tag{7}$$
$$f_t = \sigma(W_f \cdot [h_{t-1}, x_t] + b_f) \tag{8}$$
$$o_t = \sigma(W_o \cdot [h_{t-1}, x_t] + b_o) \tag{9}$$
$$c_t^* = tanh(W_c \cdot [h_{t-1}, x_t] + b_c) \tag{10}$$
$$c_t = (f_t) \times c_{t-1} + z_t \times c_t^* \tag{11}$$
$$h_t = o_t \times tanh(c_t) \tag{12}$$

This again leads to weight matrices W_z, W_f, W_o, and W_c to train as well as biases b_z, b_f, b_o, and b_c with σ being the sigmoid activation function. **BiLSTM** is the bidirectional variant of a regular LSTM, analogous to BiGRU, which is the bidirectional variant of GRU.

4.2. Advanced Models

This subsection describes the details of recent state-of-the-art models presented in [23,24] in the way they are used for the experiments in Section 5.

4.2.1. DR-CAML

DR-CAML is a CNN-based model adopted for ICD coding [23]. When an ICD code is defined by the WHO, it is accompanied by a label definition expressed in natural language to guide the model towards learning the appropriate parameter values of the model. For this purpose, the model employs a per-label attention mechanism enabling it to learn distinct document representations for each label. It has been shown that for labels for which there are very few training instances available, this approach is advantageous. The idea is that the description of a target code is itself a very good training example for the corresponding code. Similarity between the representation of a given test sample and the representation of the description of a target code gives extra confidence in assigning this label.

In general, after the convolutional layer, DR-CAML employs a per-label attention mechanism to attend to the relevant parts of text for each predicted label. An additional advantage is that the per-label attention mechanism provides the model with the ability of explaining why it decided to assign each code by showing the spans of text relevant for the ICD code.

DR-CAML consists of two modules: one for the representation of the input text, and the other for the embedding of the label's description as is visualized in Figure 5. The CAML module has a CNN at the base layer which takes a sequence of the embeddings of the text tokens as input and consequently represents the document as the matrix H. Then, the per-label attention mechanism applies. Attention in this context means learning which parts of some context (the label description vectors) are relevant for a given input vector.

After calculating the attention vector α using a softmax activation function, it is applied as a product with H. With h_l, the vector parameter for label l, the vector representation for each label is computed as

$$v_l = \sum_{n=1}^{N} \alpha_{l,n} h_n \tag{13}$$

Given the vector representation of a document and the probability for label l, $\hat{y}_l$ can be obtained as shown in Figure 5.

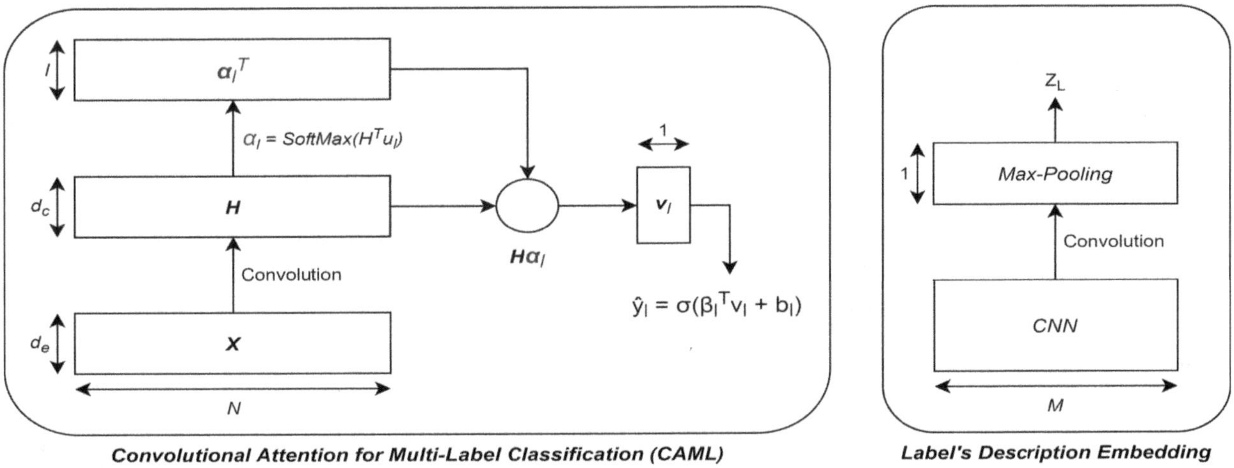

Figure 5. DR-CAML (after [23]).

The CNN modules on the left hand side try to minimize the binary cross entropy loss. The second module is a max-pooling CNN model which produces a max-pooled vector, z_l, by getting the description of code l. Assuming n_y is the number of true labels in train data, the final loss is computed by adding a regularization term to the base loss function. The loss function is explained in more detail in Section 4.2.3.

4.2.2. MVC-(R)LDA

MVC-LDA and **MVC-RLDA** can be seen as extensions of DR-CAML. Similar to that model, they are based on a CNN architecture with a label attention mechanism that considers ICD coding as a multi-task binary classification problem. The added functionality lies in the use of parallel CNNs with different kernel sizes to capture information of different granularity. MVC-LDA, the top module in Figure 6, is a multi-view CNN model stacked on an embedding layer. MVC-RLDA reintroduces the per-label attention mechanism introduced in the previous subsection.

In general, the multi-view CNNs are constructed with four CNNs that have the same number of filters but with different kernel sizes. This convolutional layer is followed by a max-pooling function across all channels to select the most relevant span of text for each filter. A separate attention layer for each label comes next, helping the model to attend to relevant parts of a document for each label. A linear layer with weight vector V_j is implemented for the jth label and CV_j is the attention for the input C and label j. This attention vector CV_j is the output of a dense layer with softmax activation function leading to a relative weighting of the input elements C.

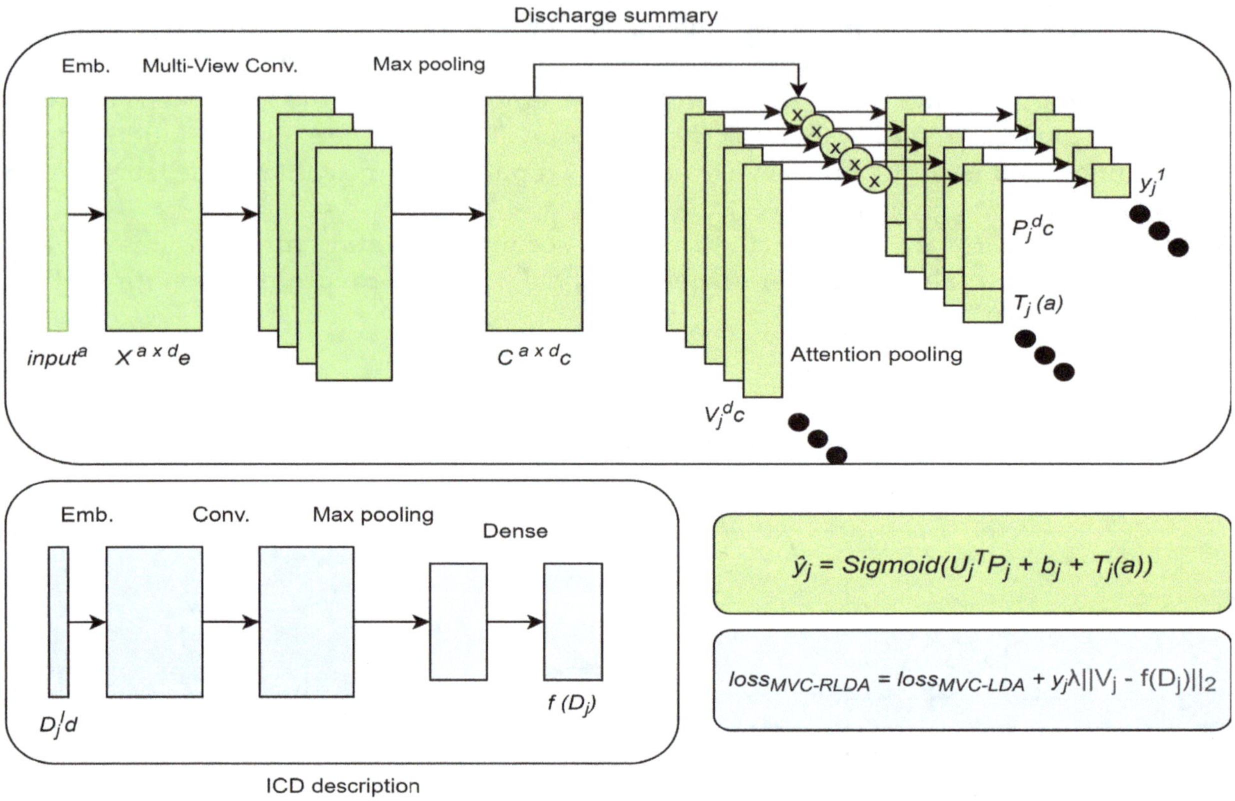

Figure 6. MVC-(R)LDA (after the work in [24]).

Then, the pooled outputs of the attention layer are computed as

$$P_j = C^T(CV_j). \tag{14}$$

At the end, a dense layer is used for each label. The length of an input document is also encoded into the output layers with embedding function

$$T_j(l) = Sigmoid(K_j l + d_j), \tag{15}$$

to decrease the problem of under-coding to some extent. This is done as in [24], which showed a statistically significant Pearson's correlation between the input length and the number of ground truth codes. Therefore, the model can derive an underlying bias that, on average, shorter input documents represent a lower amount of categories.

Parameters a, K_j, and d_j in the length embedding function respectively represent the input length, and the layer's weight and bias, respectively, for a given label j. The prediction y_j for class j is then computed as

$$y_j = Sigmoid(U_j^T P_j + b_j + T_j(a)). \tag{16}$$

Similar to DR-CAML, this model tries to minimize the binary loss function. Adding the label description embedding to MVC-LDA, the lower part of Figure 4 leads to MVC-RLDA whose loss function includes an extra weighted term as a regularizer. It guides the attention weights to avoid overfitting. In addition, this regularization forces the attention for classes with similar descriptions to be closer to each other. The loss function is again explained in more detail in Section 4.2.3.

4.2.3. Loss Function

The loss functions used to train DR-CAML and the multiview models MVD-(R)LDA are calculated in the same way. The general loss function is the binary cross entropy loss $loss_{BCE}$. This loss is extended by regularization on the long description vectors of the target categories, visualized in Figure 6 on the lower right corner.

Given N different training examples x^i. The values of $\hat{y}_l$ and max-pooled vector z_l can be calculated as represented in Figure 5 by getting the description of code l out of all L target codes. In this figure, and the following formulas, β_l is a vector of prediction weights and v_l the vector representation for code l. Assuming n_y is the number of true labels in the training data, the final loss is computed by adding regularization to the base loss function as

$$\hat{y}_l = \sigma(\beta_l^t v_l + b_l) \tag{17}$$

$$loss_{BCE}(X) = -\sum_{i=1}^{N}\sum_{l=1}^{L} y_l \log(\hat{y}_l) + (1 - y_l)\log(1 - \hat{y}_l) \tag{18}$$

$$loss_{Model}(X) = loss_{BCE} + \lambda \frac{1}{n_y} \sum_{i=1}^{N}\sum_{l=1}^{L} \|z_l - \beta_l\|_2 \tag{19}$$

4.3. *Modeling Hierarchical Dependencies*

In this section, we investigate the modeling of hierarchical dependencies as extensions of the models described above. A first part integrates the hierarchical dependencies directly into the structure of the model. This leads to **Hierarchical models**, which are layered variants of the already discussed approaches. The second way hierarchical dependencies are explicitly introduced into the model is via the use of a hierarchical loss function to penalize hierarchical inconsistencies across the model's prediction layer.

4.3.1. Hierarchical Models

Hierarchical relationships can be shaped directly into the architecture of any of the described models above. The ICD-9 taxonomy can be modeled as a tree with a general ICD root and 4 levels of depth, as already described in Section 1. This leads to a hierarchical variant of any of the models. In this variant, not 1 but 4 identical models will be trained, one for each of the different layers in the ICD hierarchy (corresponding to the length of the codes).

Such an approach is presented in [34] and is adapted to the target domain of ICD categories. An overview of the approach is given in Figure 7.

The input for each layer is partially dependent on an intermediary representation from the previous layer as well as the original input through concatenation of both. Layers are stacked from most to least specific or from leaf to root node in the taxonomy. Models corresponding to different layers will then rely on different features, or characteristics, to classify the input vectors. This way the deepest, most advanced representations, can be used for classifying the most abstract and broad categories. On the other hand, for the most specific categories, word level features can directly be used to make detailed decisions between classes that are very similar.

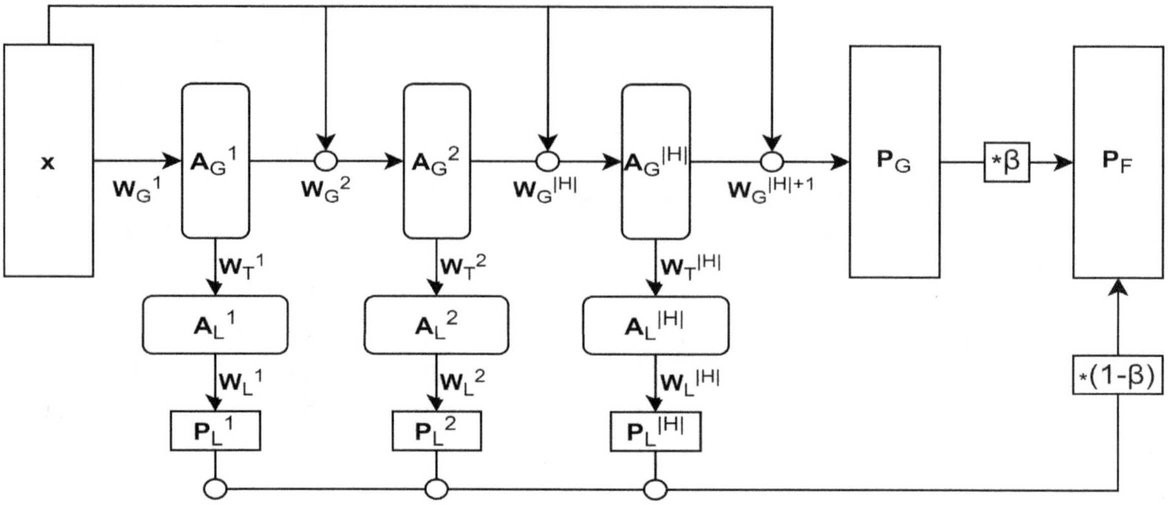

Figure 7. Overview of hierarchical variant of a model, inspired by [34].

4.3.2. Hierarchical Loss Function

To capture the hierarchical relationships in a given model, the loss function of the above models can be extended with an additional term. This leads to the definition of a **Hierarchical loss function** ($loss_H$). This loss function penalizes classifications that contradict the inherent ICD hierarchy. More specifically, when a parent category is not predicted to be true, none of its child categories should be predicted to be true. The hierarchical loss between a child and its parent in the tree is then defined as the difference between their computed probability scores, with 0 as a lower bound. More formally, for the entire loss function $loss_{H\_Model}$ for a category of layer X, combining the regular training loss $loss_{Model}$ described above and the hierarchical loss $loss_H$, is calculated as follows,

$$P(X) = Probability(X == True) \tag{20}$$

$$Par(X) = Probability(Parent(X) == True) \tag{21}$$

$$L(X) = True\,label\,of\;\;X(0\,or\;\;1) \tag{22}$$

$$loss_H(X) = Clip(P(X) - Par(X), 0, 1) \tag{23}$$

$$loss_{H\_Model}(X) = (1-\lambda)loss_{Model}(X) + \lambda loss_H(X) \tag{24}$$

which leaves a parameter λ to optimize the loss function (parameter λ is optimized over the training set).

5. Results

5.1. MIMIC-III

Results are displayed for five different models. First, results for the two baseline models, **CNN** and **BiGRU**, are shown. Because in most of the experiments, the BiGRU models performed at least on par with their BiLSTM variants, we only report the results of **BiGRU** as a recurrent neural network baseline. The reason for this good performance of GRU models compared to LSTM models most likely resides in the amount of available training data for various target categories. Then, we report on three more advanced models as discussed in the Method section: **DR-CAML, MVC-LDA,** and **MVD-RLDA**. Different hyperparameter values are considered and tested on the development set of MIMIC-III the setting giving the highest average performance on the development set is reported in Table 2.

Table 2. Optimal hyperparameter values obtained on the development set of the MIMIC-III dataset.

	CNN	BiGRU	DRCAML	MVC-LDA	MVC-RLDA
# of filters	500	-	50	6,8,10,12	6,8,10,12
Filter Sizes	4	-	10	70	90
λ	-	0.0005	-	-	0.0005
Lr	0.003	0.003	0.0001	0.001	0.001
Batch size	16	16	16	4	4
Seq. length~	2500	2500	2500	10000	10000

For all these models using their optimal hyperparameter settings, the average performance is reported in terms of Micro F1, Macro F1, Micro AUC (ROC), and Precision@X. For models that are only evaluated on the top 50 most frequent categories in the training data, results are displayed in Table 3. This experiment is then repeated over all categories, which leads to the results in Table 4. Last, Table 5 gives the results of training the models on all labels for the Full dataset.

Table 3. Results of flat models on top 50 most frequent categories of the MIMIC-III Dis-50 dataset.

		Micro F1	Macro F1	Micro AUC	P@5
Dis-50	**CNN**	63.42	59.74	91.57	62.33
	GRU	63.49	55.72	91.79	61.72
	DR-CAML	69.64	64.56	93.90	65.39
	MVC-LDA	69.07	64.17	93.69	65.15
	MVC-RLDA	69.53	64.85	93.77	64.91

Table 4. Results of flat models on all labels of the MIMIC-III Dis dataset.

		Micro F1 Proc	Micro F1 Diag	Micro F1 Both	Micro AUC	P@5
Dis	**CNN**	51.01	40.80	42.58	84.38	59.48
	GRU	53.88	40.86	43.40	85.36	61.59
	DR-CAML	48.99	59.03	50.47	89.45	68.28
	MVC-LDA	59.75	51.60	53.03	90.02	69.77
	MVC-RLDA	58.84	50.74	52.10	89.77	68.71

Table 5. Results of flat models on all labels of the MIMIC-III Full dataset.

		Micro F1 Proc	Micro F1 Diag	Micro F1 Both	Micro AUC	P@5
Full	**CNN**	46.19	41.19	42.18	83.96	57.53
	GRU	46.50	37.74	39.64	83.19	55.00
	DR-CAML	57.90	41.40	49.94	89.42	67.16
	MVC-LDA	58.12	50.70	51.97	89.93	68.53
	MVC-RLDA	57.61	49.67	50.97	89.68	67.60

This experiment is repeated for the hierarchical variants of all described models. This time, only results on the top 50 most frequent target categories are reported in Table 6. As hierarchical models introduce a large number of additional intermediate categories, the target space is too large to train these hierarchical variants in a full category setting.

Table 6. Results of hierarchical models obtained on the MIMIC-III Dis-50 dataset.

		Micro F1	Macro F1	Micro AUC	P@5
Dis-50	**CNN**	61.70	53.79	90.62	59.87
	GRU	62.38	54.88	91.77	60.03
	DR-CAML	67.68	63.74	93.47	63.48
	MVC-LDA	65.21	60.06	92.29	62.41
	MVC-RLDA	65.43	61.22	92.34	61.73

To assess the importance of the different components of the highest performing model on MIMIC-III Dis, an ablation study is conducted. The multi-view and the hierarchical component are added and the regularization on long descriptions of the target ICD-codes is removed while all other components stay the same. The difference in performance is measured and visualized in Figure 8.

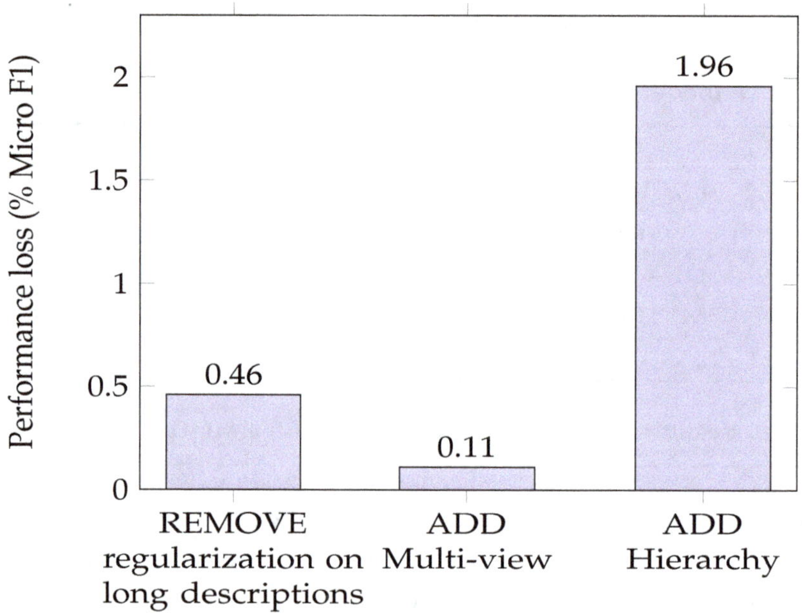

Figure 8. Ablation study on highest performing model (hierarchical MVC-RLDA) for MIMIC-III dataset.

5.2. *CodiEsp*

Similar experiments are carried out on the CodiEsp dataset, while only using the top 50 most frequent codes. The same hyperparameter settings are used as in Table 2. Results are visualized in Tables 7 and 8. Results for the full target space are not reported, as 90% of the target categories would only have 5 or less positive training examples. Furthermore, this would lead to a target space of 1767 different categories with only 500 training examples in total, which makes training of a decent model unfeasible.

Table 7. Results of flat models on top 50 codes obtained on the CodiEsp dataset.

		Micro F1	Macro F1	Micro AUC	P@5
CodiEsp	**CNN**	12.52	6.17	49.35	7.96
	GRU	11.54	11.03	50.54	7.68
	DR-CAML	9.58	8.24	48.63	7.96
	MVC-LDA	10.84	6.23	49.26	4.17
	MVC-RLDA	11.52	6.67	48.01	3.70

Table 8. Results of hierarchical models for top 50 codes obtained on the CodiEsp dataset.

		Micro F1	Macro F1	Micro AUC	P@5
CodiEsp	CNN	12.44	6.18	53.08	2.84
	GRU	11.87	11.50	50.14	7.68
	DR-CAML	10.35	3.97	53.61	5.59
	MVC-LDA	13.00	2.79	60.76	11.94
	MVC-RLDA	13.92	4.21	56.38	8.72

To assess the importance of the different components of the highest performing model on CodiEsp, an ablation study is conducted. The multi-view, the hierarchical component, and the regularization on long descriptions of the target ICD-codes are each removed while all other components stay the same. The difference in performance is measured and visualized in Figure 9.

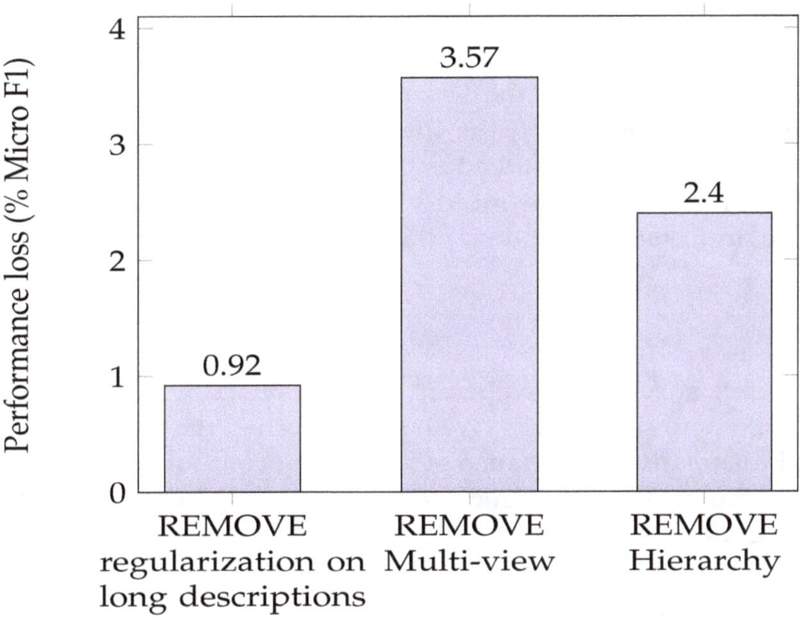

Figure 9. Ablation study on highest performing model (hierarchical MVC-RLDA) for CodiEsp dataset.

6. Discussion

A comparison between the results displayed in Tables 3 and 4 shines a light on the value of the multiview component. The micro F1 scores of the five models are in similar relationship to each other in both tables, except for the two multiview models. They outperform CAML in the full label setting of the MIMIC-III Dis dataset, where they show very similar behavior to CAML in a top-50 category setting, where for each of the categories a decent amount of training samples is available. When the target space increases and more categories have fewer training examples, the added granularity of having multiple kernel sizes in the MVC-(R)LDA model pays off. Table 5 shows results for models trained on the Full dataset. The best performing model (MVC-LDA, 58.12%) gets outperformed by the best performing model for all labels on Dis (MVD-LDA, 59, 75%). The addition of the information in other medical documents than just discharge summaries thus seems to complicate instead of facilitate the classification process.

Furthermore, comparing Tables 3 and 6, where the influence of the hierarchical parameter can be assessed in a top-50 category setting, reveals a shift in the opposite direction. While in general, the modeling of the hierarchical relationships hurts the classification process for all categories, it hinders the multiview models the most. This time, DR-CAML is clearly the best performing model. Adding multiview and simultaneously modeling the hierarchical relationships between the target categories tend to make the model overfit on the training data.

Looking at Tables 7 and 8, it is clear that the lack of a sufficient amount of training data in CodiEsp (about 100 times less than for the Dis dataset) for most categories led to lower performance of all models on this dataset. For the flat variants of the models, a regular CNN even outperforms the more complex models. As the amount of training data is low, the added complexity of the latter models hinders them generalizing well for unseen data. Comparing the results in both tables also leads to the conclusion that in contrast to the results on MIMIC-III, on average the hierarchical component increases the classification performance based on Micro F1 on CodiEsp. Where the information embedded in the ICD taxonomy is redundant and even counteracting the performance for the larger MIMIC-III dataset, it is leveraged when there is a lack of information in the training data itself, which is the case for CodiEsp.

Last, Figures 8 and 9 display the relative importance of the long description regularization, the multi-view. and the hierarchy for the top performing model on both the Dis and CodiEsp datasets. For the Dis dataset, not using the hierarchy is by far the most important component. The regularization on long descriptions still adds 0.46% and the multi-view almost does not influence the results. For CodiEsp, it shows that the multi-view component has the biggest influence, followed by the hierarchy, whose importance on this smaller dataset is already shown previously.

7. Conclusions

In this paper, we have surveyed the current methods used for classification of clinical reports based on ICD codes using neural networks. We have combined the techniques already present in the literature and assessed the relative importance of all present components. Combining a convolutional framework with self-attention as well as regularizing, the loss function with attention on the long descriptions of target ICD codes proved to be valuable. Furthermore, a hierarchical objective was integrated in all presented models. Its added value lies especially in a setting with low amounts of available training data. Last, extending the dataset with the information present in other medical documents introduced too much noise into the data, hindering the performance of the tested models.

Concerning future research directions, it would be valuable to test the techniques on a ICD-10 or ICD-11 dataset of larger size. This would give better insights into which performance these models could achieve in current hospital settings. On a similar note, tackling the problem of lack of data by finding a way to combine the available training data from different datasets (e.g., MIMIC-III and CodiEsp) and different ontologies (e.g., ICD-9, ICD-10, and MeSH) could further improve the classification performance of all models. Last, it would be interesting to investigate the use of hierarchical descriptions as an addition to the loss function, giving another use for the information inherently present in the ICD taxonomy.

Author Contributions: Conceptualization, E.M. and M.-F.M.; Methodology, E.M. and M.-F.M.; Software, E.M., A.A. and A.K.; Validation, E.M., A.A. and A.K.; Formal Analysis, E.M. and M.-F.M.; Investigation, E.M.; Resources, A.K.; Data Curation, A.K.; Writing-Original Draft Preparation, E.M. and M.-F.M.;Writing-Review Editing, E.M., A.A., A.K. and M.-F.M..; Visualization, E.M.; Supervision, M.-F.M.; Project Administration, A.A. and M.-F.M.; Funding Acquisition, M.-F.M. All authors have read and agreed to the published version of the manuscript.

References

1. Larkey, L.; Croft, W.B. *Automatic Assignment of ICD9 Codes To Discharge Summaries*; Technical Report; University of Massachusetts: Amherst, MA, USA, 1995.
2. Johnson, A.E.W.; Pollard, T.J.; Shen, L.; Lehman, L.w.H.; Feng, M.; Ghassemi, M.; Moody, B.; Szolovits, P.; Anthony Celi, L.; Mark, R.G. MIMIC-III, a freely accessible critical care database. *Sci. Data* **2016**, *3*, 1–9. [CrossRef] [PubMed]
3. Larkey, L.S.; Croft, W.B. Combining classifiers in text categorization. In Proceedings of the 19th Annual International ACM SIGIR Conference on Research and Development in Information Retrieval, Zurich, Switzerland, 18–22 August 1996; (Special Issue of the SIGIRForum); pp. 289–297.
4. Goldstein, I.; Arzumtsyan, A.; Özlem, U. Three approaches to automatic assignment of ICD-9-CM codes to radiology reports. In *Proceedings of the AMIA Annual Symposium*; American Medical Informatics Association: Washington, DC, USA, 2007; pp. 279–283.
5. Farkas, R.; Szarvas, G. Automatic construction of rule-based ICD-9-CM coding systems. *BMC Bioinform.* **2008**, *9* (Suppl. 3), S10. [CrossRef] [PubMed]
6. Marafino, B.J.; Davies, J.M.; Bardach, N.S.; Dean, M.L.; Dudley, R.A. N-gram support vector machines for scalable procedure and diagnosis classification, with applications to clinical free text data from the intensive care unit. *J. Am. Med. Inform. Assoc.* **2014**, *21*, 871–875. [CrossRef] [PubMed]
7. Stanfill, M.; Williams, M.; Fenton, S.; Jenders, R.; Hersh, W. A systematic literature review of automated clinical coding and classification systems. *J. Am. Med. Inform. Assoc. JAMIA* **2010**, *17*, 646–651. [CrossRef] [PubMed]
8. Kavuluru, R.; Rios, A.; Lu, Y. An empirical evaluation of supervised learning approaches in assigning diagnosis codes to electronic medical records. *Artif. Intell. Med.* **2015**, *65*, 155–166. [CrossRef]
9. Scheurwegs, E.; Cule, B.; Luyckx, K.; Luyten, L.; Daelemans, W. Selecting relevant features from the electronic health record for clinical code prediction. *J. Biomed. Inform.* **2017**, *74*, 92–103. [CrossRef]
10. Leo, M.; Furnari, A.; Medioni, G.G.; Trivedi, M.M.; Farinella, G.M. Deep Learning for Assistive Computer Vision. In Proceedings of the Computer Vision—ECCV 2018 Workshops—Part VI, Munich, Germany, 8–14 September 2018; pp. 3–14.
11. Shickel, B.; Tighe, P.; Bihorac, A.; Rashidi, P. Deep EHR: A survey of recent advances in deep learning techniques for electronic health record (EHR) analysis. *IEEE J. Biomed. Health Inform.* **2018**, *22*, 1589–1604. [CrossRef]
12. Kelly, L.; Suominen, H.; Goeuriot, L.; Neves, M.; Kanoulas, E.; Li, D.; Azzopardi, L.; Spijker, R.; Zuccon, G.; Scells, H.; et al. Overview of the CLEF eHealth Evaluation Lab 2019. In *International Conference of the Cross-Language Evaluation Forum for European Languages*; Springer: Cham, Switzerland, 2019; pp. 322–339.
13. Shi, H.; Xie, P.; Hu, Z.; Zhang, M.; Xing, E.P. Towards automated ICD coding using deep learning. *arXiv* **2017**, arXiv:1711.04075.
14. Duarte, F.; Martins, B.; Pinto, C.S.; Silva, M.J. Deep neural models for ICD-10 coding of death certificates and autopsy reports in free-text. *J. Biomed. Inform.* **2018**, *80*, 64–77. [CrossRef]
15. Xie, P.; Xing, E. A neural architecture for automated ICD coding. In *Proceedings of the 56th Annual Meeting of the Association for Computational Linguistics (Volume 1: Long Papers)*; ACL: Melbourne, Australia, 2018.
16. Huang, J.; Osorio, C.; Sy, L.W. An empirical evaluation of deep learning for ICD-9 code assignment using MIMIC-III clinical notes. *Comput. Methods Prog. Biomed.* **2019**, *177*, 141–153. [CrossRef]
17. Li, M.; Fei, Z.; Zeng, M.; Wu, F.; Li, Y.; Pan, Y.; Wang, J. Automated ICD-9 coding via a deep learning approach. *IEEE/ACM Trans. Comput. Biol. Bioinform.* **2019**, *16*, 1193–1202. [CrossRef] [PubMed]
18. Xu, K.; Lam, M.; Pang, J.; Gao, X.; Band, C.; Mathur, P.; Papay, F.; Khanna, A.K.; Cywinski, J.B.; Maheshwari, K.; et al. Multimodal machine learning for automated ICD coding. In *Proceedings of the 4th Machine Learning for Healthcare Conference*; Doshi-Velez, F., Fackler, J., Jung, K., Kale, D., Ranganath, R., Wallace, B., Wiens, J., Eds.; PMLR: Ann Arbor, MI, USA, 2019; Volume 106, pp. 197–215.
19. Quinlan, J.R. Induction of decision trees. *Mach. Learn.* **1986**, *1*, 81–106. [CrossRef]
20. Wang, G.; Li, C.; Wang, W.; Zhang, Y.; Shen, D.; Zhang, X.; Henao, R.; Carin, L. Joint embedding of words and labels for text classification. In *Proceedings of the 56th Annual Meeting of the Association for Computational Linguistics (Volume 1: Long Papers)*; ACL: Melbourne, Australia, 2018.

21. Zeng, M.; Li, M.; Fei, Z.; Yu, Y.; Pan, Y.; Wang, J. Automatic ICD-9 coding via deep transfer learning. *Neurocomputing* **2018**, *324*, 43–50. [CrossRef]
22. Baumel, T.; Nassour-Kassis, J.; Elhadad, M.; Elhadad, N. Multi-Label Classification of Patient Notes: A Case Study on ICD Code Assignment. In Proceedings of the Workshops at the Thirty-Second AAAI Conference on Artificial Intelligence, Hilton, NO, USA, 2–7 February 2018.
23. Mullenbach, J.; Wiegreffe, S.; Duke, J.; Sun, J.; Eisenstein, J. Explainable prediction of medical codes from clinical text. In *Proceedings of the 2018 Conference of the North American Chapter of the Association for Computational Linguistics: Human Language Technologies, Volume 1 (Long Papers)*; ACL: New Orleans, LA, USA, 2018.
24. Sadoughi, N.; Finley, G.P.; Fone, J.; Murali, V.; Korenevski, M.; Baryshnikov, S.; Axtmann, N.; Miller, M.; Suendermann-Oeft, D. Medical code prediction with multi-view convolution and description-regularized label-dependent attention. *arXiv* **2018**, arXiv:1811.01468.
25. Amin, S.; Neumann, G.; Dunfield, K.; Vechkaeva, A.; Chapman, K.A.; Wixted, M.K. MLT-DFKI at CLEF eHealth 2019: Multi-label classification of ICD-10 codes with BERT. In Proceedings of the Working Notes of CLEF 2019—Conference and Labs of the Evaluation, Forum, Lugano, Switzerland, 9–12 September 2019.
26. Campbell, S.; Giadresco, K. Computer-assisted clinical coding: A narrative review of the literature on its benefits, limitations, implementation and impact on clinical coding professionals. *Health Inf. Manag. J.* **2019**, *49*, 183335831985130. [CrossRef] [PubMed]
27. Deschacht, K.; Moens, M. Efficient hierarchical entity classifier using conditional random fields. In Proceedings of the 2nd Workshop on Ontology Learning and Population: Bridging the Gap between Text and Knowledge@COLING/ACL 2006, Sydney, Australia, 22 July 2006; pp. 33–40.
28. Babbar, R.; Partalas, I.; Gaussier, É.; Amini, M. On flat versus hierarchical classification in large-scale taxonomies. In Proceedings of the Advances in Neural Information Processing Systems 26: Proccedings of the 27th Annual Conference on Neural Information Processing Systems 2013, Lake Tahoe, NV, USA, 5–8 December 2013; pp. 1824–1832.
29. Gopal, S.; Yang, Y. *Recursive Regularization for Large-Scale Classification with Hierarchical and Graphical Dependencies*; Association for Computing Machinery: New York, NY, USA, 2013.
30. Cai, L.; Hofmann, T. Hierarchical document categorization with support vector machines. In Proceedings of the Thirteenth ACM International Conference on Information and Knowledge Management, Washington, DC, USA, 8–13 November 2004.
31. Jati, A.; Kumar, N.; Chen, R.; Georgiou, P. Hierarchy-aware loss function on a tree structured label space for audio event detection. In Proceedings of the ICASSP 2019–2019 IEEE International Conference on Acoustics, Speech and Signal Processing (ICASSP), Brighton, UK, 12–17 May 2019; pp. 6–10.
32. Perotte, A.; Pivovarov, R.; Natarajan, K.; Weiskopf, N.; Wood, F.; Elhadad, N. Diagnosis code assignment: Models and evaluation metrics. *J. Am. Med. Inform. Assoc.* **2014**, *21*, 231–237. [CrossRef]
33. Mohammed, A.A.; Umaashankar, V. Effectiveness of hierarchical softmax in large scale classification tasks. In Proceedings of the 2018 International Conference on Advances in Computing, Communications and Informatics (ICACCI), Bangalore, India, 19–22 September 2018; pp. 1090–1094.
34. Wehrmann, J.; Cerri, R.; Barros, R. Hierarchical multi-label classification networks. In Proceedings of the Thirty-Fifth International Conference on Machine Learning, Stockholm, Sweden, 10–15 July 2018; pp. 5075–5084.
35. Silla, C.N.; Freitas, A.A. A survey of hierarchical classification across different application domains. *Data Min. Knowl. Discov.* **2011**, *22*, 31–72. [CrossRef]
36. Kowsari, K.; Brown, D.E.; Heidarysafa, M.; Meimandi, K.J.; Gerber, M.S.; Barnes, L.E. HDLTex: Hierarchical Deep Learning for Text Classification. In Proceedings of the 2017 16th IEEE International Conference on Machine Learning and Applications, Cancun, Mexico, 18–21 December 2017.
37. Yang, Y.; Zhang, J.; Kisiel, B. A scalability analysis of classifiers in text categorization. In Proceedings of the 26th Annual International ACM SIGIR Conference on Research and Development in Informaion Retrieval, Toronto, ON, Canada, 28 July–1 August 2003; pp. 96–103.
38. Babbar, R.; Metzig, C.; Partalas, I.; Gaussier, E.; Amini, M.R. On power law distributions in large-scale taxonomies. *ACM Sigkdd Explor. Newsl.* **2014**, *16*, 47–56. [CrossRef]

39. Miranda-Escalada, A.; Gonzalez-Agirre, A.; Krallinger, M. CodiEsp Corpus: Spanish Clinical Cases Coded in ICD10 (CIE10)—eHealth CLEF2020. Available online: https://zenodo.org/record/3758054#.XxXGgy17E6h (accessed on 29 July 2020).
40. Chung, J.; Gulcehre, C.; Cho, K.; Bengio, Y. Empirical evaluation of gated recurrent neural networks on sequence modeling. *arXiv* **2014**, arXiv:1412.3555.
41. Yin, W.; Kann, K.; Yu, M.; Schütze, H. Comparative study of CNN and RNN for natural language processing. *arXiv* **2017**, arXiv:1702.01923.
42. Kaiser, Ł.; Sutskever, I. Neural GPUs learn algorithms. *arXiv* **2015**, arXiv:1511.08228.

3

Searching for Premature Ventricular Contraction from Electrocardiogram by Using One-Dimensional Convolutional Neural Network

Junsheng Yu [1], Xiangqing Wang [1,*], Xiaodong Chen [2] and Jinglin Guo [1]

1 School of Electronic Engineering, Beijing University of Posts and Telecommunications, Beijing 100876, China; jsyu@bupt.edu.cn (J.Y.); jinglinguo@126.com (J.G.)
2 Queen Mary University of London, London E1 4NS, UK; xiaodong.chen@qmul.ac.uk
* Correspondence: wangxiangqing@bupt.edu.cn

Abstract: Premature ventricular contraction (PVC) is a common cardiac arrhythmia that can occur in ordinary healthy people and various heart disease patients. Clinically, cardiologists usually use a long-term electrocardiogram (ECG) as a medium to detect PVC. However, it is time-consuming and labor-intensive for cardiologists to analyze the long-term ECG accurately. To this end, this paper suggests a simple but effective approach to search for PVC from the long-term ECG. The recommended method first extracts each heartbeat from the long-term ECG by applying a fixed time window. Subsequently, the model based on the one-dimensional convolutional neural network (CNN) tags these heartbeats without any preprocessing, such as denoise. Unlike previous PVC detection methods that use hand-crafted features, the proposed plan rationally and automatically extracts features and identify PVC with supervised learning. The proposed PVC detection algorithm acquires 99.64% accuracy, 96.97% sensitivity, and 99.84% specificity for the MIT-BIH arrhythmia database. Besides, when the number of samples in the training set is 3.3 times that of the test set, the proposed method does not misjudge any heartbeat from the test set. The simulation results show that it is reliable to use one-dimensional CNN for PVC recognition. More importantly, the overall system does not rely on complex and cumbersome preprocessing.

Keywords: electrocardiogram; deep learning; convolutional neural network; Premature ventricular contraction

---

1. Introduction

The heart is a vital organ of the human body and has four chambers: right atrium, right ventricle, left atrium, left ventricle. These four chambers cooperate in providing power for blood flow in the blood vessel. First, the oxygen-poor blood flows through the right atrium and right ventricle in turn, and finally reaches the lungs. Then the oxygen-poor blood absorbs oxygen from the air in the alveoli. With the left atrium and left ventricle's work, the rest organ and tissue will receive the oxygenated blood. The most intuitive feeling of this process is the heartbeat. Every heartbeat moves blood forward through the arteries. Heart rhythm, which is the heartbeat pattern, is a critical clinical indicator to assess whether the heart is working correctly. Healthy heart rhythm is orderly and uniform. Abnormal heart rhythm, also called arrhythmia, is usually closely related to cardiovascular disease (CVD). According to the World Health Organization (WHO), CVD is widespread globally. Taking America and China as examples, ten people die every 6 min in America from CVD, and nearly 20.7% of China residents suffer from CVD [1].

Although there are many origins of the arrhythmia, premature ventricular contraction (PVC) caused by an ectopic cardiac pacemaker located in the ventricle is the most common cause. Moreover,

PVC is also related to multiple conditions, such as myocardial infarction (MI), left ventricular dysfunction (LVD) [2,3]. Electrocardiogram (ECG), which can record the heart's electrical signals, is a non-invasive and effective visualization tool widely used by cardiologists [4]. A normal heartbeat generates four entities with different shapes in ECG—a P wave, a QRS complex, a T wave, and a U wave, as shown in Figure 1.

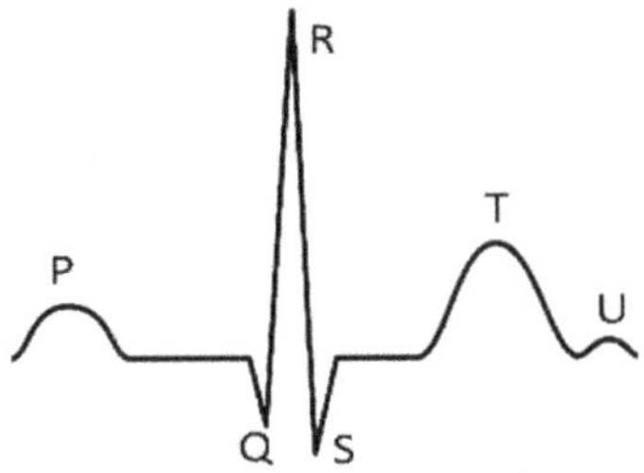

Figure 1. There is a normal heartbeat in electrocardiogram (ECG). The atria's depolarization caused the P wave; the ventricles' depolarization caused the QRS complex; the repolarization of the ventricles caused the T wave; the repolarization of the Purkinje fibers caused the U wave.

It is worth mentioning that the long-term ECG is more clinically significant for the diagnosis of PVC. However, it is time-consuming and arduous for cardiologists to analyze many long-term ECGs. Therefore, accurate and automatic searching for PVC from the long-term ECG is crucial for improving cardiology workflow efficiency.

In recent years, many researchers have developed various algorithms to search for PVC from ECG, as summarized in Table 1. Most of the algorithms manually extract morphological-based features. Manikandan et al. designed a set of temporal characteristics and proposed a decision-rule-based detection algorithm. The suggested method achieved an average sensitivity of 89.69% and specificity of 99.63% based on the MIT-BIH arrhythmia database [5]. Jun et al. extracted six features from the ECG signal and developed a classification algorithm on TensorFlow [6], an open-source machine learning platform. This algorithm used an optimized deep neural network (DNN) whose input is the six features, as the classifier. These six characteristics are R-peak amplitude, R-R interval time, QRS duration time, ventricular activation time, Q-peak, and S-peak amplitude. The experimental results based on the MIT-BIH arrhythmia database achieved 99.41% accuracy [7].

Hadia et al. not only summarized a feature extraction procedure based on the Principal Component Analysis (PCA) and waveform estimation but also combined the extracted features and k-nearest neighbor (KNN) algorithm. The classification sensitivity of this model is 93.45% [8]. Atanasoski et al. presented an unsupervised clustering method based on the R-R intervals and morphological rule. This algorithm does not rely on pre-existing labels and has an excellent overall accuracy above 99.5% and specificity above 99.6% [9]. Junior et al. developed a system based on threshold adaptive algorithm and wavelet transform for PVC detection. The result validated on the MIT-BIH arrhythmia database reported that Daubechies 2 wavelet mother is more indicated compared with Coiflets and Symlets [10]. Oliveira et al. proposed a simplified set of features extracted from geometric figures constructed over QRS complexes and selected the most suitable classifiers based on the analytic hierarchy process (AHP). The results of this method indicated that the artificial immune system (AIS) classifier with the geometrical features is the best suggestion for PVC recognition [11].

Considering that labeled ECG data is rare and precious, Lynggaarda suggested a multivariate statistical classifier that used robust designed features and a regularization mechanism. Even though this classifier's input is a very sparse amount of expert annotated ECG data, this model's average accuracy, specificity, and sensitivity are above 96% by using the MIT-BIH arrhythmia database [12]. Sokolova et al. recommended a set of weighted shape parameters from the different QRS shape metrics and designed a two-stage PVC detection rule. All these shape parameters are in the time and frequency domains. It is worth noting that this method achieved good results on the multi-lead ECG database: the St. Petersburg INCART 12-lead Arrhythmia Database [13]. Rizal and Wijayanto proposed a simple and low computation method. This method only used six characteristics obtained by the multi-order Rényi entropy and chose the support vector machine (SVM) with six kernels to detect PVC. The simulation results obtained 95.8% accuracy [14]. Chen et al. designed an algorithm to distinguish the QRS complex's peak points and proposed a PVC identification system based on the back-propagation neural network (BPNN). The system's input is a set of features obtained from the QRS complex peak points. The simulation result's average accuracy attains 97.46% on the China Physiological Signal Challenge 2018 (CPSC2018) Database [15].

Mazidi et al. evaluated three sets of ECG features and two classifiers on the field programable gate arrays (FPGAs). These three groups of characteristics come from time-domain based on the reconfiguration Pan–Tompkins algorithm, frequency-domain based on the Haar wavelet algorithm, and time-domain combination of frequency-domain based on the above two. The two classifiers are the SVM and the Naive Bayes [16]. Besides, Mazidi et al. introduced six robust features extracted by morphological assessment, polynomial curve fitting, discrete wavelet transform, and nonlinear analysis. Moreover, this literature used an SVM with a linear kernel to recognize PVC. This algorithm acquires the overall accuracy of 99.78%, with a sensitivity of 99.91% and 99.37% specificity for the MIT-BIH arrhythmia database [17]. Allami applied an artificial neural network (ANN) to classify the features extracted through morphological and statistical methods. The proposed method resulted in a sensitivity and accuracy of 98.7% and 98.6%, respectively, on the MIT-BIH arrhythmia database. Additionally, this method is computationally simple and suitable for real-time patient monitoring. [18]. Chen et al. extracted three features and provided these to a classifier based on the perceptron model. The three characteristics are the ratio of the QRS areas, the previous R-R interval, and the last R-R interval ratio to the next RR-interval. The experiments applied to the MIT-BIH arrhythmia database achieved high accuracy with a sensitivity of 98.7%. Moreover, this method's logic resources and power consumption are low, so it is suited for wearable monitoring [19]. Jeon et al. designed a model based on the error backpropagation algorithm and used four characteristics to detect PVC. These features are R-R interval, Q-S interval, Q-R amplitude, and R-S amplitude. The proposed approach's overall accuracy was above 90%, with testing on the MIT-BIH arrhythmia database [20].

With the popularity of deep learning and outstanding performance in other fields, researchers use deep learning to monitor PVC. Many experts used deep learning to detect PVC. Zhou et al. developed a reliable ECG analysis program to detect PVC. This system consists of two parts: data preprocessing and a recurrent neural network (RNN) with long short-term memory (LSTM). The accuracy of this method based on the MIT-BIH arrhythmia database is 96–99% since the RNN is good at processing time-series signals [21]. Zhao et al. combined the Modified Frequency Slice Wavelet Transform (MFSWT) and CNN, which has 25 layers, to search for PVC from 12-lead ECG data provided by the CPSC2018 Database. The MFSWT can transform one-dimensional time-series signals into two-dimensional time-frequency images as the input of the CNN. The test results of this method achieved a high accuracy of 97.89% [22].

Li et al. used three types of wavelets to convert single-channel ECG signals to wavelet power spectrums and constructed a CNN consisting of three convolutional layers, two max-pooling layers, and a rectified linear unit layer, a fully connected layer. These three wavelets are Morlet wavelet, Paul wavelet, and Gaussian derivative. The CNN receives and processes the transformed wavelet power spectrums, then labels it. It is commendable that the generalization ability of this method is excellent. The validation results on the American Heart Association (AHA) database achieved an overall F1 score of 84.96% and an accuracy of 97.36% with the training data from the MIT-BIH arrhythmia database [23]. Gordon and Williams developed a PVC detection algorithm based on autoencoder and random forest classifier. The proposed autoencoder consists of two parts. The first part is an encoder with two convolutional layers used for encoding the ECG to a latent space representation, which is low-dimensional and effective. The second part is a decoder with transposed convolutional layers for decoding the latent space representation to recover the ECG. The random forest classifier composed of 10 decision trees takes the latent space representation as input and annotate it. This algorithm achieved an overall accuracy above 97% on the MIT-BIH arrhythmia database [24]. Rahhal et al. report a model based on the Stacked Denoising Autoencoders (SDAs) networks and DNN to search PVC from the multi-lead ECG signals. The SDAs networks have the function of extracting features. The DNN classifies the ECG according to the obtained features. In the experiments with St. Petersburg INCART 12-lead Arrhythmia Database, the results are 98.6% and 91.4% respectively for accuracy and sensitivity [25]. Hoang et al. proposed a PVC detection algorithm for the multi-leads ECG and deployed it on wearable devices. The algorithm includes the Wavelet fusion method, Tucker-decomposition, and CNN, which has six layers: two convolutional layers, two max-pooling layers, a fully connected layer, and a dropout layer. Although this algorithm's accuracy is 90.84% on the 12 lead ECG St. Petersburg Arrhythmias Database, the proposed method is scalable to analyze 3-Lead to 16-Lead ECG systems [26]. Liu et al. applied deep learning to develop models that can search PVC from children's ECG. The children's ECG used in the experiment are JPEG images from the hospital. This study's experimental results show that the Inception-V3 with waveform images and one-dimensional CNN with time-series data extracted from waveform images can detect PVC in children [27].

According to Table 1, various algorithms for detecting PVC in recent years, we can quickly obtain the following conclusions. First, the amount of morphological-based literature is more than Deep Learning. Secondly, relevant researchers prefer these three classifiers: DNN, SVM, and Pattern matching. Third, the R-R interval is recognized by most research as a useful feature, but the other features do not seem to be unanimously recognized by most research. Finally, the model's performance based on morphology is slightly better than that of Deep Learning, thanks to the expertise of the person who designed the feature.

Although the morphological-based methods have achieved good results, they still have some limitations. First of all, these methods rely heavily on professional knowledge about ECG and signal processing to design the rules for extracting features. Second, these features extracted manually are biased and varies from person to person. Finally, most morphological-based methods are also limited by each wave's positioning algorithm in a heartbeat. For example, the inaccurate positioning of Q wave and S wave will directly affect the performance of detecting PVC, in literature 20.

Fortunately, some methods based on deep learning mostly avoid these limitations. The approach based on deep learning has the following three characteristics: first, it can automatically extract features, such as by convolution kernels; second, it can continuously optimize and select features during the training process to make the features non-redundant, such as by max-pooling; third, it can directly analyze the preprocessed heartbeats.

However, these existing methods based on the Deep Learning require preprocessing of the original ECG or the cooperation of other classifiers. The method proposed in the literature [21] has many preprocessing steps, such as resampling, denoising, signature detection, normalize. The studies [22,23,26] performed wavelet transform on the ECG to obtain 2-D time-frequency images. Moreover, the research [24,25] used the features extracted by a trained autoencoder to recognize PVC. There is no doubt that the above methods are computationally intensive.

Furthermore, identifying PVC is very complicated because the PVC waveform is quite uncertain, even for the same patient. Figure 2 shows some PVC waveforms from the same person. Therefore, achieving a real-time classifier with high accuracy and sensitivity is a challenging problem to address.

Table 1. Various algorithms for detecting premature ventricular contraction (PVC) in recent years.

Reference	Features	Classifier	Accuracy	Sensitivity	Specificity
[5]	Temporal characteristics.	Pattern matching	-	89.69%	99.63%
[7]	R-peak amplitude, R-R interval time, QRS duration time, ventricular activation time, Q-peak amplitude, S-peak amplitude.	DNN	99.41%	-	-
[8]	Principal Component Analysis and Waveform estimation.	KNN	-	93.45%	93.14%
[9]	R-R intervals, cross-correlation coefficient.	Pattern matching	99.5%	94.7%	99.6%
[10]	Energy wavelet coefficients.	Adaptive thresholding	-	99.18%	**99.94%**
[11]	Geometrical features.	AIS	98.04%	91.08%	98.65%
[12]	Maximal signal value in the P-Q interval; the area between the signal in the P-Q interval and zero, etc.	Multivariate statistical classier	-	96%	99%
[13]	Weighted six different QRS shape parameters.	Pattern matching	-	82.7%	98.82%
[14]	Six characteristics based on the Multiorder Rényi Entropy.	SVM	95.8%	-	-
[15]	Amplitude of R peaks; R-R interval; R-R interval ratio, etc.	DNN	97.46%	-	-
[16]	three groups of characteristics come from time-frequency domain.	SVM	99%	98.4%	99.8%
[17]	Six features extracted by several methodologies.	SVM	**99.78%**	**99.91%**	99.37%
[18]	Three morphological features and seven statistical features.	DNN	98.6%	98.7%	-
[19]	the ratio of the QRS areas; the previous R-R interval; the last R-R interval ratio to the next R-R interval.	a single neuron perceptron	98.8%	98.7%	98.9%

Table 1. *Cont.*

Reference	Features	Classifier	Accuracy	Sensitivity	Specificity
[20]	R-R interval; Q-S interval; Q-R amplitude; R-S amplitude.	DNN	Above 90%	-	-
[21]	Learned features automatically.	RNN	96–99%	99–100%	94–96%
[22]	Learned features automatically from time-frequency images	2D CNN	97.89%	98.58%	97.17%
[23]	Learned features automatically from wavelet power spectrums	2D CNN	97.96%	82.60%	99.11%
[24]	Learned features automatically by convolutional autoencoder	RF	98.55%	91.41%	99.06%
[25]	Learned features automatically by the stacked denoising autoencoders networks	DNN	98.6%	91.4%	93.9%
[26]	Learned features automatically by the Wavelet fusion method, Tucker-decomposition	2D CNN	90.84%	78.6%	99.86%
[27]	Learned features automatically from waveform images	2D CNN	88.5%	-	-

Abbreviations: deep neural network (DNN), K-nearest neighbor (KNN), artificial immune system (AIS), support vector machine (SVM), recurrent neural network (RNN), convolutional neural network (CNN), random forest (RF). Besides, "-" means that relevant information is not mentioned in the literature.

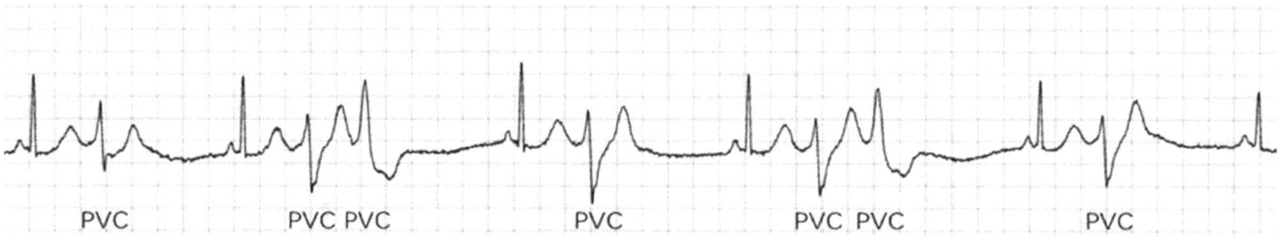

Figure 2. There are some PVC waveforms from the same person. The waveforms of these PVCs in the picture are different, especially the second and third.

In summary, considering the limitations of manually extracted features and the advantage that deep learning can automatically extract features, this study proposed a method based on one-dimensional CNN. This method can autonomously learn features from the labeled ECG data with supervised learning to avoid the manually extracted features' bias. Secondly, this method does not rely on professional knowledge that is used to design features. Third, this method does not have to preprocessing steps such as denoising and can directly process and analyze heartbeats, which will improve the efficiency of searching for PVC from ECG. Notably, the MIT-BIH arrhythmia database [28,29] will assess the validity of our proposed method. The following is the arrangement of the remainder: Section 2 describes the dataset, proposed framework, and evaluation measures; Section 3 presents and discusses the results; finally, Section 4 gives the conclusion and directions.

2. Materials and Methods

2.1. Materials

The MIT-BIH arrhythmia database is the first generally available benchmark database for the evaluation of arrhythmia detectors. The database contains 48 long-term Holter recordings obtained from 25 men subjects and 22 women subjects. Each of the 48 records numbered from 100 to 234 inclusive with some numbers missing, is slightly over half an hour-long and has two leads (the upper signal and lower signal). The upper signal in most records is a modified limb lead II (MLII), but the lower signal is occasionally V1, V2, V4, or V5. It is worth noting that recordings 201 and 202 came from the same male subject and the rest records are from a different subject. Furthermore, all records in this database are annotated by two or more cardiologists independently. Detailed annotations and a large number of records have made most researchers admire this database.

To effectively use this database, the Association for the Advancement of Medical Instrumentation (AAMI) recommends that records 102, 104, 107, and 217 are discarded because of the pacemaker or presenting complete heart block. Besides, this study designed three schemes to divide the remaining ECG records for evaluating the proposed method's effectiveness. Table 2. Splitting data into training and test sets. and Figure 3 showed the grouping schemes. It is worth mentioning that blind cross-validation cannot reasonably evaluate the performance of the model and comes with risks associated with label leakage.

Taking Scheme 1 in Table 2, splitting data into training and test sets, and Figure 3, splitting data into training and test sets, the information in Figure 3 is the same as in Table 2. As an example: the "DS1" and "DS2" represent the training set and the test set. The "101" represents the records number in the MIT-BIH arrhythmia database. The "N" and "V" respectively represent the number of the regular beat and PVC in the dataset. The "Ratio" means the ratio of the samples' number in the training set and the test set, such as (35640 + 2851)/(33868 + 2548) = 0.9778. Notably, most researchers adopt Scheme 1, which AAMI suggested and can also guarantee a reasonable comparison between our proposed method and other studies. Scheme 2 and Scheme 3 can evaluate the proposed method's performance in the situation that the number of samples in the training set is higher than the test set.

Table 2. Splitting data into training and test sets.

Scheme	Dataset	Records	N	V	Ratio
Scheme 1	Training set (DS1)	101, 106, 108, 109, 112, 114, 115, 116, 118, 119, 122, 124, 201, 203, 205, 207, 208, 209, 215, 220, 223, 230	35,640	2851	0.9778
	Test set (DS2)	100, 103, 105, 111, 113, 117, 121, 123, 200, 202, 210, 212, 213, 214, 219, 221, 222, 228, 231, 232, 233, 234	33,868	2548	
Scheme 2	Training set (DS3)	100, 103, 105, 106, 108, 109, 111, 113, 114, 116, 118, 119, 121, 123, 124, 200, 201, 202, 203, 205, 207, 208, 209, 210, 212, 213, 214, 215, 219, 222, 223, 228, 230, 231, 232, 234	53,279	4277	3.3172
	Test set (DS4)	101, 112, 115, 117, 122, 220, 221, 233	16,229	1122	
Scheme 3	Training set (DS5)	100, 101, 103, 105, 106, 108, 109, 111, 112, 113, 114, 115, 117, 118, 119, 121, 122, 123, 124, 200, 201, 202, 203, 207, 208, 209, 210, 212, 213, 214, 215, 219, 220, 222, 223, 228, 230, 231, 232, 233, 234	62,706	4862	9.2067
	Test set (DS6)	116, 205, 221	6802	537	

In this table, the 'Scheme' represents the name of the scheme for splitting data; the 'Dataset' represents the name of the training set or test set; the 'Records' represents ECG recordings in each 'Dataset'; the 'N' and 'V' respectively represent the number of the regular heartbeat and PVC in each 'Dataset'; the 'Ratio' means the ratio of the samples' number in the training set and the test set of each scheme.

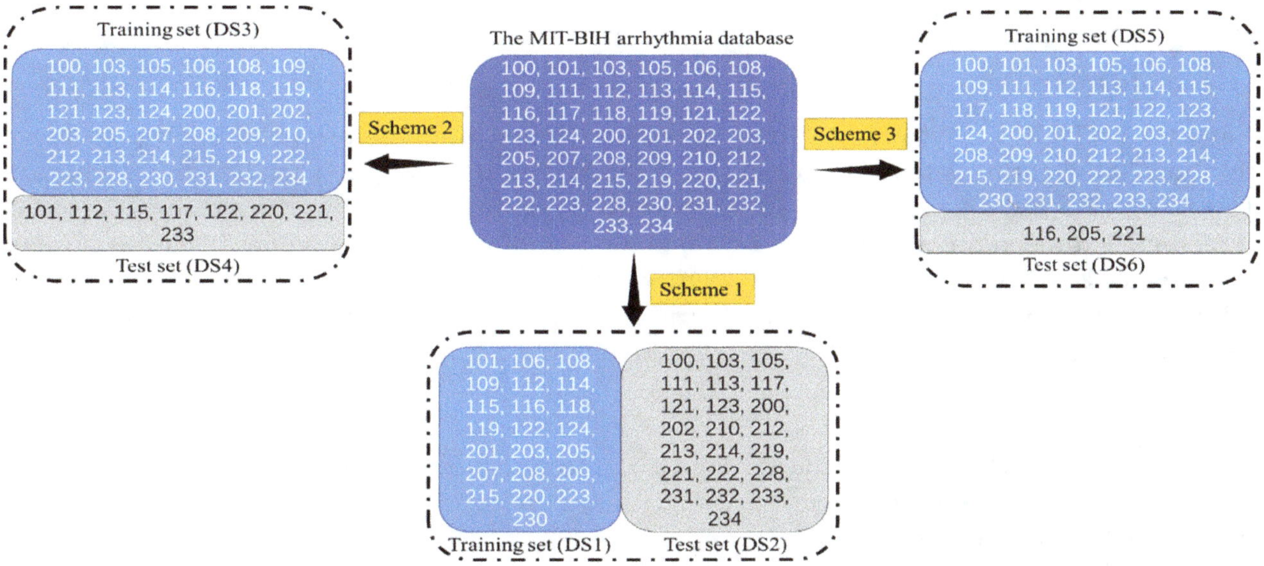

Figure 3. Splitting data into training and test sets. The information in this figure is the same as in Table 2. Splitting data into training and test sets.

2.2. Methodology

Figure 4 shows a block diagram of the proposed study, with a view showing the proposed method's flow. Initially, this research divided each ECG signal from the modified limb lead II (MLII) into separate heartbeats according to a fixed time window and an R peak detection algorithm. The duration of each heartbeat composed of 433 sampling points is 1.2 s. Then the proposed model based on the one-dimensional CNN takes these heartbeats as input to search PVC.

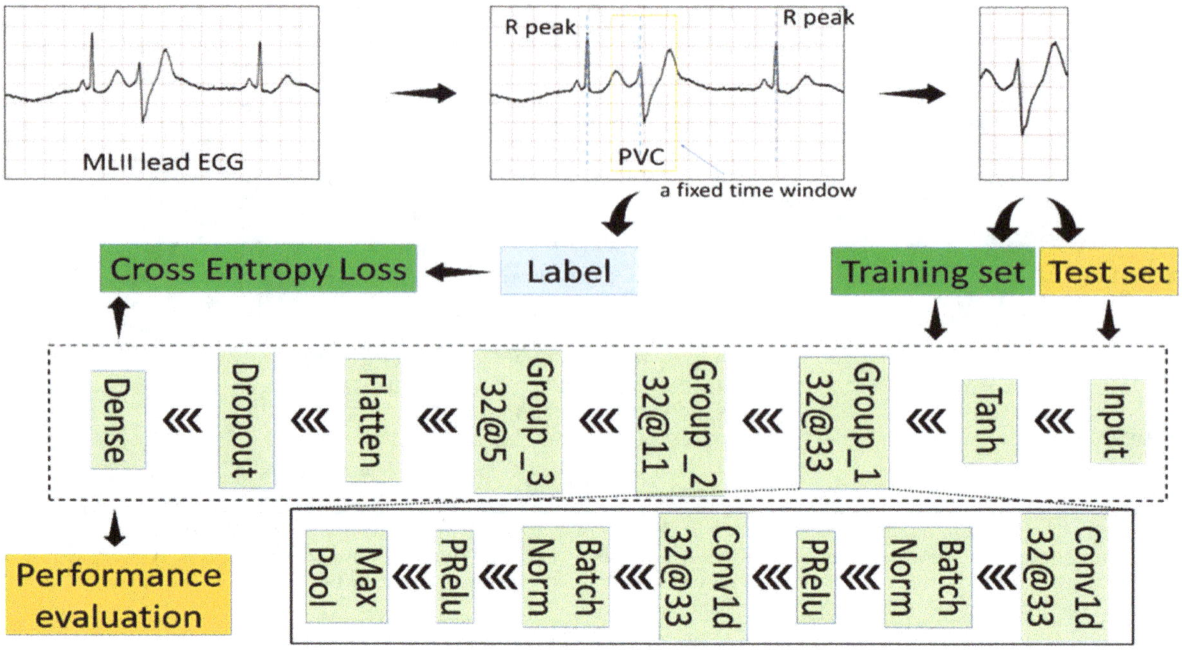

Figure 4. Block diagram of the proposed study.

2.2.1. Generate Input Data

Since the MIT-BIH arrhythmia database provides detailed annotations, including R-peak locations and rhythms' label, input data is the raw signal directly corresponding to each heartbeat without any preprocessing. We use a fixed-size window to extract the heartbeat from the MLII ECG lead since each heartbeat's dimension must be the same as the proposed classification model's input dimension. The window's size is 433, and the window's center is the location of R-peak. Because R-peak detection algorithms [30–33], such as Pan–Tompkins algorithm, can accurately find the R-peak point. We use the R-peak location in the database directly without developing a novel method to detect R-peak location.

2.2.2. Classifier Structure

First, the proposed model uses the Tanh function to transform the input data. The Tanh function can normalize the input data between −1 and 1, which is conducive to the training of the model. Equation (1) is the definition of the Tanh function.

$$\mathrm{Tanh(x)} = \frac{Sinh(x)}{Cosh(x)} = \frac{e^x - e^{-x}}{e^x + e^{-x}} \tag{1}$$

Secondly, the proposed model has three convolutional groups, as shown in Figure 4. Each convolutional group contains five layers. A one-dimensional convolutional layer is a powerful tool that results in a feature map representing a detected feature's positions and intensity in an input. Convolution is a simple operation:

(1) Flip the convolution kernel;

(2) Move the convolution kernel one data point at a time along the input vector;

(3) Calculate the dot product of two corresponding points at each position;

(4) The generated sequence is the convolution of the convolution kernel with the input vector.

For example, specifying the input vector and the convolution kernel are discrete sequences, then the definition of convolution is as follows.

$$y_j = \sum_{i=-\infty}^{\infty} x_i \times h_{j-i} \tag{2}$$

The batch normalization layer allows the neural network to complete training faster and more stably by normalizing the feature map and does the following during training time [34]:

(1) Compute the mean and variance of the layer's input;

$$\textit{Batch mean} \quad \mu_B = \frac{1}{m}\sum_{i=1}^{m} x_i \tag{3}$$

$$\textit{Batch}\ \text{variance} \quad \sigma_B^2 = \frac{1}{m}\sum_{i=1}^{m} (x_i - \mu_B)^2 \tag{4}$$

(2) Normalize the layer's input using the mean and variance;

$$\overline{x_i} = \frac{x_i - \mu_B}{\sqrt{\sigma_B^2 + \epsilon}} \tag{5}$$

(3) Obtain the output with scaling and shifting;

$$y_i = \gamma\overline{x_i} + \beta \tag{6}$$

Notice that m is the number of samples per batch, ϵ is a small constant for numerical stability. Additionally, γ and β are learnable parameters.

The Parametric Rectified Linear Unit (PReLU) is an excellent activation function and has become the default activation function for many neural networks [35]. Although PReLU will introduce slope parameters, the increase in training costs is negligible. The mathematical definition of PReLU is as follows.

$$f(y_i) = \max(0,\ y_i) + a_i \times \min(0, y_i) \tag{7}$$

The max-pooling layer can reduce the computational cost and effectively cope with the over-fitting phenomenon by down-sampling and summarizing in the feature map. Additionally, the max-pooling layer provides fundamental translation invariance.

Take 'Group_1 32@33' in the Figure 4 block diagram of the proposed study as an example to comprehend the convolution group. 'Group _1' is the convolution group's name; '32@33' represents the number and size of the one-dimensional convolutional layer's convolution kernels in the convolution group.

The proposed model also includes the Flatten layer, the Dropout layer, and the Dense layer. The Flatten layer collapses the spatial dimensions to make the multidimensional input one-dimensional. The Dropout layer refers to ignoring some neurons during a forward or backward pass to prevent over-fitting [34]. The Dense layer is a basic neural network layer and functions as a 'classifier.'

Tables 3 and 4 give the necessary parameters and the dimensional change of the proposed model's input data. The random seed in this study is 0, which can ensure that the experimental results are reproducible. Dropout in Table 3 refers to the probability of an element to be zeroed.

Table 3. Parameters of the proposed model.

Parameter Type	The Proposed Model
Batch size	512
Loss function	cross-entropy
Optimizer	Adam
Regularization rate	1
Epoch	100
Random seed	0
Dropout	0.7

Table 4. The dimensional change of the input data in the proposed model.

Layer Name	Input Shape	Out Shape
Input	None	(1, 433)
Tanh	(1, 433)	(1, 433)
Group_1	(1, 433)	(32, 216)
Group_2	(32, 216)	(32, 108)
Group_3	(32, 108)	(32, 54)
Flatten	(32, 54)	(1728)
Dropout	(1728)	(1728)
Dense	(1728)	(2)

'Batch size' refers to the number of training examples utilized in one iteration; 'Loss function' represents the category of loss function; 'Optimizer' represents how to change the parameters of the model; 'Regularization rate' means the regularization coefficient; 'Epoch' means the number of times each sample participated in training; 'Random seed' is a number used to initialize a pseudorandom number generator; 'Dropout' refers to the probability of an element to be zeroed.

2.3. *Evaluation Measures*

We chose five metrics, which have also been used in the literature [11], to measure the recognition performance of our proposed method: Accuracy (ACC), Sensitivity (Se), Specificity (Sp), Positive prediction (P_+), Negative prediction (P_-). The confusion matrix is the basis of these five metrics which can be expressed as Equation (8). Where TN, FN, TP, and FP respectively represent true negatives, false negatives, true positives, false positives. In this work, negative samples are those belonging to the regular class labeled 'N.' Additionally, this study also used the Youden's index to evaluate classification performance.

$$\text{Confusion Matrix} = \begin{bmatrix} TN & FP \\ FN & TP \end{bmatrix} \tag{8}$$

$$\text{Accuracy Acc} = \frac{\text{TP} + \text{TN}}{\text{TP} + \text{TN} + \text{FN} + \text{FP}} \tag{9}$$

$$\text{Sensitivity Se} = \frac{\text{TP}}{\text{TP} + \text{FN}} \tag{10}$$

$$\text{Specificity Sp} = \frac{\text{TN}}{\text{TN} + \text{FP}} \tag{11}$$

$$\text{Positive prediction P}_+ = \frac{\text{TP}}{\text{TP} + \text{FP}} \tag{12}$$

$$\text{Negative prediction P}_- = \frac{\text{TN}}{\text{TN} + \text{FN}} \tag{13}$$

$$\text{J} = Se + Sp - 1 \tag{14}$$

3. Results and Discussion

The size and number of kernels, number of layers, and batch size are the essential hyper-parameters in CNN. The kernels are the convolutional filters. In a convolution, the filters slide over all the points of the signal taking their dot product, which can extract some features from the input data. To quickly abstract the useful features, it is necessary to choose the size and number of kernels. The number of layers has a significant influence on the performance of CNN. Generally speaking, CNN's ability to detect PVC and the numbers of layers are positive correlations. However, more layers mean longer training time and more learnable parameters, which is very likely to cause overfitting. The batch size is the number of signals used to train a single forward and backward pass. The larger batch size can speed up the training and verification of the CNN but does not usually achieve high accuracy.

In this section, this study performed experiments on three different schemes, according to Table 2. Before anything else, we assessed the impact of varying size and number of kernels on recognizing PVC with CNN. Secondly, we evaluated the performance of CNN with a different number of layers on distinguishing PVC and regular rhythm. Immediately afterward, we tested the batch size's effect in detecting PVC. To improve the performance of the proposed model, we tried two activation functions (Sigmoid, Tanh) to normalize the input data. The data for training and verifying the above four experiments are all from Scheme 1. Finally, we checked the capabilities of the adjusted CNN to detect PVC with Scheme 2 and Scheme 3. Ubuntu 16.04.6 LTS operating system with an Nvidia GeForce RTX 2070 GPU, 32GB RAM, and Python programming language are the basis for the simulation process.

3.1. Experiment 1: Assess the Impact of Varying Size and Number of Kernels

The kernel size is usually related to the receptive field (RF), the size of the region in the input that generates the feature. In many outstanding image classification or detection algorithms, the kernel size is usually 3 × 3, 5 × 5, or 7 × 7 and decreases gradually. In this experiment, we tried multiple combinations of the size and number of kernels. The data for training and verifying are both from Scheme 1. Besides, the experimental environment is also the same. The strategy for adjusting the learning rate is multiplying the learning rate by 0.1 when the network reaches the 20th and 80th epoch. Moreover, Table 5 shows specific details and results. Figure 5 displays the receiver operating characteristic (ROC) curve about this experiment.

Table 5. The details and results of the varying size and number of kernels.

Group_1	Group_2	Group_3	Acc (%)	Se (%)	Sp (%)	P_+ (%)	P_- (%)	J (%)	Time [1]
32@43	32@11	32@5	99.47	96.35	99.71	96.12	99.73	96.06	9.68
32@33	32@11	32@5	**99.64**	96.98	**99.84**	**97.86**	99.77	96.82	9.30
32@23	32@11	32@5	99.54	**97.25**	99.72	96.27	**99.79**	**96.97**	8.82
32@33	32@7	32@5	99.62	96.94	99.82	97.63	99.77	96.76	9.15
32@11	32@7	32@5	99.54	**97.25**	99.71	96.16	**99.79**	96.96	8.20
32@7	32@5	32@3	99.37	94.31	99.75	96.66	99.57	94.06	**7.80**
64@33	64@11	64@5	99.52	96.74	99.73	96.48	99.75	96.47	14.92
16@33	16@11	16@5	99.57	96.31	99.82	97.57	99.72	96.13	7.88

[1] 'Time' refers to the duration of the training, in minutes.

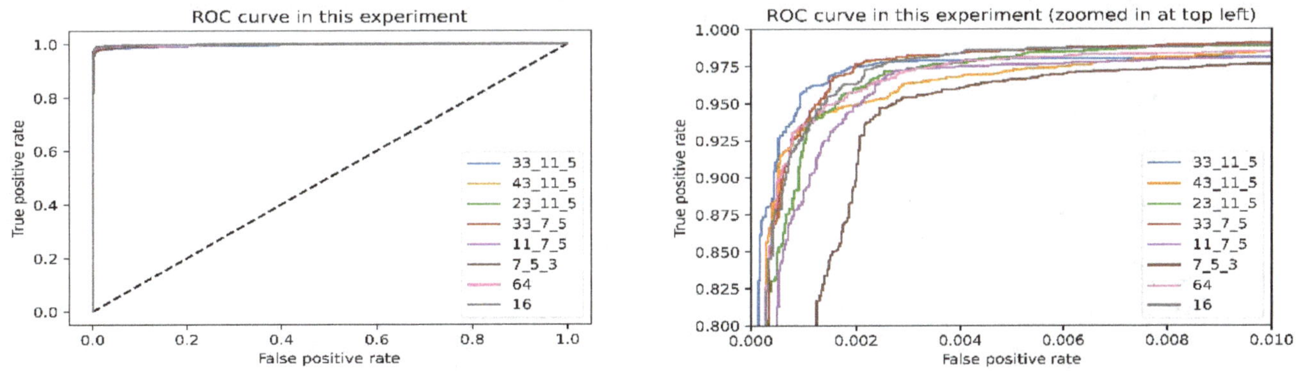

(a) (b)

Figure 5. Receiver operating characteristic (ROC) curve about this experiment: (**a**) original ROC curve; (**b**) zoomed ROC curve.

It is not difficult to find from Table 5 that although these results are not much different, the larger-sized convolution kernel's performance is slightly better in the first convolution group.

The convolution kernel size is different; the receptive field of the convolution kernel is also other. For the data used in this experiment, a larger size convolution kernel is more suitable for this task than a smaller size convolution kernel.

On the other hand, when the number of convolution kernels in each layer is 64 or 16, the model's performance has declined somewhat. The reason for this experimental phenomenon is that the number of convolution kernels is positively correlated with the learnable parameters in the model. The fewer the number of convolution kernels, the fewer the model's learnable parameters, which leads to the model not being able to extract features effectively. Also known as the underfitting state.

Furthermore, the number of convolution kernels also has a positive correlation with the time spent training the model. Especially when the number of convolution kernels in each layer is 64, the time spent training the model is nearly 15 min. Considering the accuracy, sensitivity, and Youden's index, the better combinations are the second to the fifth set of records in Table 5.

Moreover, from the ROC curves Figure 5, we can quickly know that the better combinations are the second combination in this experiment. Coincidentally, the receptive field of the convolution kernel is about 0.1 s of ECG signal when the kernel size is 33 because the sampling rate of the ECG is 360, and the QRS complexes of PVC are unusually long (typically >120 ms). In future work, we will study whether there is a relationship between the kernel size and the QRS duration of PVC.

3.2. Experiment 2: The Performance of CNN with a Different Number of Layers

With the popularity of CNN, the number of convolutional layers in each network is continually increasing, such as AlexNet (5), VGGNet16(13), ResNet50(49). The emergence of batch normalization and residual structure solves the vanishing gradient problem that makes the previous CNN challenging. Considering the marginal effects and the efficiency of the proposed model, we performed three tests. Figure 6 illustrates the basic structure of the model used in the three experiments. The configuration in this experiment is the same as the previous experiment. Moreover, Table 6 gives the results.

Table 6. The details and results of the varying size and number of kernels.

Structure	Acc (%)	Se (%)	Sp (%)	P_+ (%)	P_- (%)	J (%)	Time 1 (m) [1]
a	99.54	96.39	99.78	97.04	99.73	96.17	**5.17**
b	**99.64**	**96.98**	**99.84**	**97.86**	**99.77**	**96.82**	9.30
c	99.46	94.90	99.81	97.34	99.62	94.71	13.58

[1] 'Time 1' refers to the duration of the training.

The experimental records in Table 6 illustrate that the number of convolutional layers is not as significant as possible, which is the same as the existing prior knowledge. For example, the network with the first structure requires shorter training time than the third structure and better in some index, such as accuracy.

Besides, the number of layers is usually an essential factor that affects the complexity of the model. High-complexity models may have over-fitting problems during the training process, while low-complexity models may have under-fitting questions. Those models with too high or too low complexity have difficulty and time-consuming training. Therefore, choosing a moderately complex model can speed up the training process and make training easier.

To balance the model's efficiency and effectiveness, we choose the second structure described in Figure 6 to build the model according to the experimental results in Table 6.

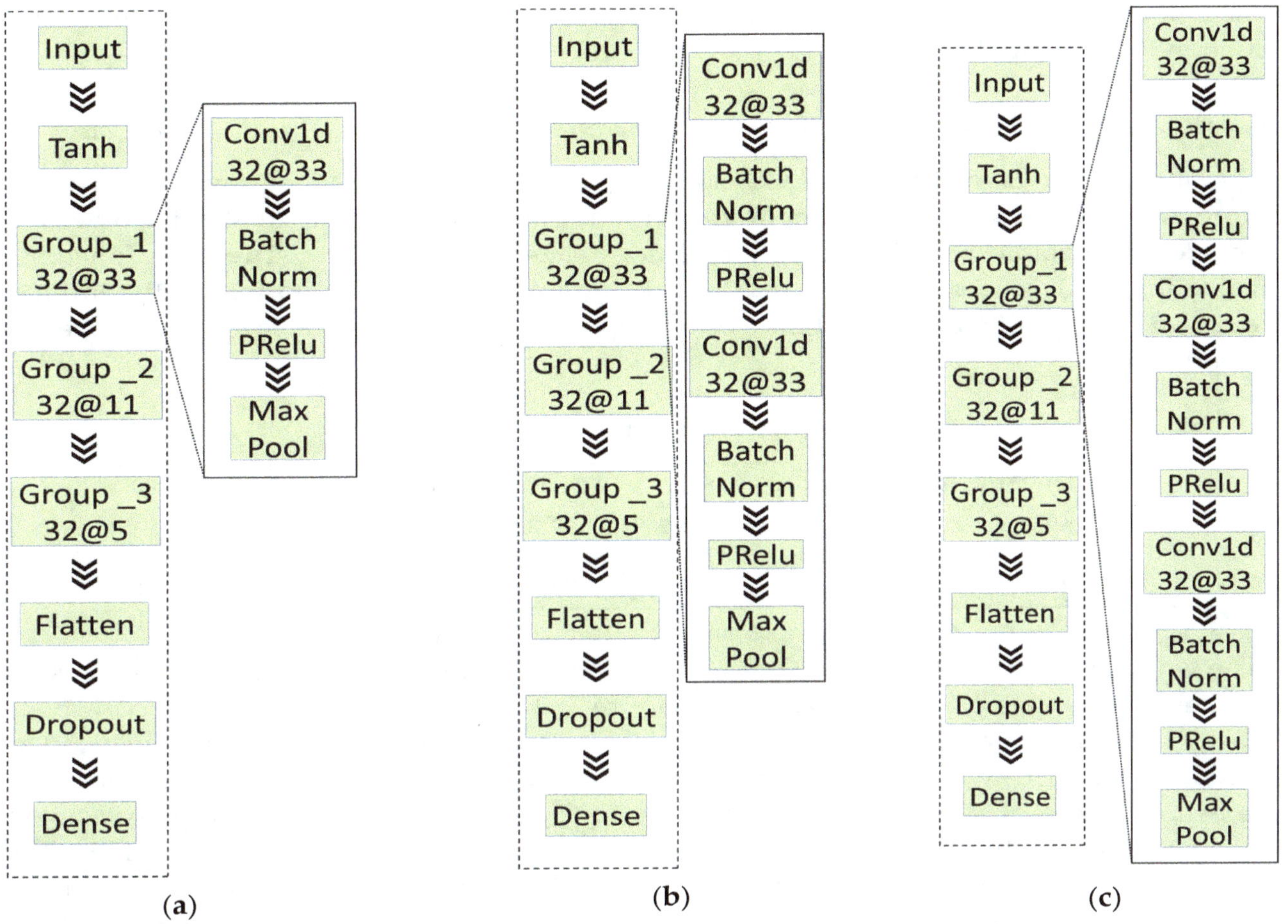

Figure 6. The basic structure of the models in experiment 2: (**a**) A convolutional layer in each convolutional; (**b**) two convolutional layers in each convolutional; (**c**) three convolutional layers in each convolutional.

3.3. Experiment 3: Test the Batch Size's Effect on Detecting PVC

Batch size is a very critical parameter and affects the performance of the neural networks. Too large or too small batch size is not appropriate. The larger batch size can reduce the training time and improve the stability of the structure. However, the smaller batch size can enhance the generalization ability of the model. To balance the generalization ability of the model and training time, we tested a series of batch sizes. Table 7 shows the results of this experiment.

Table 7. Test the batch size's effect in detecting PVC.

Batch Size	Acc (%)	Se (%)	Sp (%)	P_+ (%)	P_- (%)	J (%)	Time (m)[1]
64	99.46	95.02	99.79	97.15	99.63	94.81	22.17
128	99.43	94.82	99.78	96.95	99.61	94.60	13.63
512	**99.64**	**96.98**	**99.84**	**97.86**	**99.77**	**96.82**	9.30
1024	99.51	95.45	99.81	97.47	99.66	95.26	8.8
2048	99.47	94.86	99.82	97.54	99.61	94.68	**8.68**

[1] 'Time 1' refers to the duration of the training.

According to the experimental results in Table 7, we can find this rule that the relationship between training time and batch size is negatively correlated. Further, as the batch size keeps getting bigger, the training time is decreasing more and more slowly. Considering the training time, accuracy, and other indicators, we set the batch size in subsequent experiments to 512. After deploying the trained model, increasing the batch size can predict multiple heartbeats at the same time within the allowable range of video memory. This characteristic can significantly improve the efficiency of PVC detection in practical applications.

3.4. Experiment 4: Test the Activation Functions (Sigmoid, Tanh) Used to Normalize the Input Data

Considering the waveform of the ECG, normalizing the input data can improve the performance of the proposed model. Because the amplitude of the R wave is several times that of the other waves, we adopted the Sigmoid and Tanh function to normalize the input data. The Tanh function can normalize the input data between –1 and 1. The Sigmoid function can normalize the input data between 0 and 1. The difference is that the overall slope of Tanh is greater. Table 8 shows the results of this experiment.

Table 8. Test the activation functions.

Activation Function	Acc (%)	Se (%)	Sp (%)	P_+ (%)	P_- (%)	J (%)
None	99.56	96.74	99.77	96.97	99.75	96.51
Sigmoid	99.56	96.15	99.82	97.57	99.71	95.97
Tanh	**99.64**	**96.98**	**99.84**	**97.86**	**99.77**	**96.82**

The waveform of the ECG is very special. The amplitude of QRS complexes usually is much higher than the remaining wave. As shown in Figure 7, the points on the unnormalized waveform are mostly near the straight line with y = –1.0, and only a few moments deviate seriously. To solve this problem, we tried two activation functions (Tanh and Sigmoid) to normalize the input ECG. Figure 7 shows the normalized waveform of the ECG. The experimental results in Table 8 show that the suitable activation functions (Tanh) used to normalize the input ECG can slightly improve the model's performance. Nevertheless, inappropriate activation functions (Sigmoid) have a negative impact. The advantage of the Tanh function is that the value range of the normalized data is between –1 and 1, and the average is 0, unlike sigmoid, which is 0.5.

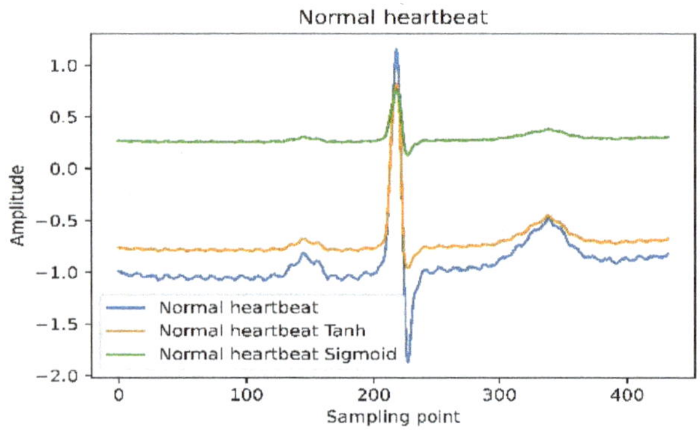

(a)

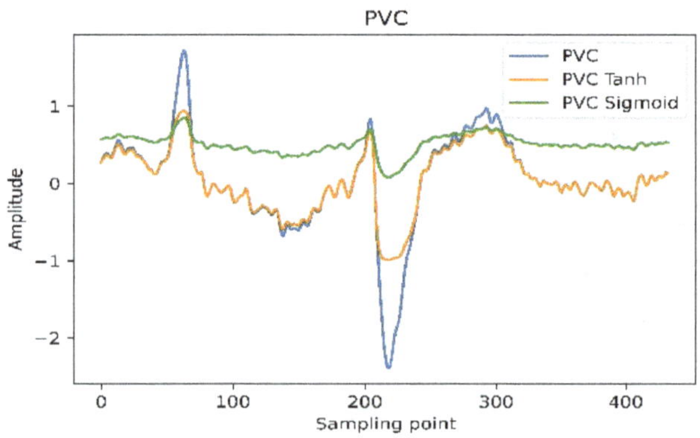

(b)

Figure 7. Tanh and Sigmoid normalize the waveform of a normal heartbeat and PVC.

3.5. Experiment 5: Employ CNN to Identify PVC with Scheme 2 and Scheme 3

As we all know, it is a common practice to distribute training and test sets in the proportion of 9:1 or 4:1 in deep learning. This experiment re-divides the data set according to Scheme 2 and Scheme 3, described in Table 2. After obtaining the training set and test set, this experiment employs the proposed model. Figure 8 shows the confusion matrix of each scheme. Table 9 shows the results of this experiment and comparisons with the consequence of Scheme 1 and previous studies.

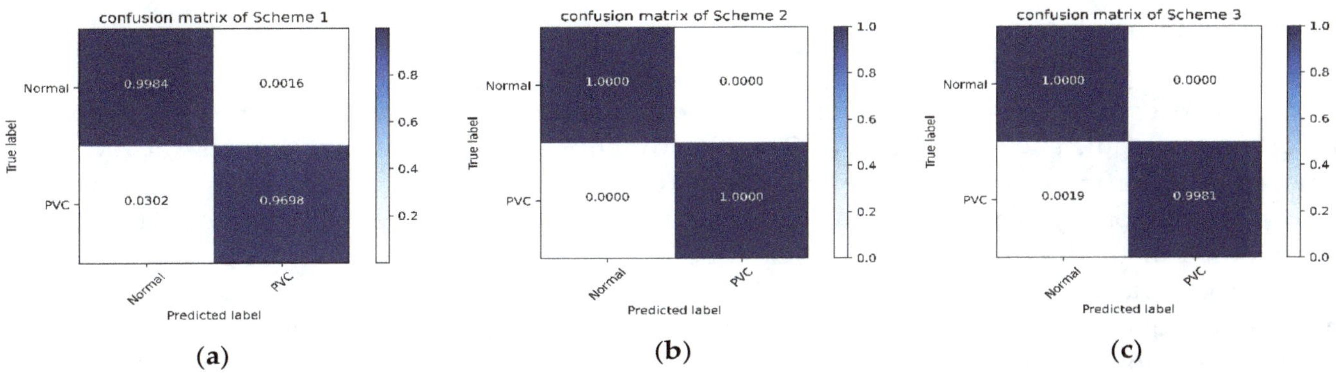

Figure 8. The confusion matrix of each scheme: (**a**) confusion matrix of Scheme 1; (**b**) confusion matrix of Scheme 2; (**c**) confusion matrix of Scheme 3.

Table 9. Employ the proposed model with Scheme 2 and Scheme 3.

Method	Acc (%)	Se (%)	Sp (%)	P_+ (%)	P_- (%)	J (%)
Scheme 1 [1]	99.64	96.98	99.84	97.86	99.77	96.82
Scheme 2 [1]	**100.00**	**100.00**	**100.00**	**100.00**	**100.00**	**100.00**
Scheme 3 [1]	99.99	99.81	100.00	100.00	99.99	99.81
Atanasoski et al. [9]	99.5%	94.7%	99.6%	-	-	94.8
Oliveira et al. [11]	98.04	91.08	98.65	85.68	99.21	89.73
Lynggaard [12]	-	96.00	99.00	93.00	99.00	95.00
Sokolova et al. [13]	-	82.70	98.82	82.97	-	81.52
Mazidi et al. [17]	99.78	99.91	99.37	-	-	99.5
Li et al. [23]	97.96	82.60	99.11	87.42	-	81.71
Gordon et al. [24]	97.61	77.81	99.02	-	-	76.83
Rahhal et al. [25]	98.6	91.4	93.9	-	-	86.7

[1] The performance of the proposed method in each Scheme.

The above experiments 1–4 confirmed the architecture and parameters of our proposed model. In Experiment 5, to evaluate the proposed model's performance in this situation: the number of samples in the training set is more than the test set. We employed the proposed model with Scheme 2 and 3. According to Table 9 and Figure 8, the proposed model's performance is unexpected, and the indicators are full marks with Scheme 2. The convolutional neural network is a class of deep learning technology. In deep learning, the number of samples used to train is generally more than that used for testing. In this case, the performance of the proposed method is remarkable.

Compared with the literature 9, 11, 12, and 13, the performance of the proposed method in Scheme 1 is better in all indicators. Additionally, the proposed method does not rely on professional knowledge to manually extract features. Next, the proposed method can directly predict the heartbeats' category in the MIT-BIH arrhythmia database without denoising.

For literature 17, the performance of the proposed method in Scheme 1 is bleak in all indicators. The literature 17 is based on a patient-independent separation approach to divide the training set and test set. This separation approach follows a principle that the same subject's heartbeats cannot appear in both training and test sets. The experiment in literature 17 considered 10% of heartbeat in the MIT-BIH arrhythmia database for training and 90% as the test set, similar to Scheme 3. The proposed method's performance in Scheme 3 is almost close to full marks and is better than literature 17.

Compared with the literature 23, 24, and 25, the proposed method's results are better. In the proposed plan, the process of extracting features and recognizing heartbeats are performed simultaneously. Finally, the proposed model can directly identify heartbeats in the MIT-BIH arrhythmia database. On the contrary, literature 23 used wavelet function to transform the heartbeat before training the model; before training the classifier model, literature 24 and 25 must first train the feature extraction network. In summary, our method has reached the most advanced level compared with other studies.

4. Conclusions

In this study, we successfully apply a model based on the one-dimensional convolutional neural network to recognize PVC and worked highly efficiently by using the raw ECG data without complex signal preprocessing such as denoising. The experimental results show that the classification effect achieved by the proposed method is significantly better than the morphological-based method and other methods. Additionally, according to Table 9, applying more ECG data can improve the performance of the proposed method. However, the annotated ECG data is hard to come by. In future works, we plan to use the generative adversarial networks (GAN) to deal with insufficient data. Next, we hope to tap the potential of our approach to classify many different types of heartbeats simultaneously. Lastly, we plan to deploy our proposed method on cloud servers or wearables to help doctors and patients in developing countries or remote regions.

Author Contributions: Conceptualization, X.C.; data curation, X.W. and J.G.; formal analysis, X.W.; methodology, J.Y., X.C. and J.G.; project administration, X.C.; resources, J.Y.; software, J.G.; visualization, J.G.; writing—original draft, X.W.; writing—review and editing, J.Y. and X.C. All authors have read and agreed to the published version of the manuscript.

References

1. Zhang, Y.; Cong, H.; Man, C.; Su, Y.; Sun, H.; Yang, H.; Guo, Z. Risk factors for cardiovascular disease from a population-based screening study in Tianjin, China: A cohort study of 36,215 residents. *Ann. Transl. Med.* **2020**, *8*, 444. [CrossRef]
2. Gerstenfeld, E.P.; De Marco, T. Premature ventricular contractions. *Circulation* **2019**, *140*, 624–626. [CrossRef] [PubMed]
3. Park, K.M.; Im, S.I.; Chun, K.J.; Hwang, J.K.; Park, S.J.; Kim, J.S.; On, Y.K. Asymptomatic ventricular premature depolarizations are not necessarily benign. *EP Eur.* **2015**, *18*, 881–887. [CrossRef] [PubMed]
4. Zipes, D.P.; Libby, P.; Bonow, R.O.; Mann, D.L.; Tomaselli, G.F. *Braunwald's Heart Disease E-Book: A Textbook of Cardiovascular Medicine*; Elsevier Health Sciences: Philadelphia, PA, USA, 2018.
5. Manikandan, M.S.; Ramkumar, B.; Choudhary, T.; Deshpande, P.S. Robust detection of premature ventricular contractions using sparse signal decomposition and temporal features. *Health Technol. Lett.* **2015**, *2*, 141–148. [CrossRef] [PubMed]
6. Abadi, M.; Barham, P.; Chen, J.; Chen, Z.; Davis, A.; Dean, J.; Devin, M.; Ghemawat, S.; Irving, G.; Isard, M. Tensorflow: A system for large-scale machine learning. *arXiv* **2016**, arXiv:1605.08695.
7. Jun, T.J.; Park, H.J.; Minh, N.H.; Kim, D.; Kim, Y. Premature ventricular contraction beat detection with deep neural networks. In Proceedings of the 15th IEEE International Conference on Machine Learning and Applications (ICMLA), Anaheim, CA, USA, 18–20 December 2016; pp. 859–864. [CrossRef]
8. Hadia, R.; Guldenring, D.; Finlay, D.D.; Kennedy, A.; Janjua, G.; Bond, R.; McLaughlin, J. Morphology-based detection of premature ventricular contractions. In *2017 Computing in Cardiology (CinC)*; IEEE: Rennes, France, 2017; pp. 1–4. [CrossRef]
9. Atanasoski, V.; Ivanovic, M.D.; Marinkovic, M.; Gligoric, G.; Bojovic, B.; Shvilkin, A.V.; Petrovic, J. Unsupervised classification of premature ventricular contractions based on R-R interval and heartbeat morphology. In Proceedings of the 14th Symposium on Neural Networks and Applications (NEUREL), Belgrade, Serbia, 20–21 November 2018; pp. 1–6. [CrossRef]
10. Junior, E.A.; Valentim, R.A.D.M.; Brandão, G.B. Real-time premature ventricular contractions detection based on Redundant Discrete Wavelet Transform. *Res. Biomed. Eng.* **2018**, *34*, 187–197. [CrossRef]
11. De Oliveira, B.R.; De Abreu, C.C.E.; Duarte, M.A.Q.; Filho, J.V. Geometrical features for premature ventricular contraction recognition with analytic hierarchy process based machine learning algorithms selection. *Comput. Methods Programs Biomed.* **2019**, *169*, 59–69. [CrossRef]
12. Lynggaard, P. Detecting premature ventricular contraction by using regulated discriminant analysis with very sparse training data. *Appl. Artif. Intell.* **2018**, *33*, 229–248. [CrossRef]

13. Sokolova, A.; Markelov, O.; Bogachev, M.; Uljanitski, Y. Multi-parametric algorithm for premature ventricular contractions detection and counting. *AIP Conf. Proc.* **2019**, *2140*, 020074. [CrossRef]
14. Rizal, A.; Wijayanto, I. Classification of Premature Ventricular Contraction based on ECG Signal using Multiorder Rényi Entropy. In Proceedings of the 2019 International Conference of Artificial Intelligence and Information Technology (ICAIIT), Yogyakarta, Indonesia, 13–15 March 2019; pp. 225–229. [CrossRef]
15. Chen, H.; Bai, J.; Mao, L.; Wei, J.; Song, J.; Zhang, R. Automatic Identification of Premature Ventricular Contraction Using ECGs. In Proceedings of the 2019 International Conference on Health Information Science (HIS), Xi'an, China, 18–20 October 2019; pp. 143–155. [CrossRef]
16. Mazidi, M.H.; Eshghi, M.; Raoufy, M.R. FPGA implementation of wearable ECG system for detection premature ventricular contraction. *Int. J. COMADEM* **2019**, *22*, 51–59.
17. Mazidi, M.H.; Eshghi, M.; Raoufy, M.R. Detection of premature ventricular contraction (PVC) using linear and nonlinear techniques: An experimental study. *Clust. Comput.* **2019**, *23*, 759–774. [CrossRef]
18. Allami, R. Premature ventricular contraction analysis for real-time patient monitoring. *Biomed. Signal. Process. Control.* **2019**, *47*, 358–365. [CrossRef]
19. Chen, Z.; Xu, H.; Luo, J.; Zhu, T.; Meng, J. Low-power perceptron model based ECG processor for premature ventricular contraction detection. *Microprocess. Microsyst.* **2018**, *59*, 29–36. [CrossRef]
20. Jeon, E.; Jung, B.K.; Nam, Y.; Lee, H. Classification of premature ventricular contraction using error back-propagation. *KSII Trans. Internet Inf. Syst.* **2018**, *12*, 988–1001. [CrossRef]
21. Zhou, X.; Zhu, X.; Nakamura, K.; Mahito, N.P. Premature ventricular contraction detection from ambulatory ECG using recurrent neural networks. In Proceedings of the 40th Annual International Conference of the IEEE Engineering in Medicine and Biology Society (EMBC), Honolulu, HI, USA, 18–21 July 2018; pp. 2551–2554. [CrossRef]
22. Zhao, Z.; Wang, X.; Cai, Z.; Li, J.; Liu, C.P. PVC Recognition for wearable ECGs using modified frequency slice wavelet transform and convolutional neural network. In Proceedings of the 2019 Computing in Cardiology (CinC), Biopolis, Singapore, 8–11 September 2019; pp. 1–4. [CrossRef]
23. Li, Q.; Liu, C.; Li, Q.; Shashikumar, S.P.; Nemati, S.; Shen, Z.; Clifford, G.D. Ventricular ectopic beat detection using a wavelet transform and a convolutional neural network. *Physiol. Meas.* **2019**, *40*, 055002. [CrossRef] [PubMed]
24. Gordon, M.G.; Williams, C.M. PVC detection using a convolutional autoencoder and random forest classifier. In Proceedings of the Pacific Symposium on Biocomputing 2019, Kohala Coast, HI, USA, 3–7 January 2019; pp. 42–53. [CrossRef]
25. Rahhal, M.M.A.; Ajlan, N.A.; Bazi, Y.; Hichri, H.A.; Rabczuk, T. Automatic premature ventricular contractions detection for multi-lead electrocardiogram signal. In Proceedings of the IEEE International Conference on Electro/Information Technology (EIT), Rochester, MI, USA, 3–5 May 2018; pp. 169–173. [CrossRef]
26. Hoang, T.; Fahier, N.; Fang, W.C. Multi-leads ECG premature ventricular contraction detection using tensor decomposition and convolutional neural network. In Proceedings of the BioCAS 2019—Biomedical Circuits and Systems Conference, Nara, Japan, 17–19 October 2019; pp. 1–4. [CrossRef]
27. Liu, Y.; Huang, Y.; Wang, J.; Liu, L.; Luo, J. Detecting premature ventricular contraction in children with deep learning. *J. Shanghai Jiaotong Univ.* **2018**, *23*, 66–73. [CrossRef]
28. Moody, G.; Mark, R. The impact of the MIT-BIH arrhythmia database. *IEEE Eng. Med. Biol. Mag.* **2001**, *20*, 45–50. [CrossRef] [PubMed]
29. Goldberger, A.L.; Amaral, L.A.N.; Glass, L.; Hausdorff, J.M.; Ivanov, P.C.; Mark, R.G.; Mietus, J.E.; Moody, G.B.; Peng, C.K.; Stanley, H.E. PhysioBank, PhysioToolkit, and PhysioNet: Components of a new research resource for complex physiologic signals. *Circulation* **2000**, *101*, e215–e220. [CrossRef]
30. Pan, J.; Tompkins, W. A Real-Time QRS Detection Algorithm. *IEEE Trans. Bio-Med. Eng.* **1985**, *32*, 230–236. [CrossRef]
31. Lin, C.C.; Chang, H.Y.; Huang, Y.H.; Yeh, C.Y. A novel wavelet-based algorithm for detection of QRS complex. *Appl. Sci.* **2019**, *9*, 2142. [CrossRef]
32. Chen, C.L.; Chuang, C.T. A QRS detection and R point recognition method for wearable single-lead ECG devices. *Sensors* **2017**, *17*, 1969. [CrossRef] [PubMed]
33. Chen, A.; Zhang, Y.; Zhang, M.; Liu, W.; Chang, S.; Wang, H.; He, J.; Huang, Q. A real time QRS detection algorithm based on ET and PD controlled threshold strategy. *Sensors* **2020**, *20*, 4003. [CrossRef] [PubMed]

34. Garbin, C.; Zhu, X.; Marques, O. Dropout vs. batch normalization: An empirical study of their impact to deep learning. *Multimedia Tools Appl.* **2020**, *79*, 12777–12815. [CrossRef]
35. He, K.; Zhang, X.; Ren, S.; Sun, J. Delving Deep into Rectifiers: Surpassing Human-Level Performance on ImageNet Classification. In Proceedings of the 2015 IEEE International Conference on Computer Vision (ICCV), Santiago, Chile, 7–13 December 2015; pp. 1026–1034. [CrossRef]

4

A Decision Support System for Elective Surgery Scheduling under Uncertain Durations

Daniel Clavel [1], Cristian Mahulea [1,*], Jorge Albareda [2] and Manuel Silva [1]

[1] Department of Computer Science and Systems Engineering, University of Zaragoza, 50018 Zaragoza, Spain; clavel@unizar.es (D.C.); silva@unizar.es (M.S.)

[2] "Lozano Blesa" Hospital of Zaragoza, 50009 Zaragoza, Spain; jcalbareda@salud.aragon.es

* Correspondence: cmahulea@unizar.es

Featured Application: A software tool for helping doctors in the automatic scheduling of elective patients is proposed. The tool has been developed considering the organizational structure of Spanish hospitals. However, it may be easily extended to any hospital (public or private) working under operation room block booking criterion.

Abstract: The *operation room* (OR) is one of the most expensive material resources in hospitals. Additionally, the demand for surgical service is increasing due to the aging population, while the number of surgical interventions performed is stagnated because of budget reasons. In this context, the importance of improving the efficiency of the surgical service is accentuated. The main objective of this work is to propose and to evaluate a *Decision Support System* (DSS) for helping medical staff in the automatic scheduling of elective patients, improving the efficiency of medical teams' work. First, the scheduling criteria are fixed and then the scheduling problem of elective patients is approached by a mathematical programming model. A heuristic algorithm is proposed and included in the DSS. Moreover, other different features are implemented in a software tool with a friendly user interface, called CIPLAN. Considering realistic data, a simulation comparison of the scheduling obtained using the approach presented in this paper and other similar approaches in the bibliography is shown and analyzed. On the other hand, a case study considering real data provided by the Orthopedic Surgical Department (OSD) of the "Lozano Blesa" hospital in Zaragoza (HCU) is proposed. The simulation results show that the approach presented here obtains similar occupation rates and similar confidence levels of not exceeding the available time than approaches in the bibliography. However, from the point of view of respecting the order of the patients in the waiting list, the approach in this paper obtains scheduling much more ordered. In the case of the Orthopedic Surgical Department of the "Lozano Blesa" hospital in Zaragoza, the occupation rate may be increased by 2.83%, which represents a saving of 110,000 euros per year. Moreover, medical doctors (who use this tool) consider CIPLAN as an intuitive, rapid and efficient software solution that can make easier the corresponding task.

Keywords: decision support system; heuristic approach; surgery scheduling; software tool; case study

---

1. Introduction

The *Operation Room* (OR) is one of the most expensive material resources of the hospitals (in Spain being about 40% of the total hospitalization cost [1]) and approximately 60% of patients need it at some point during their hospital stay [2]. On the other hand, the demand for surgical services is increasing due to the aging population. In Spain, the average life expectancy is about 81.8 years being one of the highest in Europe [3].

Moreover, as a result of the economic crisis in 2008, the number of surgical interventions performed annually in Spanish public hospitals has stagnated at 3.5 million. This situation has also contributed to a continuous increment in the number of patients in the surgical waiting lists, reaching 600,000 in 2017 [4]. In some cases, these huge lists lead into waiting times greater than six months, which is becoming a serious problem for the healthcare system. Being difficult to increase the surgical resources, the importance of improving the efficiency is accentuated. New management techniques, scheduling methods, and specific information systems could help to improve the efficiency of the surgical services and, consequently, could reduce the surgical waiting lists.

The main objective of this work is to provide a DSS for managing surgical services in hospitals. In particular, a software tool (called CIPLAN from the Spanish words *PLANificación de CIrugías*) is presented that may be used by medical doctors to automatically perform a scheduling of the patients. It is assumed that the uncertain parameters (surgery duration and cleaning time) follow a normal distribution and, consequently, the expected total duration of a surgical block also follows a normal distribution. In this way, the probability of exceeding the working time can be introduced as a capacity chance constraint. Even if the lognormal distribution may give better approximations of the surgery times [5], the optimization problem has nonlinear constraints, being difficult to solve. Since, in general, acceptable error is obtained for normal distribution, this work assumes this type of distribution.

The following three criteria have been considered for the scheduling problem.

C1. Maximize the occupation of the ORs. Since the ORs with their associated cost constitute the bottleneck of the system (they can be open only during a given period of time every working day and their cost is high), the first scheduling criterion is to maximize the occupation of the ORs. In this way, the underutilization of the ORs is prevented and the use of resources is maximized.

C2. Ensure with a minimum confidence level that the total available time in a time block is not going to be exceeded. On contrary to *C1*, an over-scheduling of the ORs is not desired since the last scheduled surgeries can be canceled if the medical personnel believes that the time of the time block will be exceeded. Among other problems, such cancellations reduce the *real* occupation rate in the ORs.

C3. Respect as much as possible the order of the patients in the waiting list. Due to ethical and common sense reasons, patients with the same urgency level should spend a similar time in the waiting list. For that, once the patients in a waiting list are ordered depending on the urgency level and the admission date, the third scheduling criterion is to respect as much as possible the order of the patients in the waiting list. For example, in the Orthopedic Department of the HCU, each team has assigned two time blocks per week for the elective patients, so the difference of scheduling a patient in the first time block with the sixth one is 21 days.

Mathematical programming is an optimization technique [6] commonly used in managing hospitals [7], not only for surgery scheduling problems [8], but also for other problems such as bed management [9], nurse scheduling [10], or management policy decisions [11]. This paper proposes first an *Mixed Integer Quadratic Constrained Programming* problem for performing the scheduling of patients based on the three criteria presented before. It is well known that the computational complexity to obtain the optimal solution is high and a heuristic method is proposed called *Specific Heuristic Algorithm* (SHA) [12]. The software tool, in addition to helping doctors in the scheduling task, has also been developed for managing medical doctors, medical teams, OR timetable, and patients.

A preliminary version of this work has been reported in [12] where a first version of the SHA has been proposed. In this paper, the heuristic SHA is improved by adding a post arranging of the time scheduled blocks. This improvement provides solutions respecting the order of the patients in the waiting list more. Additionally, the DSS is explained (not only the part related to surgery scheduling but also related to management tasks), and the solution is compared using real data from the HCU with two other methods in literature.

2. Related Work

In literature, many researchers studied the problem of planning and scheduling of elective patients (see [8,13] and the references herein for an overview while for an overview of the problems see [14]). Almost all the works consider criterion *C1* presented before. Criterion *C2* (of using chance constraints for the scheduling) is considered also in some contributions presented in the last years. For example, in [15], integer stochastic formulations are proposed for two sub-problems in which the original problem is decomposed. The approach to solve them is based on neighborhood search techniques and Monte Carlo simulation. In [16], a two-stage robust optimization model is proposed that is solved based on a column-and-constraint generation method. A similar method is used by the authors in [17] to deal with uncertain surgery duration and emergency demand, while, in [18], the authors use particle swarm optimization for the scheduling of surgeries.

The approaches presented in [19,20] are the most related to the one presented in this paper. The authors in [19] present an optimization framework for batch scheduling within a block booking system that maximizes the expected utilization of ORs subject to a set of probabilistic capacity constraints. They propose an algorithm that iteratively solves a series of mixed-integer programs that are based on a normal approximation of cumulative surgery duration. In [20], constructive and local search heuristics for maximization of ORs utilization and minimization of the overcoming risk are proposed. In their model, to address the randomness of surgery processing times, a planned time slack is reserved in each scheduling block, which is a function of total mean and variance of surgeries assigned to the corresponding block. When determining an appropriate size of the planned slacks, the authors assume that the sum of surgery duration follows a normal distribution.

Both approaches in [19,20] require setting in advance the patients that are going to be scheduled in the next blocks. Therefore, in these approaches, all considered patients must be scheduled in one of the available blocks. For this, both approaches start with an initial scheduling obtained through the scheduling rule: *first-fit probabilistic*. Following this rule, sequentially each surgery is assigned to the first available block for which the probabilistic capacity constraint is satisfied after the assignment. Once the initial scheduling is obtained, the expected occupation rate of the first blocks is improved by rescheduling the surgeries. In this way, the last blocks are totally or partially released.

Unlike [19,20], the approach presented in this paper does not require to know in advance the set of patients that should be scheduled in the next surgical blocks, since any patient on the waiting list may or may not be scheduled. Another big difference with [19,20] consists of the usage of two balanced terms in the cost function that favor patients to be scheduled in an orderly manner at the same time that the expected occupation rate of the OR is maximized. An exhaustive numerical comparison using realistic data is performed and analyzed showing that the approach presented in this manuscript provides better solutions to the considered problem than the one in [19,20]. In particular, even if the results show similar occupation rates and similar confidence levels, the approach presented in this paper respect the preference order of the patients in the waiting list more. Therefore, criterion *C3* is better considered. In the case of the hospital in which the approach is implemented, the number of available time blocks per week for each medical team is equal to two, while, on average, three patients are scheduled in a time block, making it very important to keep, if possible, the order of patients in the waiting lists. This is one of the main differences of the approach presented in this paper with the other approaches.

DSS are used for managing tasks in different fields of applications, as for example in stormwater management [21], dental manufacturing production line [22], offshore wind farms [23] and healthcare systems [24,25]. Moreover, a DSS for OR scheduling was proposed in [26] based on a Mixed Integer Linear Programming (MILP) problem [27,28] that takes into account the preference order of the patients. However, this approach does not consider the variability on the uncertain parameters (surgery duration, cleaning time, etc.) and consequently can not manage the risk of exceeding the total time. The DSS proposed in this work uses an heuristic algorithm allowing to impose a minimum confidence level of not exceeding the total time in a surgical block. In this way, doctors not only can manage the risk but also can know in advance the probability that each block exceeds the available time. The DSS proposed in this paper can also perform the management of medical teams and OR time table. Moreover, it is possible to perform iterative scheduling which is useful if, for example, after obtaining a first scheduling, some patients can not attend the day of their surgeries. Furthermore, after a surgery is performed, the DSS automatically updates and customizes the average and standard deviation of the surgery duration. Finally, in order to provide a safe environment to work and better security of the medical data, different access levels are provided to every user.

The second main contribution of this paper is the presentation of a DSS that can help medical doctors not only for scheduling of surgeries, but also it can be used for management tasks of patients, medical teams, hospital resources, etc. Finally, the scheduling approach presented is compared with real historical data from the studied hospital, this being a third contribution of this manuscript.

3. Preliminaries and Problem Definition

Let us assume that each surgical team of a hospital department has some surgical blocks booked for performing the surgeries of their elective patients list. Thus, the problem of scheduling can be divided into different independent sub-problems: one for each medical team. In this process, some patients are assigned from the waiting list to the next time blocks previously booked. Currently, in many Spanish hospitals, the scheduling is performed manually, so the schedulers (normally medical doctors) are guided by their own intuition and experience to assign the patients.

3.1. Scheduling Problem Statement

In this subsection, the **Scheduling problem** is introduced formally. First, the notation, terminology, and assumptions are fixed and then the scheduling criteria are transformed to cost function and constraints.

Let $\mathcal{S} = \{s_1, s_2, \ldots, s_{|\mathcal{S}|}\}$ be the set of surgery types that can be performed in the medical department and let us assume that the duration $d(s_k)$ of each type of surgery $s_k \in \mathcal{S}$ is a random variable with normal probability density function (pdf) $d(s_k) = N(\mu_{d(s_k)}, \sigma_{d(s_k)})$, where $\mu_{d(s_k)}$ is the average and $\sigma_{d(s_k)}$ is the standard deviation.

On the other hand, let Dt be the delay with respect to the starting time of a block and let Ct be the cleaning time duration of the OR after a surgery is performed. It is assumed that Dt and Ct are also random variables with normal pdf, i.e., $Dt = N(\mu_{Dt}, \sigma_{Dt})$ and $Ct = N(\mu_{Ct}, \sigma_{Ct})$.

Furthermore, let us consider $\mathcal{W} = \{w_1, w_2, \ldots, w_{|\mathcal{W}|}\}$ an ordered list of patients such that, if $w_j \in \mathcal{W}$, j is the preference order of the patient w_j in the waiting list.

In addition, let us assume an ordered set of time blocks $\mathcal{B} = \{b_1, ..., b_{|\mathcal{B}|}\}$ to schedule, where $b_{|\mathcal{B}|}$ is the block corresponding to the latest date. Each block $b_i \in \mathcal{B}$ has a fixed duration denoted by $l(b_i)$.

For each time block $b_i \in \mathcal{B}$ to schedule, there exists a binary decision vector $\mathbf{S}_i \in \{0,1\}^{1\times|\mathcal{W}|}$ with a dimension equal to the number of the patients in the waiting list. If $\mathbf{S}_i[j] = 1$, then surgery of patient w_j should be performed in working day $i \leq |\mathcal{B}|$.

Let S_{b_i} be the set of surgeries scheduled in the time block b_i; then, the total duration T_{b_i} of the time block b_i can be computed by Equation (1). That is the sum of: (i) the delay with respect to the starting time (i.e., Dt), (ii) the duration of the surgeries scheduled in the time block b_i, and (iii) the cleaning time duration Ct between two consecutive surgeries. Notice that the cleaning time after the last surgery is not considered:

$$T_{b_i} = Dt + (|S_{b_i}| - 1) \cdot Ct \sum_{s_k \in S_{b_i}} [d(s_k)] \,. \tag{1}$$

Because all these variables are assumed to follow a normal distribution, the total duration T_{b_i} of the time block b_i also follows a normal distribution $T_{b_i} = N(\mu_{T_{b_i}}, \sigma_{T_{b_i}})$.

The goal of the scheduling problem is the assignment of the patients from the waiting list $\mathcal{W}$ to the set of time blocks $\mathcal{B}$ considering the scheduling criteria C1, C2 and C3. Let us define the following further notations:

- $\boldsymbol{\mu_w}$ be a row vector containing the average duration of surgeries of the patients in the waiting list $\mathcal{W}$. For example, $\boldsymbol{\mu_w}(j)$ represents the average duration of the surgery corresponding to the patient w_j.
- $\boldsymbol{Po}$ be a row vector containing the preference order of the patients. Assuming that patients are ordered according to their priority, then $\boldsymbol{Po}(j) = j$.
- Cl is the minimum confidence level of not exceeding the total time.

then:

Criterion C1 is formalized by objective **O1** given by Equation (2). This equation maximizes the expected surgery time in each block ($\boldsymbol{\mu_w} \cdot \mathbf{S}_i$) giving more importance to the first ones ($(|\mathcal{B}| + 1 - i)$:

$$max \sum_{i=1}^{|\mathcal{B}|} [\boldsymbol{\mu_w} \cdot \mathbf{S}_i \cdot (|\mathcal{B}| + 1 - i)] \, . \tag{2}$$

Criterion C2 is imposed by the chance probability constraint given by Equation (3). It ensures with a minimum confidence level Cl that the total duration T_{b_i} in each time block $b_i \in \mathcal{B}$ does not exceed the available time $l(b_i)$:

$$P[T_{b_i} \leq l(b_i)] \geq Cl, \forall i = 1, 2, \ldots, |\mathcal{B}|. \tag{3}$$

Finally, criterion C3 is formalized by the objective **O2** given by Equation (4). Here, by minimizing the sum of the preference order of the patients scheduled in each time block ($\boldsymbol{Po} \cdot \mathbf{S}_i$), preference to the first patients in the waiting list is given. Moreover, multiplying by the term $(|\mathcal{B}| + 1 - i)$, first patients should be scheduled in the first time blocks:

$$min \sum_{i=1}^{|\mathcal{B}|} [\boldsymbol{Po} \cdot \mathbf{S}_i \cdot (|\mathcal{B}| + 1 - i)] \, , \tag{4}$$

3.2. *Optimal Mathematical Programming Model*

A Mixed-Integer Quadratic Constrained Programming (MIQCP) model is proposed (5) for solving the patients **Scheduling problem**. In this model, the objectives given in Equations (2) and (4) are mixed in a linear cost function with two terms balanced by the value of the parameter β:

$$\begin{aligned} \min \quad & \sum_{i=1}^{|\mathcal{B}|} [-\boldsymbol{\mu_w} \cdot \mathbf{S}_i \cdot (|\mathcal{B}| - i + 1) \; + \\ & \quad \beta \cdot \boldsymbol{P_o} \cdot \mathbf{S}_i \cdot (|\mathcal{B}| - i + 1)] \\ & \text{Subject to:} \\ & \begin{cases} P[T_{b_i} \leq l(b_i)] & \geq \; Cl, \quad \forall i = 1, 2, \ldots, |\mathcal{B}|. \\ \sum_{i=1}^{|\mathcal{B}|} \mathbf{S}_i[j] & \leq \; 1, \quad \forall j = 1, 2, \ldots, |\mathcal{W}| \\ \mathbf{S}_i \in \{0, 1\}^{1 \times |\mathcal{W}|}, & \qquad\quad \forall i = 1, 2, \ldots, |\mathcal{B}|. \end{cases} \end{aligned} \tag{5}$$

The MIQCP model has two sets of constraints. The first one is related to the chance probability constraint given in Equation (3), while the second one imposes that each patient in the waiting list is scheduled at most once. Development of the chance constraint (3) quadratic constraints is obtained [29].

Moreover, the decision variables S_i are binary, so the computational complexity of the MIQCP model is really high. In order to obtain scheduling in a reasonable time, heuristic approaches are needed.

4. Proposed Solution

4.1. Specific Heuristic Algorithm

Two heuristic approaches have been discussed for implementation in the DSS. The first one is a *Receding Horizon Strategy* (RHS) which obtains a sub-optimal solution sequentially (similar to [30]), while the second one is a *Specific Heuristic Algorithm* (SHA) based on list scheduling techniques [31–33].

The SHA for the scheduling of patients problem is composed of three parts: (i) a previous data analysis; (ii) the scheduling of the time blocks; and (iii) a re-assignment of time blocks.

Part (i): A previous data analysis. This part is composed of two steps executed sequentially once at the beginning of the scheduling.

Step 1. Classify the set of surgeries $\mathcal{S}$ in a given number t of disjoint subsets such that $\mathcal{S} = \overline{S_1} \cup \ldots \cup \overline{S_t}$, t being an input parameter. This classification is done based on two conditions: (1) the average duration of all surgeries in a subset $\overline{S_i} \in \mathcal{S}, i = 1, 2, \ldots, t-1$ must be less than or equal to the average duration of all surgeries in subset $\overline{S_{i+1}} \in \mathcal{S}$, and (2) the expected number of patients in each subset $S_i \in \mathcal{S}$ should be similar. In order to compute the expected number of patients for each $\overline{S_i} \in \mathcal{S}$, the probability of occurrence of all surgeries in $\mathcal{S}$ should be known, and it is obtained using historical data of the studied department.

For example, if there exist three types of surgeries $\mathcal{S} = \{s_1, s_2, s_3\}$ with $\mu_d(s_1) < \mu_d(s_2) < \mu_d(s_3)$ and the occurrence probabilities are 0.25 for s_1 and s_2 and 0.5 for s_3, a valid classification for $t = 2$ is $\mathcal{S} = \{\overline{S_1}, \overline{S_2}\}$ where $\overline{S_1} = \{s_1, s_2\}$ and $\overline{S_2} = \{s_3\}$. However, if $\mu_d(s_1) < \mu_d(s_3) < \mu_d(s_2)$, a valid classification could be $\overline{S_1} = \{s_1, s_3\}$ and $\overline{S_2} = \{s_2\}$ but also $\overline{S_1} = \{s_1\}$ and $\overline{S_2} = \{s_2, s_3\}$ is a valid solution.

Step 2: Obtain the set of possible scheduling types for each time block $b_i \in \mathcal{B}$. In this step, all multisets from set $\mathcal{S} = \{\overline{S_1}, \overline{S_2}, \ldots, \overline{S_t}\}$ are obtained from the possible scheduling type for the time block b_i. Formally, a possible scheduling type is a tuple $(\mathcal{S}, m)$, where $\mathcal{S}$ is the underlying set of the multiset and $m : \mathcal{S} \rightarrow \mathbb{N}_{\geq 1}$ is a function giving the multiplicity of the elements in the multiset. A multiset belonging to the possible scheduling type of block b_i should satisfy the chance constraint (3). In order to check that the chance constraint (3) is satisfied, the surgeries with lower average duration are considered.

For example, a possible scheduling type for time block b_i could be $\{\overline{S_k}, \overline{S_k}, \overline{S_j}\}$ meaning that, in block b_i, two surgeries from set $\overline{S_k}$ may be scheduled and another one from set $\overline{S_j}$. If s_k^1 is the surgery type with the lowest average duration from $\overline{S_k}$ and s_j^1 is the surgery type with the lowest average duration from $\overline{S_j}$, according to the total duration in (1), the minimum total duration of the time block b_i is

$$T_{b_i} = \left(Dt + s_k^1 + s_k^1 + s_j^1 + 2 \cdot Ct\right),$$

where Dt is the delay with respect to the starting time and Ct is the cleaning time duration after each surgery.

As observed before, T_{b_i} is following a normal distribution with mean

$$\mu_{T_{b_i}} = \mu_{Dt} + 2 \cdot \mu_d(s_k^1) + \mu_d(s_j^1) + 2 \cdot \mu_{Ct}$$

and standard deviation

$$\sigma_{T_{b_i}} = \sqrt{(\sigma_{Dt})^2 + 2 \cdot (\sigma_d(s_k^1))^2 + \left(\sigma_d(s_j^1)\right)^2 + 2 \cdot (\sigma_{Ct})^2}.$$

Since $\{\overline{S_k}, \overline{S_k}, \overline{S_j}\}$ is a possible scheduling type, the chance constraint (3) is satisfied. In order to check this equation, based on normal distribution property [34], the following inequality

$$P[T_{b_i} \leq l(b_i)] \geq Cl$$

is equivalent to

$$\frac{l(b_i) - \mu_{T_{b_i}}}{\sigma_{T_{b_i}}} \geq V_{Cl},$$

where V_{Cl} is the value corresponding to the normal variable ($x \sim N(0,1)$) with a cumulative distribution function Cl, i.e., $P[x \leq V_{Cl}] = Cl$ and this value is tabulated.

Part (ii): Scheduling of the time blocks, consisting of the following four steps executed sequentially for each time block b_i to schedule.

Step 3: For each possible scheduling type of time block b_i, obtain the sets of real scheduling. Given a possible scheduling type, a real scheduling is composed by a set of patients with the types of surgeries equal to the possible scheduling types.

For example, considering the scheduling type $\{\overline{S_k}, \overline{S_k}, \overline{S_j}\}$, a real scheduling is composed from two patients w' and w'' on which a surgery $s_k \in \overline{S_k}$ should be performed and one patient w''' on which a surgery $s_j \in \overline{S_j}$ should be performed. The first real scheduling corresponding to $\{\overline{S_k}, \overline{S_k}, \overline{S_j}\}$ is chosen by taking the patients with a lower number of preference order (corresponding to the higher preference). However, all other combinations of patients satisfying the chosen scheduling type having no patients with preference order greater than the maximum preference order of the patient in the first real scheduling will be considered.

Let us assume, for example, the list of patients given in Table 1 with $\mathcal{W} = \{w_1, w_2, w_3, w_4, w_5, w_6\}$ such that patients w_1, w_3, and w_5 have assigned the surgery s_1, the patient w_2 has assigned the surgery s_2, the patient w_4 the surgery s_3, and the patient w_6 the surgery s_4. Assuming the set of surgeries $\mathcal{S} = \{\overline{S_1}, \overline{S_2}, \overline{S_3}\}$ with $\overline{S_1} = \{s_1, s_2\}$, $\overline{S_2} = \{s_3\}$ and $\overline{S_3} = \{s_4\}$ and two possible scheduling types $\{\overline{S_1}, \overline{S_1}, \overline{S_2}\}$ and $\{\overline{S_1}, \overline{S_2}, \overline{S_3}\}$, the first real scheduling considered for $\{\overline{S_1}, \overline{S_1}, \overline{S_2}\}$ is $\{w_1, w_2, w_4\}$. The maximum order of patients in this real scheduling is 4 (corresponding to w_4), hence the following real scheduling will be considered as well: $\{w_1, w_3, w_4\}$ and $\{w_2, w_3, w_4\}$. For the scheduling type $\{\overline{S_1}, \overline{S_2}, \overline{S_3}\}$, the first real scheduling is $\{w_1, w_4, w_6\}$. Since the maximum preference order of patients is 6, the following real scheduling will be considered as well: $\{w_2, w_4, w_6\}$, $\{w_3, w_4, w_6\}$ and $\{w_4, w_5, w_6\}$. All of this real scheduling is shown in Table 2.

Table 1. Surgery data and waiting list of patients used for explaining part 2 of the SHA.

Surgeries Data			**Waiting List**						
S	**Types**	**Average Duration**							
$\overline{S_1}$	s_1	90	**Patient**	w_1	w_2	w_3	w_4	w_5	w_6
	s_2	110	**Surgery type**	s_1	s_2	s_1	s_3	s_1	s_4
$\overline{S_2}$	s_3	125							
$\overline{S_3}$	s_4	135							

Table 2. Motivation example for explaining part 2 of the SHA.

Possible Scheduling Types	**Real Scheduling**	***r* (%)**	***Ap***	**H (Step 4)**	**H (Step 5)**
	$w_1w_2w_4$	77.38	2.33	0	10.71
$\overline{S_1}\ \overline{S_1}\ \overline{S_2}$	$w_1w_3w_4$	72.61	2.66	5.62	-
	$w_2w_3w_4$	77.38	3	1.74	-
	$w_1w_4w_6$	83.33	3.66	4.76	-
$\overline{S_1}\ \overline{S_2}\ \overline{S_3}$	$w_2w_4w_6$	88.09	4	**0.88**	**4.34**
	$w_3w_4w_6$	83.33	4.33	6.50	-
	$w_4w_5w_6$	83.33	5	8.24	-

Step 4: Evaluate the real scheduling and select the best one for each scheduling type. First, the real scheduling not fulfilling the chance constraint (3) is removed and the check is similar to the one in Step 2. For the remaining real scheduling, the expected occupation rate r is computed by summing the average duration of all surgeries in the real scheduling divided by the time block duration $l(b_i)$ (multiplied by 100 if percentage). Furthermore, the average preference order Ap is computed by summing the preference order of all patients in the real scheduling divided by the number of patients in the real scheduling. The real scheduling with the minimum value of the following fitness function is chosen:

$$H = (Ap - Min_{Ap}) \cdot \beta + (Max_r - r), \tag{6}$$

where Min_{Ap} is the minimum average preference order of all real scheduling; Max_r is the maximum occupation rate r of all real scheduling; and β is a balancing parameter between the two terms (one for preference order and one for occupation rate).

For example, in Table 2, the computations of the occupation rates are given, preference order, and fitness function (fifth column) for the set of real scheduling considered before. In this example, a value of $\beta = 2.6$ is used and the time block duration are assumed to be $l(b_i) = 420$ (min), corresponding to 7 h. In this step, the real scheduling $w_1w_2w_4$ is chosen for the possible scheduling type $\overline{S_1S_1S_2}$ and $w_2w_4w_6$ is chosen for $\overline{S_1S_2S_3}$.

Step 5: Evaluate the best real scheduling chosen in Step 4 (one for each scheduling type) and select the best one for the current time block b_i. From the set of selected real scheduling in the previous step, the one with minimum value of the fitness function (6) is chosen. Notice that the value of the fitness function of a real scheduling in this step is, in general, different by the one computed in step 4. In particular, Min_{Ap} and Max_r have different values since are computed based only on the best real scheduling computed in step 4.

The sixth column of Table 2 is showing the computation of the fitness function on the two selected real scheduling instances on the previous step. Hence, in this step, $Min_{Ap} = 2.33$ corresponding to $w_1w_2w_4$ while $Max_r = 88.09$ corresponding to $w_2w_4w_6$. According to them, patients $w_2w_4w_6$ are selected for the time block $l(b_i)$.

Step 6: Remove the scheduled patients. The patients scheduled in Step 5 are removed from the waiting list, and the procedure is iterated for time block b_{i+1} from Step 3.

By using the case study in the HCU hospital, it has been observed that values of $t = 3$ and of $\beta = 2.6$ are appropriate. However, for different medical departments, a previous study is necessary in order to better choose these design parameters.

Part (iii): Sorting the time blocks with the same available time. First, the time blocks are grouped depending on their available time $l(b_i)$. Then, the time blocks of each group are sorted in ascending order according to the average preference order of the scheduled patients (indicator Ap). At the end, for each date, a time block is assigned sequentially starting with the closest one.

4.2. Decision Support System

In this section, the main features of the proposed DSS are discussed. Each doctor in the hospital department has his own list of patients and the waiting list of a team is composed by the merged list of doctors belonging to the team. Each team must schedule the patients from its waiting list during the time blocks previously booked by the head of the department. Thus, the main objective of the DSS is to help medical doctors perform a fast efficient and dynamic scheduling of the elective patients. The DSS uses as a core for the scheduling of patients the SHA approach presented in the previous subsection. However, other features are also included which enable (a) managing the medical teams and the OR time-table; (b) updating the waiting lists; (c) dynamic planning; and (d) improving the problem parameter by updating the surgeries duration.

Manage medical team and OR time-table. Normally, the medical teams are composed of the same medical doctors. However, sometimes medical doctors could move from one team to another. The head of the department is responsible for updating the medical teams and including this information in the DSS. Moreover, the head of the department should define the ORs time-table in the DSS. The OR, the date, the starting time, and the ending time of each time block assigned to each team is the information that must be included in the DSS.

Updating the waiting list. Generally, the new arrived patients are included at the end of the waiting list. However, depending on medical criteria, the surgeon could decide to advance the patient into a higher position in the waiting list. The DSS automatically orders the waiting list of patients. There are two parameters influencing directly the position of the patient in the waiting list.

1. The first parameter is related to the waiting time for surgery. A score S_1 of 10 is given to the patient with the highest number of waiting days, while the newest patient has a score of 0. A proportional score between 10 and 0 is given to other patients. In the calculation of total score (denoted S_T), the score S_1 has a weight of p.
2. The second parameter has to do with the surgery priority. Although non-urgent surgeries are scheduled with the DSS, three levels of priorities 1, 2, and 3 are considered by doctors depending on the urgency. A corresponding score (S_2) of 0, 5, and 10 is associated respectively.

The final score is obtained as follows:

$$S_T = p \cdot S_1 + S_2 \tag{7}$$

Finally, the patients are ordered according to their total score. The patient with the highest total score will be the first, while the patient with the lowest punctuation will be the last one.

Iterative planning. The scheduler of each medical team performs the scheduling for the next $|\mathcal{B}|$ time blocks (this is done by using the SHA). The secretary calls the patients scheduled and asks them for their availability on the scheduled date. The secretary gives back this information to the team scheduler who should schedule the empty gaps again. This process is repeated until the $|\mathcal{B}|$ time blocks are completely scheduled with all patients confirmed.

During the iterative scheduling, if a patient confirms the attendance, she/he is fixed in the corresponding time block. However, in the case that a patient cannot be contacted or she/he cannot be hospitalized, then the patient is not considered for the scheduling of the next $|\mathcal{B}|$ time blocks.

Thus, in the next iteration, the patients previously confirmed and the patients who cannot be hospitalized are not considered in the waiting list. The SHA schedules new patients in the gaps of the uncompleted time blocks.

Updating and customizing the average duration. The average duration and standard deviation of each type of surgery should be computed using historical data from the hospital department. Considering two years, a sufficiently high number of surgeries of each type is obtained, and the average duration is representative. However, depending on the skills and experience of the surgeons, significant differences could exist between their average duration. Moreover, for the same medical doctor, a continuous decrease of the average duration, due to the experience occurring, so these input values should be dynamically updated.

When a surgery is finished, the name of the surgeon and the time spent are introduced in the DSS. The DSS registers this information in a database and updates the average duration.

Overview of the DSS. All the previously explained features are integrated into the DSS whose flowchart is given in Figure 1.

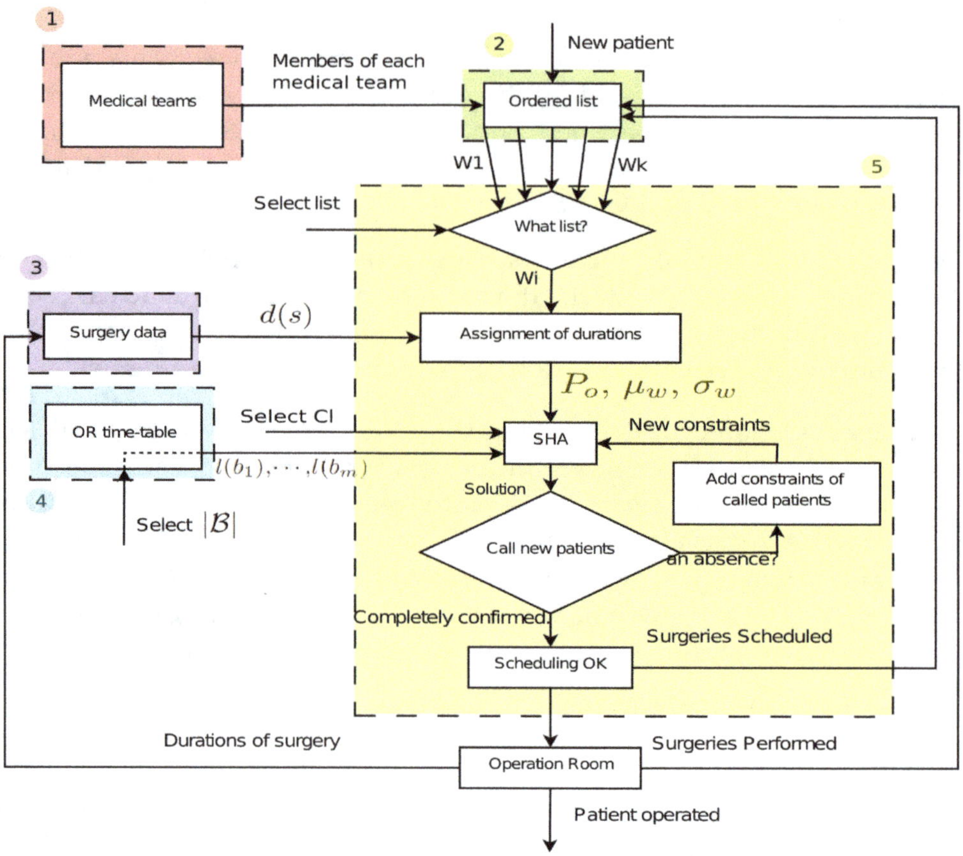

Figure 1. Flowchart of the DSS. The steps form the moment when a patient arrives until she/he is surgically operated are shown. The discontinuous colored boxes reference the five main panels included in the developed software tool: (1) Medical teams; (2) Patients; (3) Surgeries; (4) OR timetable; and (5) Scheduling.

When a new patient arrives at the service, she/he is introduced into the waiting list of a medical doctor. Each surgeon is responsible for including their patients in the system. The DSS recognizes the surgeon (using a personal password) and she/he must enter some personal information of the patient, the pathology and the priority of the surgery. Additionally, the DSS saves the actual date (to compute the waiting time in the list) and the surgeon to whom the patient belongs. When a team scheduler wants to perform a scheduling, she/he is recognized by the DSS and automatically composes the ordered waiting list of his patients.

The DSS has a database, which is updated every time that a surgery is performed. The pathology and its surgery durations are saved in the database. Thus, considering this information, the tool assigns average theoretical duration and standard deviation to each surgery in the waiting list. In this way, the vectors $\boldsymbol{\mu}_w$ and $\boldsymbol{\sigma}_w$ are generated. On the other hand, the DSS saves the OR time-table introduced previously by the head of the department—that is, the time blocks booked for each team as well as their duration defined as $l(b_i)$. The DSS performs an operation scheduling in an iterative way. The input data that the team's manager has to introduce in the DSS to schedule the next time blocks are: (i) the minimum confidence level Cl and (ii) the number of time blocks to schedule $|\mathcal{B}|$.

When a patient has been scheduled, his/her state changes from "pending" to "scheduled". Once a specific surgery is performed, the surgeon indicates this situation in the DSS and the corresponding patient is removed from the waiting list. Additionally, the surgeon introduces the operating time in the tool and these new input data are used to update the average duration. If finally a scheduled surgery is not performed, the DSS changes the state of this surgery from "scheduled" to "pending".

Based on the previously described DSS, a Software tool for scheduling elective patients in Spanish Hospitals called CIPLAN has been developed. A first version of this software was described in [12].

CIPLAN has been developed in JAVA language and has a SQL database. Moreover, in order to provide a safe work environment and a better security of the medical data, different access levels are provided to the users. The preferences and concerns of medical doctors in the OSD have been considered not only at the surgery scheduling level but also at the user interface level. Thus, a friendly interface divided into six main panels was proposed. These panels are based on the DSS and the first five are shown with color boxes in the flowchart of Figure 1: (1) *Medical teams*, (2) *Patients*, (3) *Surgeries*, (4) *OR timetable*, (5) *Scheduling*, and (6) *User*. Figure 2 shows the interface of the scheduling panel.

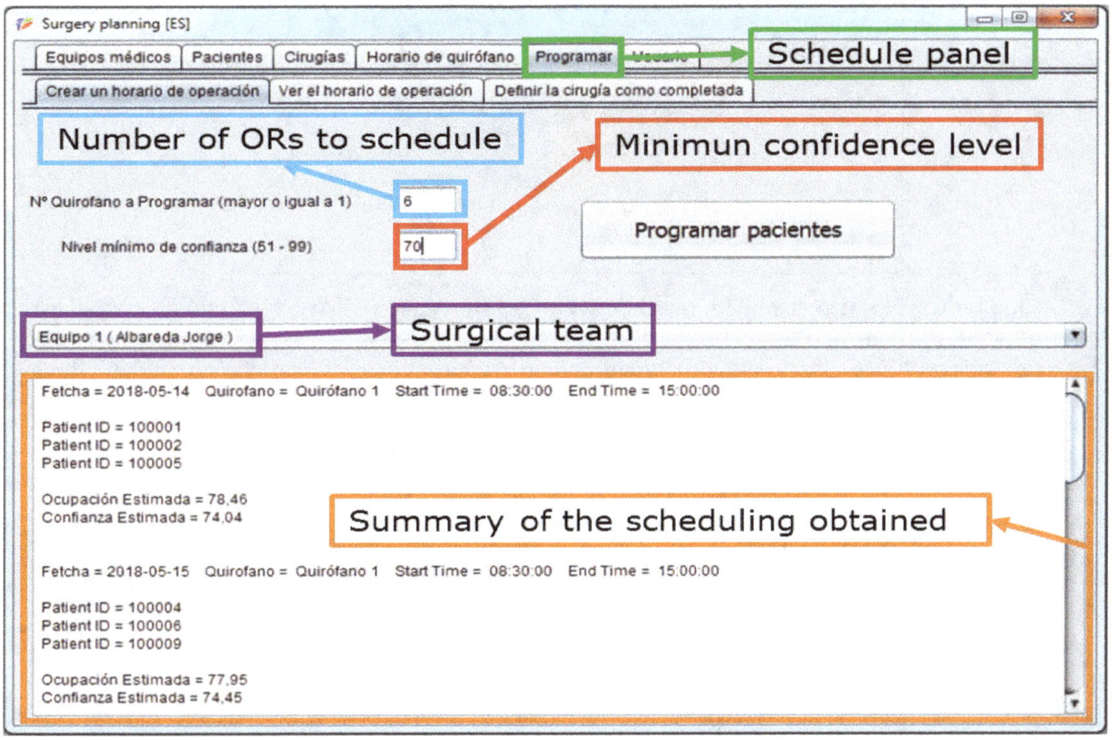

Figure 2. Scheduling panel. The main interface of the software tool is shown. Particularly, the scheduling panel where once the number of blocks to schedule, the minimum confidence level, and the surgical team are introduced, a summary of the scheduling performed is shown at the bottom part.

5. Simulations

In this section, some scheduling results derived of simulation are described and analyzed. The approach presented here is compared with two approaches in literature.

5.1. Simulation Methodology

In order to test the SHA and to compare it with the approaches proposed in [19,20], a discrete event simulation model of the scheduling has been implemented. It is used to simulate scheduling decision for a medical team in the Orthopedic Surgery Department (OSD) at the HCU. One year and the half length (78 weeks) is set for each simulation run. The new patients are assumed to arrive according to a Poisson distribution with an average of six per week. We assume initially a waiting list of 100 patients and every week the new arrived patients are added to the list.

During the last two years, considering historical data in the OSD, the occurrence probability of each surgery type and their duration have been computed. These values are considered in the simulation for generating the surgery of the arrival patients. Figure 3 shows the occurrence of the most common surgeries performed in the OSD while Table 3 indicates their average and standard deviation. Notice that seven types of surgeries represent around 73% of the total surgeries performed; however, all of them are used in the simulations.

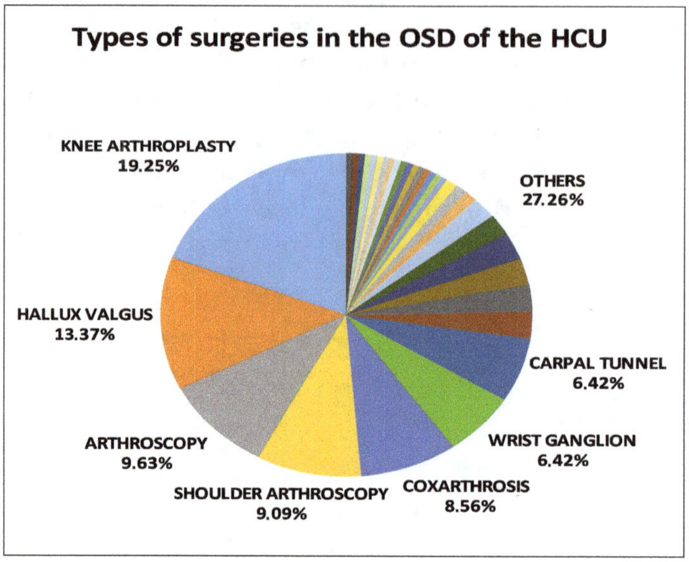

Figure 3. Occurrence of surgeries. The occurrence of some types of surgery that can be performed in the OSD of the LBH are shown.

Table 3. Duration of the surgeries performed in the OSD of the LBH.

Surgery Type	Avg. Duration [min]	Std. Deviation [min]
Knee arthroplasty	123.3	20.95
Hallux Valgus	99.4	17.67
Arthroscopy	79.8	17.97
Shoulder Arthroscopy	115.2	24.76
Coxarthrosis	125.9	32.10
Wrist Ganglion	47.5	21.16
Carpal Tunnel	32.9	7.53

For each set of simulations, 50 replications are performed. Each replication is a schedule of 156 time blocks (78 weeks $\times$ 2 time blocks per week) all of them having the same time duration of $l(b_i) = 390$ min (6.5 h). The average values of the probability of not exceeding the total time (confidence level) and the occupation rate are computed. Moreover, the total overtime and the total number of treated patients per year are considered.

In order to be able to compare two different schedules from the point of view of the order of the patients, indicator Ω is defined. This indicator measures the disorder of the patients in the obtained scheduling, so, the smaller it is, the more ordered are the patients. To compute this value, for each time block, an interval $[f_i, l_i]$ is defined. If the preference order of the surgeries scheduled in the time block b_i belongs to the interval $[f_i, l_i]$, Ω is not increased. On the contrary, each patient w_j with a preference order j outside the interval increases the value of Ω. The formal calculation of Ω is given in Algorithm 1, where Np is the total number of patients scheduled and $Pd = \frac{Np}{|B|}$ is the average number of patients scheduled per time block.

Algorithm 1 computes first the lower (f_i) and upper (l_i) preference orders of the patients that should be ideally scheduled in the time block b_i. However, we allow one block before and one block after without any penalization and, for this reason, $f_i = Pd \cdot (i - 2)$ and $l_i = Pd \cdot (i + 1)$. Then, for all patients scheduled in b_i, if their preference order in the waiting list does not belong to $[f_i, l_i]$, Ω parameter is increased with a value depending on the deviation (step 4).

Algorithm 1 Calculation of Ω parameter in a scheduling of $|\mathcal{B}|$ time blocks

Input: $\mathcal{B}, Pd$
Output: Ω
$\Omega := 0$
forall $b_i \in \mathcal{B}$ **do**
  $f_i := (1, \lfloor Pd \cdot (i-2) \rfloor)$;
  $l_i := \lceil Pd \cdot (i+1) \rceil$;
  forall *patient* (w_j) *scheduled in block* b_i **do**
    if *the preference order* $(j) \notin [f_i, l_i]$ **then**
      $\Omega := \Omega + \min(|j - f_i|, |j - l_i|)$

5.2. Simulation Results

Table 4 shows a comparison between the scheduling obtained by using: (1) the first-fit probabilistic rule (commonly used in hospitals), (2) the batch scheduling approach in [19], (3) the constructive algorithm proposed in [20], and (4) the SHA approach presented in this paper. The scheduling is obtained following the simulation methodology explained in the previous subsection for a minimum confidence level $Cl = 70\%$. The average value of probability of not exceeding the total time, occupation rate, and the order of the patients (Ω) are analyzed. Moreover, the total overtime and the total number of treated patients per year are shown.

Table 4. Comparison of the one and the half years scheduling using different chain-constrained approaches with a minimum confidence level of 70%.

Approach	Avg. Confidence Level	OVERTIME (Total) [min]	Avg. Occupation Rate (%)	Total # of Surgeries	Average Ω
first-fit rule	81.98	806.41	76.12	429.9	1935.9
Constructive Alg. [20]	80.43	922	76.69	432.02	2840
Batch Scheduling [19]	75	1183	79.06	447.78	3993.1
SHA (this paper)	77.31	1059	78.28	438.3	395.4

The three approaches analyzed in Table 4 improve the occupation rates obtained by using the first-fit probabilistic rule. However, the improvement in the occupation rate of the time block implies a decrement in the confidence level. For example, the Batch Scheduling approach [19] achieves the highest occupation rate (79.06%) and the highest number of treated patients (447.78), and, consequently, the lower confidence level (75%) and the highest total overtime (1183 [min]) are obtained. Taking into account the pairs of values occupation rate and confidence level, the Batch Scheduling approach obtains the better solution with: (1) the highest occupation rate and (2) a confidence level within the allowed.

The SHA approach presented in this paper obtains a little worse occupation rate (78.28%) than the Batch Scheduling (79.06%). However, considering the order of the patients given by the indicator Ω, it can be checked that the SHA approach by far obtains the best scheduling ($\Omega = 395$). Medical doctors of the OSD consider that the scheduling obtained using the SHA approach is the best one since it maintains the order of the waiting list better. Due to patients having more orders with SHA scheduling, it is possible to provide an estimation period for the patients in the list and this is a possible extension.

6. Case Study Results

This section presents a comparison between a scheduling obtained manually in the OSD and the scheduling obtained by using CIPLAN.

6.1. Case Study Description

Hospital Description. The HCU is a public hospital located in Zaragoza, Spain providing health services to around 325,000 people, and it is a reference center of specialized attention of a population over 1 million inhabitants. The hospital has 800 beds and 15 ORs for major surgery, which is performed by eight different surgical departments. The case study considers the Orthopedic Surgical Department (OSD).

The OSD is composed of five medical teams and has assigned 3 ORs (OR_1, OR_2 and OR_3) from 8:30 a.m. to 3:00 p.m. every day. Although there are other time blocks available for the department, the case study considers only these three ORs because the other ones have a variable time-table depending on the urgent surgeries. OR_1 and OR_2 are used to perform surgeries of elective patients, while OR3 is assigned to perform urgent surgeries. Table 5 shows an example of the weekly OR time-table of this OSD.

Table 5. OR time-table in the Orthopedic Surgical Department of the HCU.

	OR 1	OR 2	OR 3
Mon	team 1	team 2	team 3
Tue	team 4	team 5	team 1
Wed	team 2	team 3	team 4
Thu	team 5	team 1	team 2
Fri	team 3	team 4	team 5

According to Table 5, each medical team has two time blocks per week for performing surgeries on the elective patients.

Methodology of the case study. The main objective of the developed software tool is to improve the efficiency and quality of the surgical service. Thus, in the case study, the scheduling obtained manually is compared with the scheduling obtained by using CIPLAN. The methodology is as follows:

1. Analysis of manual scheduling. Considering historical data of one medical team of the OSD, 36 consecutive OR time blocks of elective patients are analyzed. For each time block, the following information is obtained:

- the type of surgeries performed,
- the starting and ending time of each surgery (real duration),
- the expected and real occupation rate,
- the confidence level of not exceeding the available time,
- the real ending time of each block.

The effective time in a surgery block is the time of using the OR for surgeries; therefore, the occupation rate in a time block is computed as the effective time divided by the total time.

2. Create the waiting list. The manual scheduling and consequently the surgery types in the waiting list are known. However, the preference order of each surgery in the waiting list is unknown. In order to be able to obtain an ordered waiting list from which the scheduling using CIPLAN is performed, it is assumed that the position of the patients (surgeries) in the list corresponds to the order in which they were operated by using the manual scheduling. That is, the first patient in the waiting list is the first patient operated in the first time block. Thus, considering the surgeries performed in the 36 time blocks, an ordered waiting list containing 111 patients is created.

3. Scheduling using CIPLAN. The data necessary to perform the scheduling using CIPLAN are included in the tool and then the scheduling is performed:

- All elective surgery types are added to CIPLAN including their average duration and standard deviation (computed considering historical data of the team during last two years).
- A new medical team (team 1) is added to the tool. Moreover, a new doctor is added to the team.

- All patients in the waiting list constructed using the 36 time blocks are assigned to the doctor.
- For the next three months, two time blocks are booked weekly from 8:30 a.m. to 3:00 p.m., in total being 24 time blocks.
- Using CIPLAN, the 24 time blocks previously booked are scheduled considering a minimum confidence level of not exceeding the total time equal to 69%. This value is fixed by doctors.

4. Analysis of the scheduling performed using CIPLAN. For each time block scheduled, the following parameters are obtained:

- the expected occupation rate,
- the confidence level of not exceeding the total time,
- the real occupation rate,
- the real ending time.

The scheduling obtained by using CIPLAN has not been applied in practice. Thus, to compute the real occupation rate, the time spent when the surgeries were performed (manual scheduling) has been considered. Moreover, in order to obtain the real ending time, 20 min of cleaning time between two consecutive surgeries and 10 min of delay with respect the starting time have been considered.

6.2. Real Case Study

Figure 4a shows the *expected occupation rate* in each time block. The average value obtained using CIPLAN (77.44%) is greater than using the manual method (75%). Moreover, in the scheduling obtained using CIPLAN, the values of the expected occupation rate in each time block are more concentrated around the average value ($\sigma = 3.61$) than using the manual scheduling ($\sigma = 7.42$).

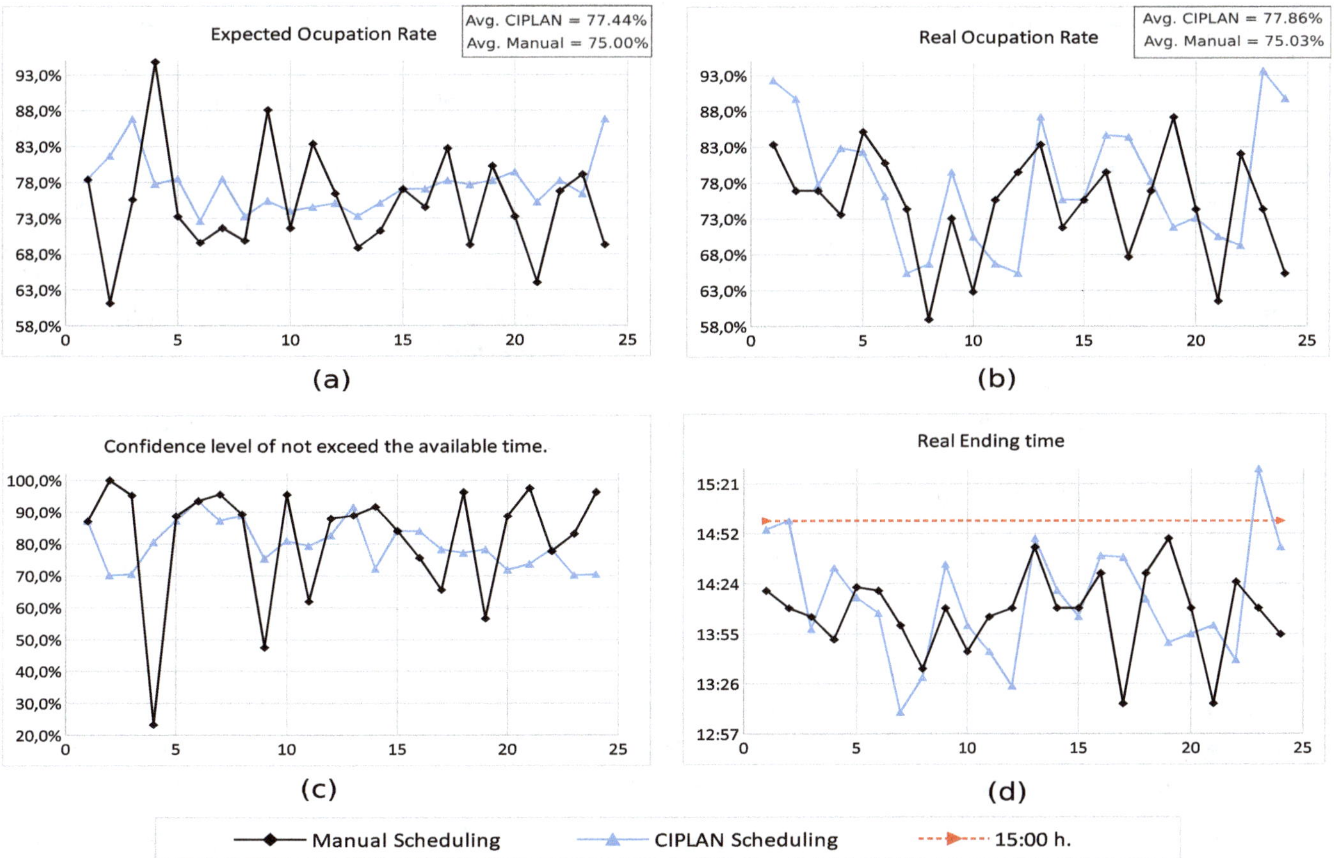

Figure 4. Comparison of manual and CIPLAN scheduling. A set of 24 time blocks has been scheduled manually and using CIPLAN. The following values are shown: (**a**) expected occupation rate; (**b**) real occupation rate; (**c**) confidence level of not exceeded the available time; (**d**) ending time.

In Figure 4b, the *real occupation rate* obtained in each time block is shown. Again, the average value obtained using CIPLAN (77.86%) is greater than the average value using the manual method (75.03%). Using CIPLAN, the improvement in the occupation rate with respect to use the manual method is 2.83%.

In Figure 4b, it is also possible to see that using CIPLAN there are some time blocks (1, 2, 23, and 24) with occupation rates too high (about 90%) and could lead to exceeding the available time. This does not happen in manual scheduling. Analyzing the results, it has been observed that it happens because the scheduler (in the manual method) knows the surgery skill of the surgeon and can estimate better the expected duration of the surgery depending on the surgeon. However, the CIPLAN scheduling algorithm initially uses the average duration of the surgeries. These average durations are computed considering historical data, independently from the surgeon. As the tool is used, the time spent in each surgery as well as the surgeon who performs it will be registered in CIPLAN. Thus, the surgery duration will be more and more customized depending on the surgeon and better results will be obtained.

In Figure 4c, the confidence level of not exceeding the available time is shown. The corresponding values are computed by considering the average duration and the standard deviation of each surgery. It can be seen that using CIPLAN does not exist time blocks with a confidence level lower than 69%. However, using the manual method, there are several time blocks with a really low confidence level. For example, in time block 4, the confidence level of not exceeding the available time is only 23.3%. Again, these low values are obtained since the scheduler knows the surgery skills of the surgeon. Particularly, in time block 4, three knee arthroplasties have been scheduled. Considering the average duration and the standard deviation based on historical data, the expected occupation rate is 94.8% and the confidence level that will not exceed the available time is 23.3%. However, the scheduler knows that the surgeon who has to perform the knee arthroplasties needs 25 min less than the average duration of the team. Consequently, the real occupation rate obtained is 73.3% and the time block ends at 13:52.

Figure 4d shows the ending time of each block. It can be observed that, using CIPLAN, there are four time blocks (1, 2, 13, and 24) ending around 3:00 p.m. and the time block 23 exceeding the available time 30 min (ending 15:30). This situation does not happen in manual scheduling.

According to the results obtained in the case study, the quality of the service decreases, because some blocks exceed the available time. However, this situation will be solved when the average duration and standard deviation of the surgeries will be customized depending on the surgeon. This customization will allow that the real occupation rate will be more similar to the expected one and, consequently, not only the number of blocks exceeding the available time will decrease, but also the total exceeding time.

In Figure 5, the time execution of the manual (a) and automatic (b) scheduling are shown by two bar-graphs.

Each row is composed by boxes that represent different actions in one surgical time block. Colored boxes represent surgeries while white boxes are idle times. The idle time could be: (i) delay regarding the starting time if the box is at the beginning or (ii) cleaning time if the box is between two surgeries. On the other hand, to check how much the order of patients in the waiting list is respected, the preference order of the patients inside the colored boxes has been included. Since the waiting list of patients has been constructed considering real surgeries, in Figure 5a, the patients are perfectly ordered. However, considering the automatic method (Figure 5b), although the SHA tries to make the scheduling respecting as much as possible, the order of the patients in the waiting list results in being a little disorderly. In order to see it visually, three colors have been used with a different meaning:

- The patients delayed or advanced at most a time block respect to the manual scheduling (perfectly ordered) are given in green boxes.
- The patients delayed or advanced two or three time blocks with respect to the manual scheduling are shown in orange or red boxes, respectively.

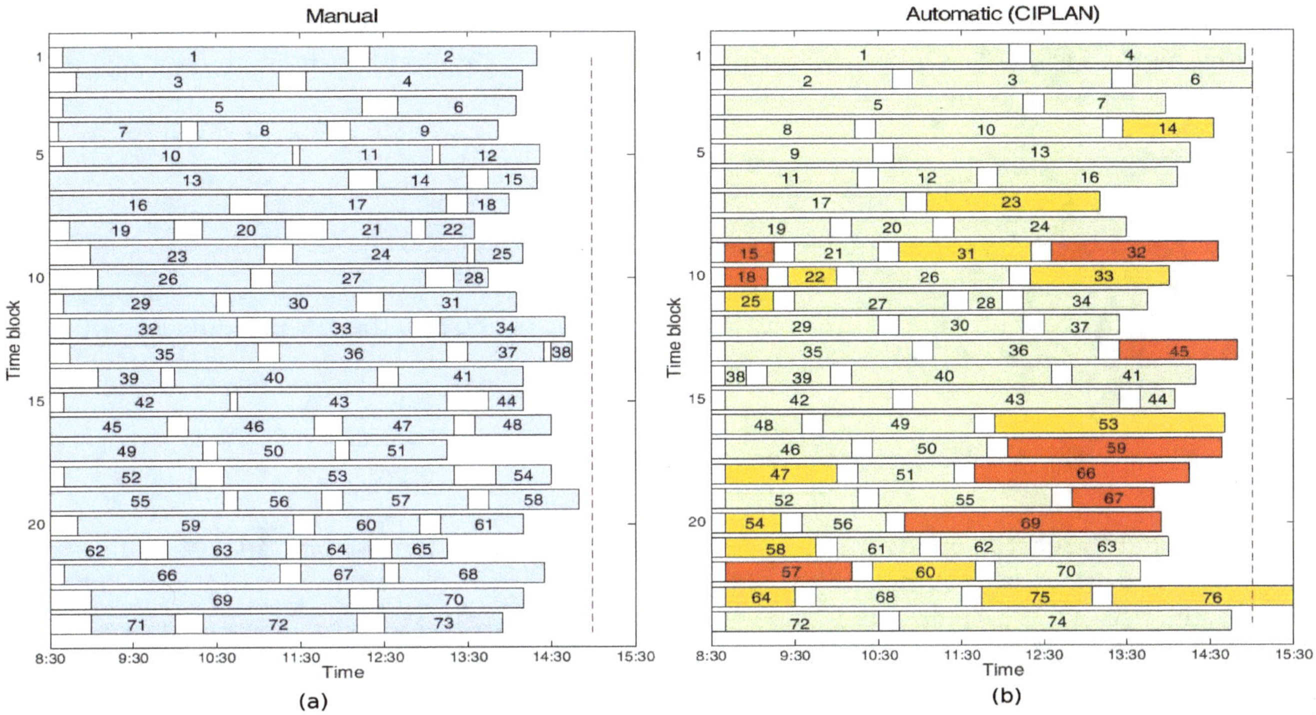

Figure 5. Comparison of the time execution of the surgical blocks. The time execution of the 24 time blocks scheduled (**a**) manually and (**b**) using CIPLAN are compared. Numbers inside the boxes represent the preference order of the patients. In case (**b**) color green/orange/red means that the patient has been advanced or delayed at most 1/2/3 time blocks with respect to the manual scheduling.

Remember that the waiting list has been constructed considering the real surgeries performed in 36 surgical blocks, obtaining a waiting list composed of 111 patients. Considering the manual scheduling, patients with preference order from 1 to 73 have been scheduled in the first 24 time blocks. Using CIPLAN, patients with preference order from 1 to 76 (except 65 and 71) have been scheduled in 24 time blocks. The number of patients advanced or delayed two time blocks (orange) is 14 while the number of patients advanced or delayed three time blocks (red) is 9. However only three patients (15, 18, and 57) have been delayed three time blocks and seven patients (22, 25, 47, 54, 58, 60, and 64) have been delayed two time blocks. This means:

- 4.05% of the patients are delayed three time blocks with respect to the preference order;
- 9.45% of the patients are delayed two time blocks with respect to the preference order.

7. Discussion

7.1. The Use and Experiences with the Scheduling Software Tool

Medical doctors who have used CIPLAN consider it an intuitive, rapid, and efficient software solution that can make easier the scheduling task. With the manual method, the confidence level of not exceeding the available time is unknown before building the schedule. However, with CIPLAN, they find an important advantage that the input parameter is the confidence level and the tool maximizes the occupation rate respecting this confidence level. Moreover, they said that the time spent for scheduling is drastically reduced, a check of the obtained solution being necessary.

Using CIPLAN, from an economic point of view, the improvement in the occupation rate using the manual method is 2.83%. Only considering the OSD, this 2.83% implies an increment Δ_{Oc} of 95.65 effective hours per year in the use of the ORs:

$$\begin{aligned}\Delta_{Oc} &= 0.0283 \cdot 6.5 \left[\frac{hours}{block}\right] \cdot 2 \left[\frac{block}{team \cdot week}\right] \\ &\cdot 52 \left[\frac{week}{year}\right] \cdot 5[team] = 95.65 \left[\frac{effe.\ hours}{year}\right]\end{aligned} \tag{8}$$

Assuming an occupation rate of 77.86% and time blocks of 6.5 h, these 95.65 effective hours are equivalent to an increment Δ_{Tb} of 18.89 blocks per year:

$$\Delta_{Tb} = \frac{95.65 \left[\frac{effe.\ h}{year}\right]}{0.7786 \left[\frac{effe.\ h}{h}\right] \cdot 6.5 \left[\frac{h}{block}\right]} = 18.89 \left[\frac{blocks}{year}\right] \tag{9}$$

Considering that the cost to open an OR during 6.5 h is 5850 euros, the use of CIPLAN in the surgical scheduling could suppose a saving of about 110,000 euros per year. The savings could be really greater extending the use of CIPLAN to other Departments.

7.2. Future Work

Doctors propose two new features that could improve significantly the tool. The first one is a new panel to give the possibility of performing virtual scheduling in which all patients included in a waiting list are scheduled. These provisional scheduling will allow doctors to give patients an estimated date of surgery from the moment when he/she is included in the waiting list. On the other hand, the virtual scheduling allows the head of the department to know the number of time blocks necessary to schedule all patients in the waiting list. Thus, he/she will be able to demand from the health administration the exact blocks needed to operate all patients in a certain period of time.

The second feature proposed is to include a new panel in the tool that, once a time block has finished and the starting and ending time of each surgery performed has been introduced in the tool; a comparison between the expected scheduling and the real execution of the time block is shown. In this way, it will be possible to detect the causes of time deviation between the expected and the real durations.

8. Conclusions

In Spanish hospitals, doctors are responsible for scheduling of elective patients. Currently, this task is performed manually and has three main problems: (i) doctors need to spend their time in the administrative task (scheduling); (ii) usually under or overutilization of the ORs is obtained; and (iii) objectivity can be questioned due to fact that the scheduling is done by a human. This paper presents a *Decision Support System* (DSS) that uses a *specific heuristic algorithm* SHA, in order to help the hospital managers in the scheduling of the elective patients.

Considering the duration of the surgeries and of the cleaning time as random variables with normal probability density function, the SHA with some statistics concepts can be used to schedule the elective patients from the waiting list to the next time blocks in such a way that: (i) the occupation rate of the time block is maximized; (ii) ensures a minimum confidence level of not exceeding the available time; and (iii) respect as much as possible the order of the patients in the waiting list. In addition, the DSS also includes features enabling the management of the medical teams and the OR time-table, updating the waiting list of patients, iterative planning, and automatic improvement of the input data.

In collaboration with the Orthopedic Surgery Department of the "*Lozano Blesa*" Hospital in Zaragoza, a software tool (CIPLAN) based on the proposed DSS has been developed. The preferences and concerns of doctors have been considered not only at the surgery scheduling level, but also at the user interface level. Thus, a friendly interface divided into six main panels is proposed in CIPLAN. It has been developed in Java language and uses a SQL database. Moreover, in order to provide a safe environment to work and better security of the medical data, different access levels are provided to every user.

Finally, in order to check the impact of the software tool in the efficiency and the quality of the surgical service, a case study considering real data from the Orthopedic Department of the HCU has been discussed. The results show that, using CIPLAN, an improvement in the occupation rate of the ORs can be reached.

However, it has been observed that there are significant differences in the surgery duration depending on the experience and on the surgery skill of the surgeon. Thus, if the SHA works with general average duration, over and under occupation rates are obtained more frequently than if it works with customized data. It would be convenient to customize the data of the surgical durations depending on each specific surgeon. In this way, the expected occupation rate and the expected ending time will be more similar to the real ones improving the quality of the service.

As future work, a new panel in CIPLAN can be developed that, once a time block has been finished, allows doctors to compare in a visual way the expected scheduling and the real execution. On the other hand, a new feature in CIPLAN can be included that enables them to perform virtual scheduling in which all patients in the waiting list are scheduled. In this way, an approximated date could be given to patients from the moment when they are included in the system. Moreover, other extensions can be developed—among others, an app connected to CIPLAN allowing patients to know the approximated date of their surgeries.

9. Patents

The developed software tool has been registered by the Office of Transfer of Research Result (OTRI) at the University of Zaragoza.

Author Contributions: All authors contributed to the design of the mathematical model and the conceptual design of the decision support system. J.A. was responsible for collecting the necessary surgical data to analyze the mathematical models and perform the case study. D.C., C.M. and M.S. were involved in the development of the proposed heuristic method as well as the implementation of the DSS. All authors have read and agreed to the published version of the manuscript.

Acknowledgments: We would like to acknowledge with much appreciation Lidia Castan's help in the collection of the necessary surgical data.

Abbreviations

The following abbreviations are used in this manuscript:

OR	Operation Room
DSS	Decision Support System
SHA	Specific Heuristic Algorithm
RHS	Receding Horizon Strategy
HCU	"Lozano Blesa" Hospital in Zaragoza
MIQCP	Mixed Integer Quadratic Constrained Programming
Ap	Average Preference Order
OSD	Orthopedic Surgery Department
CIPLAN	Developed Software Tool
MILP	Mixed Integer Linear Programming.

References

1. Antares Consulting. Libro Blanco de la Actividad y Gestion del Bloque Quirurgico en España. Available online: https://www.antares-consulting.com/uploads/TPublicaciones/356f8ea46ff1e222fbcdcdafb4415c0363c9c9aa.pdf (accessed on 11 March 2020).
2. OECD. *Health Data 2005—Statistics and Indicators for 30 Countries*; OECD: Paris, France, 2005.
3. C.I.A. The World Factbook. 2017. Available online: https://www.cia.gov/~library/publications/the-world-factbook/ (accessed on 11 March 2020).
4. Ministerio de Sanidad, Consumo y Bienestar Social. *Crisis Económica y Salud en España*; Informes, Estudios e Investigación; Ministerio de Sanidad, Consumo y Bienestar Social: Madrid, Spain, 2018.
5. Spangler, W.E.; Strum, D.P.; Vargas, L.G.; May, J.H. Estimating Procedure Times for Surgeries by Determining Location Parameters for the Lognormal Model. *Health Care Manag. Sci.* **2004**, *7*, 97–104. [CrossRef] [PubMed]
6. Boyd, S.; Vandenberghe, L. *Convex Optimization*; Cambridge University Press: Cambridge, MA, USA, 2004.
7. Capan, M.; Khojandi, A.; Denton, B.T.; Williams, K.D.; Ayer, T.; Chhatwal, J.; Kurt, M.; Lobo, J.M.; Roberts, M.S.; Zaric, G.; et al. From Data to Improved Decisions: Operations Research in Healthcare Delivery. *Med. Decis. Mak.* **2017**, *37*, 849–859. doi:10.1177/0272989X17705636. [CrossRef] [PubMed]
8. Cardoen, B.; Demeulemeester, E.; Belien, J. Operating room planning and scheduling: A literature review. *Eur. J. Oper. Res.* **2010**, *201*, 921–932. [CrossRef]
9. Schmidt, R.; Geisler, S.; Spreckelsen, C. Decision support for hospital bed management using adaptable individual length of stay estimations and shared resources. *BMC Med. Inform. Decis. Mak.* **2013**, *13*, 3. [CrossRef] [PubMed]
10. Miller, H.E.; Pierskalla, W.P.; Rath, G.J. Nurse scheduling using mathematical programming. *Oper. Res.* **1976**, *24*, 857–870. [CrossRef]
11. Epstein, D.M.; Chalabi, Z.; Claxton, K.; Sculpher, M. Efficiency, Equity, and Budgetary Policies: Informing Decisions Using Mathematical Programming. *Med. Decis. Mak.* **2007**, *27*, 128–137. [CrossRef] [PubMed]
12. Clavel, D.; Botez, D.; Mahulea, C.; Albareda, J. Software Tool for Operating Room Scheduling in a Spanish Hospital Department. In Proceedings of the 22nd International Conference on System Theory, Control and Computing, Sinaia, Romania, 10–12 October 2018.
13. Zhu, S.; Wenjuan, F.; Shanlin, Y.; Jun, P.; Panos, M.P. Operating room planning and surgical case scheduling: A review of literature. *J. Comb. Optim.* **2019**, *37*, 757–805. [CrossRef]
14. Samudra, M.; Van-Riet, C.; Demeulemeester, E.; Cardoen, B.; Vansteenkiste, N.; Rademakers, F.E. Scheduling operating rooms: Achievements, challenges and pitfalls. *J. Sched.* **2016**, *19*, 493–525. [CrossRef]
15. Landa, P.; Aringhieri, R.; Soriano, P.; Tanfani, E.; Testi, A. A hybrid optimization algorithm for surgeries scheduling. *Oper. Res. Health Care* **2016**, *8*, 103–114. [CrossRef]
16. Neyshabouri, S.; Berg, B.P. Two-stage robust optimization approach to elective surgery and downstream capacity planning. *Eur. J. Oper. Res.* **2017**, *260*, 21–40. [CrossRef]
17. Wang, Y.; Tang, J.; Fung, R.Y.K. A column-generation-based heuristic algorithm for solving operating theater planning problem under stochastic demand and surgery cancellation risk. *Int. J. Prod. Econ.* **2014**, *158*, 28–36. [CrossRef]
18. Wang, Y.; Tang, J.; Pan, Z.; Yan, C. Particle swarm optimization-based planning and scheduling for a laminar-flow operating room with downstream resources. *Soft Comput.* **2015**, *19*, 2913–2926. [CrossRef]
19. Shylo, O.V.; Prokopyev, O.A.; Schaefer, A.J. Stochastic operating room scheduling for high-volume specialties under block booking. *INFORMS J. Comput.* **2012**, *25*, 682–692. [CrossRef]
20. Hans, E.; Wullink, G.; Van Houdenhoven, M.; Kazemier, G. Robust surgery loading. *Eur. J. Oper. Res.* **2008**, *185*, 1038–1050. [CrossRef]
21. Kazak, J.; Chruściński, J.; Szewrański, S. The Development of a Novel Decision Support System for the Location of Green Infrastructure for Stormwater Management. *Sustainability* **2018**, *12*, 4388. [CrossRef]
22. Cheng, Y.J.; Chen, M.H.; Cheng, F.C.; Cheng, Y.C.; Lin, Y.S.; Yang, C.J. Developing a Decision Support System (DSS) for a Dental Manufacturing Production Line Based on Data Mining. In Proceedings of the 2018 IEEE International Conference on Applied System Invention (ICASI), Chiba, Japan, 13–17 April 2018; Volume 7.
23. Seyr, H.; Muskulus, M. Decision Support Models for Operations and Maintenance for Offshore Wind Farms: A Review. *Appl. Sci.* **2019**, *9*, 278. [CrossRef]

24. Bernardi, S.; Mahulea, C.; Albareda, J. Toward a decision support system for the clinical pathways assessment. *Discret. Event Dyn. Syst. Theory Appl.* **2019**, *29*, 91–125. [CrossRef]
25. Mahulea, C.; Mahulea, L.; Garcia-Soriano, J.M.; Colom, J.M. Modular Petri Net Modeling of Healthcare Systems. *Flex. Serv. Manuf. J.* **2018**, *30*, 329–357. [CrossRef]
26. Dios, M.; Molina-Pariente, J.M.; Fernandez-Viagas, V.; Andrade-Pineda, J.L.; Framinan, J.M. A Decision Support System for Operating Room scheduling. *Comput. Ind. Eng.* **2015**, *88*, 430–443. [CrossRef]
27. Karlof, J. *Integer Programming: Theory and Practice*; Operations Research Series; CRC Press: Boca Raton, FL, USA, 2005.
28. Apt, K. *Principles of Constraint Programming*; Cambridge University Press: Cambridge, MA, USA, 2003.
29. Clavel, D.; Mahulea, C.; Albareda, J.; Silva, M. *Robust Scheduling of Elective Patients under Block Booking by Chance Constrained Approaches*; Technical Report RR-18-01; Universidad de Zaragoza: Zaragoza, Spain, 2018. Available online: http://webdiis.unizar.es/~cmahulea/papers/rr_2018.pdf (accessed on 11 March 2020).
30. Camacho, E.; Bordons, C. *Model Predictive Control*; Advanced Textbooks in Control and Signal Processing; Springer: London, UK, 2004.
31. Johnson, D.S. Near-Optimal Bin Packing Algorithms. Ph.D. Thesis, Massachusetts Institute of Technology, Cambridge, MA, USA, 1973.
32. Klement, N.; Grangeon, N.; Gourgand, M. Medical Imaging: Exams Planning and Resource Assignment: Hybridization of a Metaheuristic and a List Algorithm. In Proceedings of the 10th International Joint Conference on Biomedical Engineering Systems and Technologies (BIOSTEC 2017), Porto, Portugal, 21–23 February 2017; pp. 260–267.
33. Arabnejad, H.; Barbosa, J.G. List Scheduling Algorithm for Heterogeneous Systems by an Optimistic Cost Table. *IEEE Trans. Parallel Distrib. Syst.* **2014**, *25*, 682–694. doi:10.1109/TPDS.2013.57. [CrossRef]
34. Siegel, A.F. (Ed.) *Practical Business Statistics*, 7th ed.; Academic Press: Cambridge, MA, USA, 2016; pp. 549–552.

5

Integrating Enhanced Sparse Autoencoder-Based Artificial Neural Network Technique and Softmax Regression for Medical Diagnosis

Sarah A. Ebiaredoh-Mienye, Ebenezer Esenogho * and Theo G. Swart

Center for Telecommunication, Department of Electrical and Electronic Engineering Science, University of Johannesburg, Johannesburg 2006, South Africa; snabofa@yahoo.com (S.A.E.-M.); ebenic4real@gmail.com (T.G.S.)

* Correspondence: ebenezere@uj.ac.za

Abstract: In recent times, several machine learning models have been built to aid in the prediction of diverse diseases and to minimize diagnostic errors made by clinicians. However, since most medical datasets seem to be imbalanced, conventional machine learning algorithms tend to underperform when trained with such data, especially in the prediction of the minority class. To address this challenge and proffer a robust model for the prediction of diseases, this paper introduces an approach that comprises of feature learning and classification stages that integrate an enhanced sparse autoencoder (SAE) and Softmax regression, respectively. In the SAE network, sparsity is achieved by penalizing the weights of the network, unlike conventional SAEs that penalize the activations within the hidden layers. For the classification task, the Softmax classifier is further optimized to achieve excellent performance. Hence, the proposed approach has the advantage of effective feature learning and robust classification performance. When employed for the prediction of three diseases, the proposed method obtained test accuracies of 98%, 97%, and 91% for chronic kidney disease, cervical cancer, and heart disease, respectively, which shows superior performance compared to other machine learning algorithms. The proposed approach also achieves comparable performance with other methods available in the recent literature.

Keywords: sparse autoencoder; unsupervised learning; Softmax regression; medical diagnosis; machine learning; artificial neural network; e-health

---

1. Introduction

Medical diagnosis is the process of deducing the disease affecting an individual [1]. This is usually done by clinicians, who analyze the patient's medical record, conduct laboratory tests, and physical examinations, etc. Accurate diagnosis is essential and quite challenging, as certain diseases have similar symptoms. A good diagnosis should meet some requirements: it should be accurate, communicated, and timely. Misdiagnosis occurs regularly and can be life-threatening; in fact, over 12 million people get misdiagnosed every year in the United States alone [2]. Machine learning (ML) is progressively being applied in medical diagnosis and has achieved significant success so far.

In contrast to the shortfall of clinicians in most countries and expensive manual diagnosis, ML-based diagnosis can significantly improve the healthcare system and reduce misdiagnosis caused by clinicians, which can be due to stress, fatigue, and inexperience, etc. Machine learning models can also ensure that patient data are examined in more detail and results are obtained quickly [3]. Hence, several researchers and industry experts have developed numerous medical diagnosis models using machine learning [4]. However, some factors are hindering the growth of ML in the medical domain, i.e., the imbalanced nature of medical data and the high cost of labeling data. Imbalanced data are a classification problem in which the number of instances per class is not uniformly distributed. Recently, unsupervised feature learning methods have received massive attention since they do not entirely rely on labeled data [5], and are suitable for training models when the data are imbalanced.

There are various methods used to achieve feature learning, including supervised learning techniques such as dictionary learning and multilayer perceptron (MLP), and unsupervised learning techniques which include independent component analysis, matrix factorization, clustering, unsupervised dictionary learning, and autoencoders. An autoencoder is a neural network used for unsupervised feature learning. It is composed of input, hidden, and output layers [6]. The basic architecture of a three-layer autoencoder (AE) is shown in Figure 1. When given an input data, autoencoders (AEs) are helpful to automatically discover the features that lead to optimal classification [7]. There are diverse forms of autoencoders, including variational and regularized autoencoders. The regularized autoencoders have been mostly used in solving problems where optimal feature learning is needed for subsequent classification, which is the focus of this research. Examples of regularized autoencoders include denoising, contractive, and sparse autoencoders. We aim to implement a sparse autoencoder (SAE) to learn representations more efficiently from raw data in order to ease the classification process and ultimately, improve the prediction performance of the classifier.

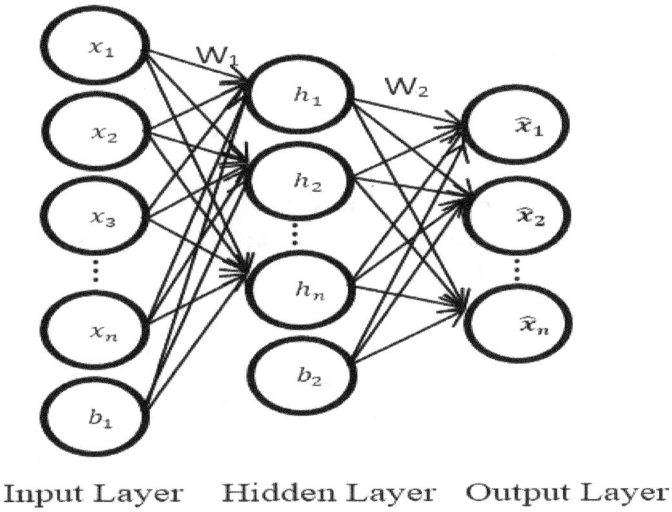

Figure 1. The structure of an autoencoder.

Usually, the sparsity penalty in the sparse autoencoder network is achieved using either of these two methods: L1 regularization or Kullback–Leibler (KL) divergence. It is noteworthy that the SAE does not regularize the weights of the network; rather, the regularization is imposed on the activations. Consequently, suboptimal performances are obtained with this type of structure where the sparsity makes it challenging for the network to approximate a near-zero cost function [8]. Therefore, in this paper, we integrate an improved SAE and a Softmax classifier for application in medical diagnosis. The SAE imposes regularization on the weights, instead of the activations as in conventional SAE, and the Softmax classifier is used for performing the classification task.

To demonstrate the effectiveness of the approach, three publicly available medical datasets are used, i.e., the chronic kidney disease (CKD) dataset [9], cervical cancer risk factors dataset [10], and Framingham heart study dataset [11]. We also aim to use diverse performance evaluation metrics to assess the performance of the proposed method and compare it with some techniques available in the recent literature and other machine learning algorithms such as logistic regression (LR), classification and regression tree (CART), support vector machine (SVM), k-nearest neighbor (KNN), linear discriminant analysis (LDA), and conventional Softmax classifier. The rest of the paper is structured as follows: Section 2 reviews some related works, while Section 3 introduces the methodology and provides a detail background of the methods applied. The results are tabulated and discussed in Section 4, while Section 5 concludes the paper.

2. Related Works

This section discusses some recent applications of machine learning in medical diagnosis. Glaucoma is a vision condition that develops gradually and can lead to permanent vision loss. This condition destroys the optic nerve, the health of which is essential for good vision and is usually caused by too much pressure inside one or both eyes. There are diverse forms of glaucoma, and they have no warning signs; hence, early detection is difficult yet crucial. Recently, a method was developed for the early detection of glaucoma using a two-layer sparse autoencoder [7]. The SAE was trained using 1426 fundus images to identify salient features from the data and differentiate a normal eye from an affected eye. The structure of the network comprises of two cascaded autoencoders and a Softmax layer. The autoencoder network performed unsupervised feature learning, while the Softmax was trained in a supervised fashion. The proposed method obtained excellent performance with an F-measure of 0.95.

In another research, a two-stage approach was proposed for the prediction of heart disease using a sparse autoencoder and artificial neural network (ANN) [12]. Unsupervised feature learning was performed with the help of the sparse autoencoder, which was optimized using the adaptive moment estimation (Adam) algorithm, whereas the ANN was used as the classifier. The method achieved an accuracy of 90% on the Framingham heart disease dataset and 98% on the cervical cancer risk factors dataset, which outperformed some ML algorithms. In a similar research, Verma et al. [13] proposed a hybrid technique for the classification of heart disease, where optimal features were selected via the particle swarm optimization (PSO) search technique and k-means clustering. Several supervised learning methods, including decision tree, MLP, and Softmax regression, were then utilized for the classification task. The method was tested using a dataset containing 335 cases and 26 attributes, and the experimental results revealed that the hybrid model enhanced the accuracy of the various classifiers, with the Softmax regression model obtaining the best performance with 88.4% accuracy.

Tama et al. [14] implemented an ensemble learning method for the diagnosis of heart disease. The ensemble method was developed via a stacked structure, whereby the base learners were also ensembles. The base learners include gradient boosting, random forest (RF), and extreme gradient boosting (XGBoost). Additionally, feature ranking and selection were conducted using correlation-based feature selection and PSO, respectively. When tested on different heart disease datasets, the proposed method outperformed the conventional ensemble methods. Furthermore, Ahishakiye et al. [15] developed an ensemble learning classifier to detect cervical cancer risk. The model comprised of CART, KNN, SVM, and naïve Bayes (NB) as base learners, and the ensemble model achieved an accuracy of 87%.

The application of sparse autoencoders in the medical domain has been widely studied, especially for disease prediction [12]. Furthermore, sparse autoencoders have been utilized for classifying Parkinson's disease (PD). Recently, Xiong and Lu [16] proposed an approach which involved a feature extraction step using a sparse autoencoder, to classify PD efficiently. Prior to the feature extraction, the data were preprocessed and an appropriate input subset was selected from the vocal features via the adaptive grey wolf optimization method. After feature extraction by the SAE, six ML classifiers were then applied to perform the classification task, and the experimental results signaled improved performance compared to other related works.

From the above-related works, we observed that most of the studies have some limitations: firstly, most of the authors utilized a single medical dataset to validate the performance of their models and not many studies experimented on more than two different diseases. By training and testing the model on two or more datasets, appropriate and more reliable conclusions can be drawn, and this can further validate the generalization ability of the ML method. Secondly, some recent research works have implemented sparse autoencoders for feature learning; however, most of these methods achieved sparsity by regularizing the activations [17], which is the norm. However, in this paper, sparsity is achieved via weight regularization. Additionally, poor generalization of ML algorithms resulting from imbalanced datasets, which is common in medical data, can be easily addressed using an effective feature learning method such as this.

3. Methodology

The sparse autoencoder (SAE) is an unsupervised learning method which is used to automatically learn features from unlabeled data [14]. In this type of autoencoder, the training criterion involves a sparsity penalty. Generally, the loss function of an SAE is constructed by penalizing activations within the hidden layers. For any particular sample, the network is encouraged to learn an encoding by activating only a small number of nodes. By introducing sparsity constraints on the network, such as limiting the number of hidden units, the algorithm can learn better relationships from the data [18]. An autoencoder consists of two functions: an encoder and decoder function. The encoder maps the d-dimensional input data to obtain a hidden representation. In contrast, the decoder maps the hidden representation back to a d-dimensional vector that is as close as possible to the encoder input [12,19]. Assuming m denotes the input features and n represents the neurons of the hidden layer, the encoding and decoding process can be represented with the following equations:

$$a^1 = \begin{bmatrix} a_1^1 \\ \vdots \\ a_n^1 \end{bmatrix} = \begin{bmatrix} w_{1,1}^1 & w_{1,2}^1 & \cdots & w_{1,m}^1 \\ \vdots & \vdots & \ddots & \vdots \\ w_{n,1}^1 & w_{n,2}^1 & \cdots & w_{n,m}^1 \end{bmatrix} \begin{bmatrix} x_1 \\ x_2 \\ \vdots \\ x_m \end{bmatrix} + \begin{bmatrix} b_1^1 \\ \vdots \\ b_n^1 \end{bmatrix}, \tag{1}$$

$$a^2 = \begin{bmatrix} a_1^2 \\ a_2^2 \\ \vdots \\ a_m^2 \end{bmatrix} = \begin{bmatrix} w_{1,1}^2 & \cdots & w_{1,n}^2 \\ \vdots & \ddots & \vdots \\ w_{m,1}^2 & \cdots & w_{m,n}^2 \end{bmatrix} \begin{bmatrix} a_1^1 \\ \vdots \\ a_n^1 \end{bmatrix} + \begin{bmatrix} b_1^2 \\ \vdots \\ b_m^2 \end{bmatrix}, \tag{2}$$

where $w^1 \in R^{n,m}$ and $w^2 \in R^{m,n}$ represent the weight matrices of the hidden layer and output layer, respectively; $b^1 \in R^{n,1}$ and $b^2 \in R^{m,1}$ denotes the bias matrices of the hidden layer and output layer, respectively; the vector $a^1 \in R^{n,1}$ denotes the inputs of the output layer; the vector $a^2 \in R^{m,1}$ represents the output of the sparse autoencoder, which is fed into the Softmax classifier for classification. The mean squared error function E_{MSE} is used as the reconstruction error function between the input x_i and reconstructed input a_i^2. Additionally, we introduce a regularization function $\Omega_{sparsity}$ to the error function in order to achieve sparsity by penalizing the weights $w^1 \in R^{n,m}$ and $w^2 \in R^{m,n}$. Therefore, the cost function E_{SAE} of the sparse autoencoder can be represented as:

$$E_{SAE} = E_{MSE} + \Omega_{sparsity}, \tag{3}$$

The mean squared error function and the regularization function can be expressed as:

$$E_{MSE} = \frac{1}{m}\sum_{i=1}^{m}\left(x_i - a_i^2\right)^2, \tag{4}$$

$$\Omega_{sparsity} = \frac{1}{m}\sum_{i=1}^{m}\left((x_i + 10)log\frac{x_i + 10}{a_i^2 + 10} + (10 - x_i)log\frac{10 - x_i}{10 - a_i^2}\right), \tag{5}$$

Once the data have been transmitted from input to output of the sparse autoencoder, the next stage involves evaluating the cost function and fine-tuning the model parameters for optimal performance. Meanwhile, the cost function E_{SAE} does not explicitly relate the weights and bias of the network; hence, it is necessary to define a sensitivity measure to sensitize the changes in E_{SAE} and transmit the changes backwards via the backpropagation learning method [8]. To achieve this, and iteratively optimize the loss function, stochastic gradient descent is employed. The stochastic gradient descent to update the bias and weights of the output layer can be written as:

$$b^2 = b^2 - \eta^2 \frac{\partial E_{SAE}}{\partial b^2}, \tag{6}$$

$$w^2 = w^2 - \eta^2 \frac{\partial E_{SAE}}{\partial w^2}, \tag{7}$$

where η^2 represents the learning rate in relation to the output layer. The derivative of the loss function E_{SAE} measures the sensitivity to change of the function value with respect to a change in its input value. Furthermore, the gradient indicates the extent to which the input parameter needs to change to minimize the loss function. Meanwhile, the gradients are computed using the chain rule. Therefore, (6) and (7) can be rewritten as:

$$b^2 = b^2 - \eta^2 \frac{\partial E_{SAE}}{\partial a^2} \times \frac{\partial a^2}{\partial b^2}, \tag{8}$$

$$w^2 = w^2 - \eta^2 \frac{\partial E_{SAE}}{\partial a^2} \times \frac{\partial a^2}{\partial w^2}, \tag{9}$$

The sensitivity at the output layer of the SAE is represented and defined as $S^2 = \frac{\partial E_{SAE}}{\partial a^2}$. Therefore, (8) and (9) can be rewritten as:

$$b^2 = b^2 - \eta^2 s^2, \tag{10}$$

$$w^2 = w^2 - \eta^2 s^2 \left(a^1\right)^T, \tag{11}$$

where

$$S^2 = \begin{bmatrix} s_1^2 \\ s_2^2 \\ \vdots \\ s_m^2 \end{bmatrix} = \begin{bmatrix} \frac{-(x_1+10)}{\log(10)\left(a_1^2+10\right)} + \frac{(10-x_1)}{\log(10)\left(10-a_1^2\right)} - \left(x_1 - a_1^2\right) \\ \frac{-(x_2+10)}{\log(10)\left(a_2^2+10\right)} + \frac{(10-x_2)}{\log(10)\left(10-a_2^2\right)} - \left(x_2 - a_2^2\right) \\ \vdots \\ \frac{-(x_m+10)}{\log(10)\left(a_m^2+10\right)} + \frac{(10-x_m)}{\log(10)\left(10-a_m^2\right)} - \left(x_m - a_m^2\right) \end{bmatrix}, \tag{12}$$

Using the same method for computing S^2, the sensitivities can be transmitted back to the hidden layer

$$b^1 = b^1 - \eta^1 s^1, \tag{13}$$

$$w^1 = w^1 - \eta^1 s^1 (x)^T, \tag{14}$$

where η^1 denotes the learning rate with respect to the hidden layer, whereas s^1 is defined as:

$$s^1 = \begin{bmatrix} s_1^1 \\ \vdots \\ s_n^1 \end{bmatrix} = \begin{bmatrix} s_1^2 w_{1,1}^2 + s_2^2 w_{2,1}^2 + \cdots + s_m^2 w_{m,1}^2 \\ \vdots \\ s_1^2 w_{1,n}^2 + s_2^2 w_{2,n}^2 + \ldots + s_m^2 w_{m,n}^2 \end{bmatrix}, \tag{15}$$

Furthermore, the Softmax classifier is employed for the classification task. The learned features from the proposed SAE are used to train the classifier. Though, Softmax regression, otherwise called multinomial logistic regression (MLR), is a generalization of logistic regression that can be utilized for multi-class classification [20]. However, in the literature, the Softmax classifier has been applied for several binary classification tasks and has obtained excellent performance [21]. The Softmax function provides a method to interpret the outputs as probabilities and is expressed as:

$$f(x_i) = \frac{e^{x_i}}{\sum_{j=1}^{k} e^{x_j}} \; (i = 1, 2, \ldots, N), \tag{16}$$

where $x_1, x_2, \ldots, x_N$ represent the input values and the output $f(x_i)$ is the probability that the sample belongs to the ith label [22]. For N input samples, the error at the Softmax layer is measured using the cross-entropy loss function:

$$L(w) = \frac{1}{N}\sum_{n=1}^{N} H(p_n, q_n) = -\frac{1}{N}\sum_{n=1}^{N}[y_n log\hat{y}_n + (1 - y_n)\log(1 - \hat{y}_n)], \tag{17}$$

where the true probability p_n is the actual label and q_n is the predicted value. $H(p_n, q_n)$ is a measure of the dissimilarity between p_n and q_n. Furthermore, neural networks can easily become stuck in local minima, whereby the algorithm assumes it has reached the global minima, thereby resulting in non-optimal performance. To prevent the local minima problem and further enhance classifier performance, the mini-batch gradient descent with momentum is applied to optimize the cross-entropy loss of the Softmax classifier. This optimization algorithm splits the training data into small batches which are then used to compute the model error and update the model parameters [23]. The momentum [24] ensures better convergence is obtained.

The flowchart to visualize the proposed methodology is shown in Figure 2. The initial dataset is preprocessed; then, it is divided into training and testing sets. The training set is utilized for training the sparse autoencoder in an unsupervised manner. Meanwhile, the testing set is transformed and inputted into the trained model to obtain the low-dimensional representation dataset. The low-dimensional training set is used to train the Softmax classifier, and its performance is tested using the low-dimensional test set. Hence, there is no possible data leakage since the classifier sees only the low-dimensional training set.

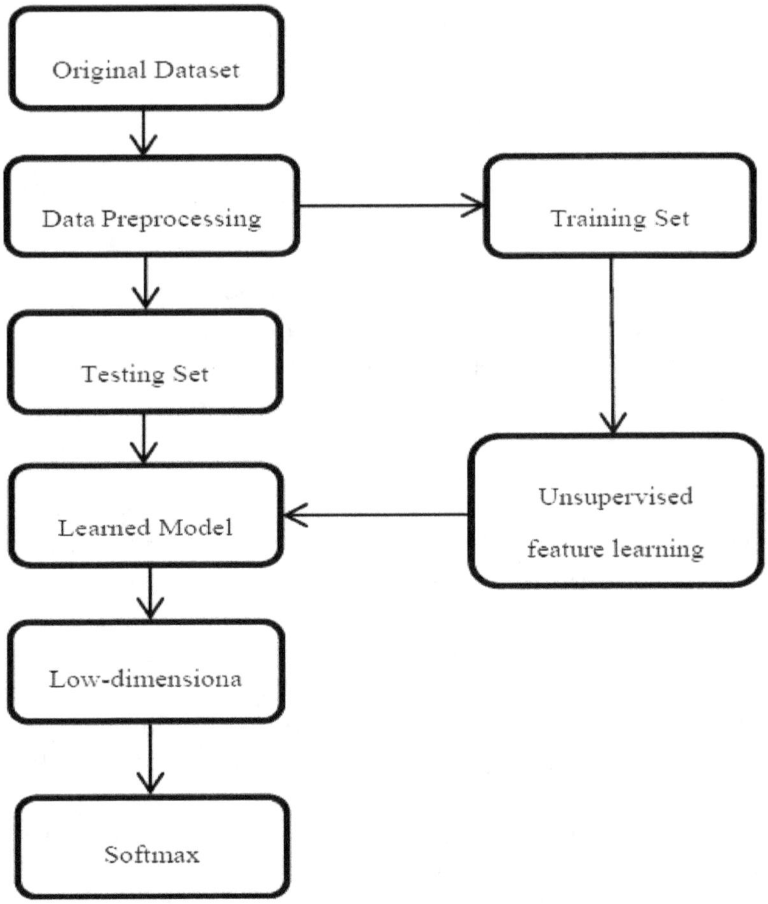

Figure 2. Flowchart of the methodology.

4. Results and Discussion

The proposed method is applied for the prediction of three diseases in order to show its performance in diverse medical diagnosis situations. The datasets include the Framingham heart study [11], which was obtained from the Kaggle website, and it contains 4238 samples and 16 features. The second dataset is the cervical cancer risk factors dataset [10], which was obtained from the University of California, Irvine (UCI) ML repository, and it contains 858 instances and 36 attributes. Thirdly, the CKD dataset [9] was also obtained from the UCI ML repository, and it contains 400 samples and 25 features. We used mean imputation to handle missing variables in the datasets.

The training parameters of the SAE include: $\eta^1 = 0.01$, $\eta^2 = 0.1$, $n = 25$, and number of epochs = 200. The hyperparameters of the Softmax classifier include learning rate = 0.01, number of samples in mini batches = 32, momentum value = 0.9, and number of epochs = 200. These parameters were obtained from the literature [12,23], as they have led to optimal performance in diverse neural network applications.

The effectiveness of the proposed method is evaluated using the following performance metrics: accuracy, precision, recall, and F1 score. Accuracy is the ratio of the correctly classified instances to the total number of instances in the test set, and precision measures the fraction of correctly predicted instances among the ones predicted to have the disease, i.e., positive [25]. Meanwhile, recall measures the proportion of sick people that are predicted correctly, and F1 score is a measure of the balance between precision and recall [26]. The following equations are used to determine these metrics:

$$Classification\ accuracy = \frac{TP + TN}{TP + TN + FP + FN}, \tag{18}$$

$$Precision = \frac{TP}{TP + FP}, \tag{19}$$

$$Recall = \frac{TP}{TP + FN}, \tag{20}$$

$$F1\ score = \frac{2 * Precision * Recall}{Precision + Recall} = \frac{2TP}{2TP + FP + FN}, \tag{21}$$

where

- True positive (TP): Sick people correctly predicted as sick.
- False-positive (FP): Healthy people wrongly predicted as sick.
- True negative (TN): Healthy people rightly predicted as healthy.
- False-negative (FN): Sick people wrongly predicted as healthy.

To demonstrate the efficacy of the proposed method, it is benchmarked with other algorithms, such as LR, CART, SVM, KNN, LDA, and conventional Softmax regression. In order to show the improved performance of the proposed method, no parameter tuning was performed on these algorithms; hence, their default parameter values in scikit-learn were used, which are adequate for most machine learning problems. The K-fold cross-validation technique was used to evaluate all the models. Tables 1–3 show the experimental results when the proposed method is tested on the Framingham heart study, cervical cancer risk factors, and CKD datasets, respectively. Meanwhile, Figures 3–5 show the receiver operating characteristic (ROC) curves comparing the performance of the conventional Softmax classifier and the proposed approach for the various disease prediction models. The ROC curve illustrates the diagnostic ability of binary classifiers, and it is obtained by plotting the true positive rate (TPR) against the false positive rate (FPR).

Table 1. Performance of the proposed method and other classifiers on the Framingham dataset.

Algorithm	Accuracy (%)	Precision (%)	Recall (%)	F1 Score (%)
LR	83	84	86	84
CART	75	74	75	74
SVM	82	78	82	80
KNN	81	75	81	77
LDA	83	81	83	82
Softmax classifier	86	84	88	86
Proposed SAE + Softmax	91	93	90	92

Table 2. Performance of the proposed method and other classifiers on the cervical cancer dataset.

Algorithm	Accuracy (%)	Precision (%)	Recall (%)	F1 Score (%)
LR	94	96	91	93
CART	90	93	96	94
SVM	94	90	93	91
KNN	93	98	95	96
LDA	95	93	91	92
Softmax classifier	94	97	91	94
Proposed SAE + Softmax	97	98	95	97

Table 3. Performance of the proposed method and other classifiers on the chronic kidney disease (CKD) dataset.

Algorithm	Accuracy (%)	Precision (%)	Recall (%)	F1 Score (%)
LR	98	93	97	95
CART	95	97	95	96
SVM	96	94	96	95
KNN	94	93	89	91
LDA	96	97	93	95
Softmax classifier	96	95	97	96
Proposed SAE + Softmax	98	97	97	97

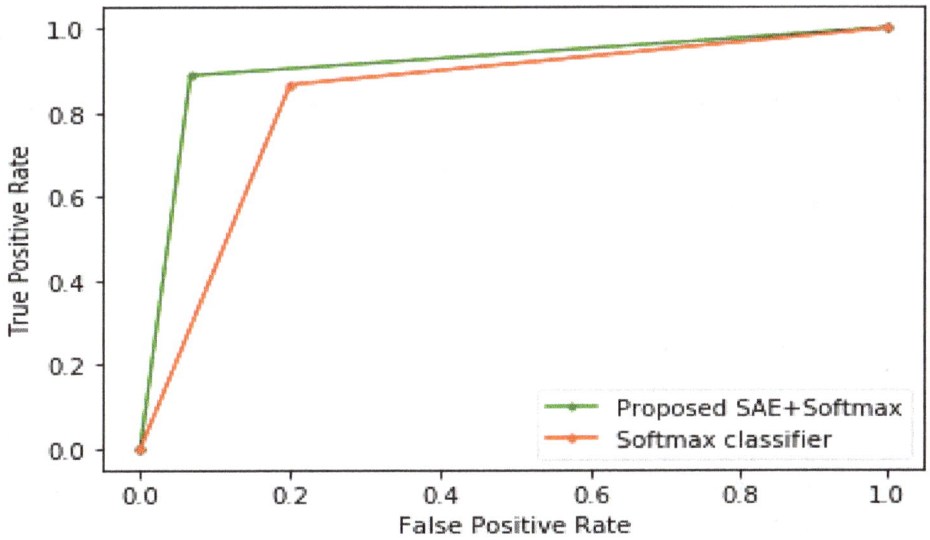

Figure 3. Receiver operating characteristic (ROC) curve of the heart disease model.

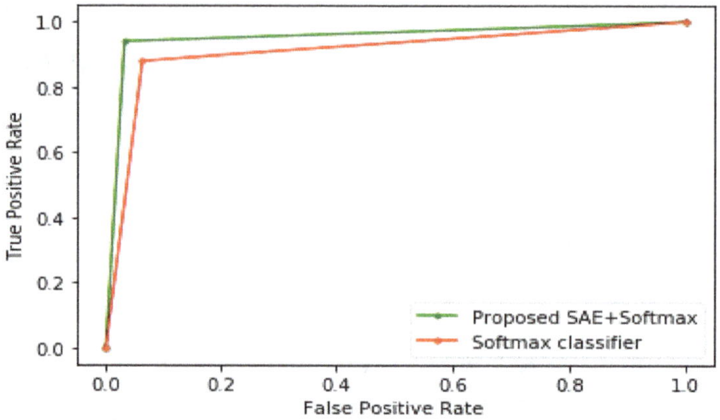

Figure 4. ROC curve of the cervical cancer model.

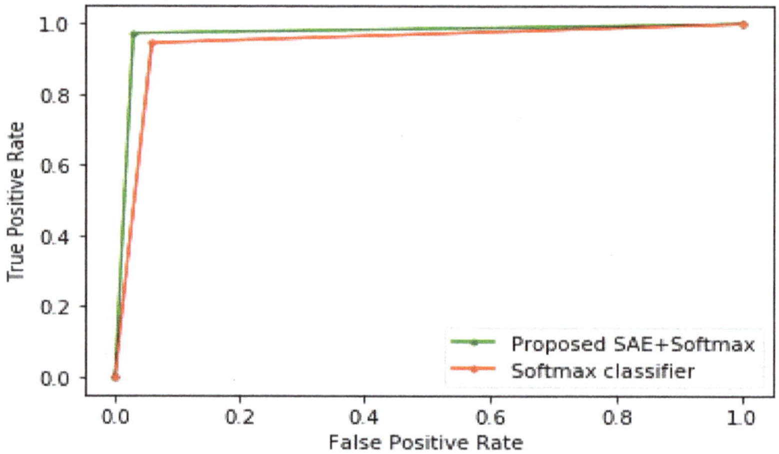

Figure 5. ROC curve of the CKD model.

From the experimental results, it can be seen that the sparse autoencoder improves the performance of the Softmax classifier, which is further validated by the ROC curves of the various models. The proposed method also performed better than the other machine learning algorithms. Furthermore, the misclassifications obtained by the model in the various disease predictions are also considered. For the prediction of heart disease, the proposed method recorded an FPR of 7% and a false-negative rate (FNR) of 10%. In addition, the model specificity, which is the true negative rate (TNR), is 93%, and the TPR is 90%. For the cervical cancer dataset, the following were obtained: FPR = 3%, FNR = 5%, TNR = 97%, and TPR = 95%. For the CKD prediction: FPR = 0, FNR = 3%, TNR = 100%, and TPR = 97%.

Additionally, to further validate the performance of the proposed method, we compare it with some models for heart disease prediction available in the recent literature, including a feature selection method using PSO and Softmax regression [13], a two-tier ensemble method with PSO-based feature selection [14], an ensemble classifier comprising of the following base learners: NB, Bayes Net (BN), RF, and MLP [27], a hybrid method of NB and LR [28], and a hybrid RF with a linear model (HRFLM) [29]. The other techniques include a combination of LR and Lasso regression [30], an intelligent heart disease detection method based on NB and advanced encryption standard (AES) [31], a combination of ANN and Fuzzy analytic hierarchy method (Fuzzy-AHP) [32], and a sparse autoencoder feature learning method combined ANN classifier [12]. This comparison is tabulated in Table 4. Meanwhile, in order to give a fair comparison, only the accuracies of the various techniques were considered because some authors did not report the values for other performance metrics.

Table 4. Comparison of the proposed method with the recent literature that used the heart disease dataset.

Algorithm	Method	Accuracy (%)
Verma et al. [13]	PSO and Softmax regression	88.4
Tama et al. [14]	Ensemble and PSO	85.71
Latha and Jeeva [27]	An Ensemble of NB, BN, RF, and MLP	85.48
Amin et al. [28]	A hybrid NB and LR	87.4
Mohan et al. [29]	HRFLM	88.4
Haq et al. [30]	LASSO-LR Model	89
Repaka et al. [31]	NB-AES	89.77
Samuel et al. [32]	ANN-Fuzzy-AHP	91
Mienye et al. [12]	SAE+ANN	90
Our approach	Improved SAE + Softmax	91

In Table 5, we compare the proposed approach with some recent scholarly works that used the cervical cancer dataset, including principal component analysis (PCA)-based SVM [33], a research work where the dataset was preprocessed and classified using numerous algorithms, in which LR and SVM had the best accuracy [34], a C5.0 decision tree [35]. The other methods include a multistage classification process which combined isolation forest (iForest), synthetic minority over-sampling technique (SMOTE), and RF [36], a sparse autoencoder feature learning method combined ANN classifier [12], and a feature selection method combined with C5.0 and RF [37].

Table 5. Comparison of the proposed method with the recent literature that used the cervical cancer dataset.

Algorithm	Method	Accuracy (%)
Wu and Zhou [33]	SVM-PCA	94.03
Abdullah et al. [34]	SVM	93.4884
	LR	93.4884
Chang et al. [35]	C5.0	96
Ijaz et al. [36]	iForest+SMOTE+RF	98.925
Mienye et al. [12]	SAE+ANN	98
Nithya and Ilango [37]	C5.0	97
	RF	96.9
Our approach	Improved SAE + Softmax	97

In Table 6, we compare the proposed method with other recent CKD prediction research works, including an optimized XGBoost method [38], a probabilistic neural network (PNN) [39], and a method using adaptive boosting (AdaBoost) [40]. The other research works include a hybrid classifier of NB and decision tree (NBTree) [41], XGBoost [42], and a 7-7-1 MLP neural network [43].

Table 6. Comparison of the proposed method with the recent literature that used the cervical CKD dataset.

Algorithm	Method	Accuracy (%)
Ogunleye and Qing-Guo [38]	Optimized XGBoost	100
Rady and Anwar [39]	PNN	96.7
Gupta et al. [40]	AdaBoost	88.66
Khan et al. [33]	NBTree	98.75
Raju et al. [42]	XGBoost	99.29
Aljaaf et al. [43]	MLP	98.1
Our approach	Improved SAE + Softmax	98

From the tabulated comparisons, the proposed sparse autoencoder with Softmax regression obtained comparable performance with the state-of-the-art methods in various disease predictions. Additionally, the experimental results show an improved performance obtained due to efficient feature representation by the sparse autoencoder. This further demonstrates the importance of training classifiers with relevant data, since they can significantly affect the performance of the prediction model. Lastly, this research also showed that excellent classification performance could be obtained not only by performing hyperparameter tuning of algorithms but also by employing appropriate feature learning techniques.

5. Conclusions

In this paper, we developed an approach for improved prediction of diseases based on an enhanced sparse autoencoder and Softmax regression. Usually, autoencoders achieve sparsity by penalizing the activations within the hidden layers, but in the proposed method, the weights were penalized instead. This is necessary because by penalizing the activations, it makes approximating near-zero loss function challenging for the network. The proposed method was tested on three different diseases, including heart disease, cervical cancer, and chronic kidney disease, and it achieved accuracies of 91%, 97%, and 98%, respectively, which outperformed conventional Softmax regression and other algorithms. By experimenting with different datasets, we aimed to demonstrate the effectiveness of the method in diverse conditions. We also conducted a comparative study with some prediction models available in the recent literature, and the proposed approach obtained comparable performance in terms of accuracy. Thus, it can be concluded that the proposed approach is a promising method for the detection of diseases and can be further developed into a clinical decision support system to assist health professionals as in [44]. Meanwhile, future research will apply the method studied in this paper for the prediction of more diseases, and also employ other performance metrics such as training time, classification time, computational speed, and other metrics, which could be beneficial for the performance evaluation of the model.

Author Contributions: Conceptualization, S.A.E.-M.; methodology, S.A.E.-M., E.E., T.G.S.; software, S.A.E.-M., E.E.; validation, S.A.E.-M., E.E.; formal analysis, S.A.E.-M., E.E., T.G.S.; investigation, S.A.E.-M., E.E., T.G.S.; resources, E.E., T.G.S.; data curation, E.E., T.G.S.; writing—original draft preparation, S.A.E.-M., E.E.; writing—review and editing, E.E., T.G.S.; visualization, E.E.; supervision, E.E., T.G.S.; project administration, E.E., T.G.S.; funding acquisition, E.E., T.G.S. All authors have read and agreed to the published version of the manuscript.

Acknowledgments: This work is supported by the Center of Telecommunications, University of Johannesburg, South Africa.

References

1. Stanley, D.E.; Campos, D.G. The Logic of Medical Diagnosis. *Perspect. Biol. Med.* **2013**, *56*, 300–315. [CrossRef] [PubMed]
2. Epstein, H.M. The Most Important Medical Issue Ever: And Why You Need to Know More About It. Society to Improve Diagnosis in Medicine. 2019. Available online: https://www.improvediagnosis.org/dxiq-column/most-important-medical-issue-ever/ (accessed on 30 August 2020).
3. Liu, N.; Li, X.; Qi, E.; Xu, M.; Li, L.; Gao, B. A novel Ensemble Learning Paradigm for Medical Diagnosis with Imbalanced Data. *IEEE Access* **2020**, *8*, 171263–171280. [CrossRef]
4. Ma, Z.; Ma, J.; Miao, Y.; Liu, X.; Choo, K.K.R.; Yang, R.; Wang, X. Lightweight Privacy-preserving Medical Diagnosis in Edge Computing. *IEEE Trans. Serv. Comput.* **2020**, 1. [CrossRef]
5. Li, X.; Jia, M.; Islam, M.T.; Yu, L.; Xing, L. Self-supervised Feature Learning via Exploiting Multi-modal Data for Retinal Disease Diagnosis. *IEEE Trans. Med. Imaging* **2020**, 1. [CrossRef] [PubMed]
6. Chen, Z.; Guo, R.; Lin, Z.; Peng, T.; Peng, X. A data-driven health monitoring method using multi-objective optimization and stacked autoencoder based health indicator. *IEEE Trans. Ind. Inform.* **2020**, 1. [CrossRef]
7. Raghavendra, U.; Gudigar, A.; Bhandary, S.V.; Rao, T.N.; Ciaccio, E.J.; Acharya, U.R. A Two Layer Sparse Autoencoder for Glaucoma Identification with Fundus Images. *J. Med. Syst.* **2019**, *43*, 299. [CrossRef]

8. Musafer, H.; Abuzneid, A.; Faezipour, M.; Mahmood, A. An Enhanced Design of Sparse Autoencoder for Latent Features Extraction Based on Trigonometric Simplexes for Network Intrusion Detection Systems. *Electronics* **2020**, *9*, 259. [CrossRef]
9. Rubini, L.J.; Eswaran, P. UCI Machine Learning Repository: Chronic_Kidney_Disease Data Set. 2015. Available online: https://archive.ics.uci.edu/ml/datasets/chronic_kidney_disease (accessed on 26 June 2020).
10. UCI Machine Learning Repository: Cervical cancer (Risk Factors) Data Set. Available online: https://archive.ics.uci.edu/ml/datasets/Cervical+cancer+%28Risk+Factors%29 (accessed on 27 January 2020).
11. Framingham Heart Study Dataset. Available online: https://kaggle.com/amanajmera1/framingham-heart-study-dataset (accessed on 24 January 2020).
12. Mienye, I.D.; Sun, Y.; Wang, Z. Improved sparse autoencoder based artificial neural network approach for prediction of heart disease. *Inform. Med. Unlocked* **2020**, *18*, 100307. [CrossRef]
13. Verma, L.; Srivastava, S.; Negi, P.C. A Hybrid Data Mining Model to Predict Coronary Artery Disease Cases Using Non-Invasive Clinical Data. *J. Med. Syst.* **2016**, *40*, 178. [CrossRef]
14. Tama, B.A.; Im, S.; Lee, S. Improving an Intelligent Detection System for Coronary Heart Disease Using a Two-Tier Classifier Ensemble. *BioMed. Res. Int.* **2020**. Available online: https://www.hindawi.com/journals/bmri/2020/9816142/ (accessed on 28 August 2020). [CrossRef]
15. Ahishakiye, E.; Wario, R.; Mwangi, W.; Taremwa, D. Prediction of Cervical Cancer Basing on Risk Factors using Ensemble Learning. In Proceedings of the 2020 IST-Africa Conference (IST-Africa), Kampala, Uganda, 6–8 May 2020; pp. 1–12.
16. Xiong, Y.; Lu, Y. Deep Feature Extraction from the Vocal Vectors Using Sparse Autoencoders for Parkinson's Classification. *IEEE Access* **2020**, *8*, 27821–27830. [CrossRef]
17. Daoud, M.; Mayo, M.; Cunningham, S.J. RBFA: Radial Basis Function Autoencoders. In Proceedings of the 2019 IEEE Congress on Evolutionary Computation (CEC), Wellington, New Zealand, 10–13 June 2019; pp. 2966–2973. [CrossRef]
18. Ng, A. Sparse Autoencoder. 2011. Available online: https://web.stanford.edu/class/cs294a/sparseAutoencoder.pdf (accessed on 6 June 2020).
19. İrsoy, O.; Alpaydın, E. Unsupervised feature extraction with autoencoder trees. *Neurocomputing* **2017**, *258*, 63–73. [CrossRef]
20. Kayabol, K. Approximate Sparse Multinomial Logistic Regression for Classification. *IEEE Trans. Pattern Anal. Mach. Intell.* **2020**, *42*, 490–493. [CrossRef]
21. Herrera, J.L.L.; Figueroa, H.V.R.; Ramírez, E.J.R. Deep fraud. A fraud intention recognition framework in public transport context using a deep-learning approach. In Proceedings of the 2018 International Conference on Electronics, Communications and Computers (CONIELECOMP), Cholula Puebla, Mexico, 21–23 February 2018; pp. 118–125. [CrossRef]
22. Wang, M.; Lu, S.; Zhu, D.; Lin, J.; Wang, Z. A High-Speed and Low-Complexity Architecture for Softmax Function in Deep Learning. In Proceedings of the 2018 IEEE Asia Pacific Conference on Circuits and Systems (APCCAS), Chengdu, China, 26–28 October 2018; pp. 223–226. [CrossRef]
23. Ruder, S. An overview of gradient descent optimization algorithms. *arXiv* **2017**, arXiv:1609.04747.
24. Qian, N. On the momentum term in gradient descent learning algorithms. *Neural Netw.* **1999**, *12*, 145–151. [CrossRef]
25. Mienye, I.D.; Sun, Y.; Wang, Z. An improved ensemble learning approach for the prediction of heart disease risk. *Inform. Med. Unlocked* **2020**, *20*, 100402. [CrossRef]
26. Abdulhammed, R.; Musafer, H.; Alessa, A.; Faezipour, M.; Abuzneid, A. Features Dimensionality Reduction Approaches for Machine Learning Based Network Intrusion Detection. *Electronics* **2019**, *8*, 322. [CrossRef]
27. Latha, C.B.C.; Jeeva, S.C. Improving the accuracy of prediction of heart disease risk based on ensemble classification techniques. *Inform. Med. Unlocked* **2019**, *16*, 100203. [CrossRef]
28. Amin, M.S.; Chiam, Y.K.; Varathan, K.D. Identification of significant features and data mining techniques in predicting heart disease. *Telemat. Inform.* **2019**, *36*, 82–93. [CrossRef]
29. Mohan, S.; Thirumalai, C.; Srivastava, G. Effective Heart Disease Prediction Using Hybrid Machine Learning Techniques. *IEEE Access* **2019**, *7*, 81542–81554. [CrossRef]
30. Haq, A.U.; Li, J.P.; Memon, M.H.; Nazir, S.; Sun, R. A Hybrid Intelligent System Framework for the Prediction of Heart Disease Using Machine Learning Algorithms. *Mob. Inf. Syst.* **2018**, *2018*, 3860146. [CrossRef]

31. Repaka, A.N.; Ravikanti, S.D.; Franklin, R.G. Design and Implementing Heart Disease Prediction Using Naives Bayesian. In Proceedings of the 2019 3rd International Conference on Trends in Electronics and Informatics (ICOEI), Tirunelveli, India, 23–25 April 2019; pp. 292–297. [CrossRef]
32. Samuel, O.W.; Asogbon, G.M.; Sangaiah, A.K.; Fang, P.; Li, G. An integrated decision support system based on ANN and Fuzzy_AHP for heart failure risk prediction. *Expert Syst. Appl.* **2017**, *68*, 163–172. [CrossRef]
33. Wu, W.; Zhou, H. Data-Driven Diagnosis of Cervical Cancer with Support Vector Machine-Based Approaches. *IEEE Access* **2017**, *5*, 25189–25195. [CrossRef]
34. Abdullah, F.B.; Momo, N.S. Comparative analysis on Prediction Models with various Data Preprocessings in the Prognosis of Cervical Cancer. In Proceedings of the 2019 10th International Conference on Computing, Communication and Networking Technologies (ICCCNT), Kanpur, India, 6–8 July 2019; pp. 1–6. [CrossRef]
35. Chang, C.-C.; Cheng, S.-L.; Lu, C.-J.; Liao, K.-H. Prediction of Recurrence in Patients with Cervical Cancer Using MARS and Classification. *Int. J. Mach. Learn. Comput.* **2013**, *3*, 75–78. [CrossRef]
36. Ijaz, M.F.; Attique, M.; Son, Y. Data-Driven Cervical Cancer Prediction Model with Outlier Detection and Over-Sampling Methods. *Sensors* **2020**, *20*, 2809. [CrossRef]
37. Nithya, B.; Ilango, V. Evaluation of machine learning based optimized feature selection approaches and classification methods for cervical cancer prediction. *SN Appl. Sci.* **2019**, *1*, 641. [CrossRef]
38. Ogunleye, A.A.; Qing-Guo, W. XGBoost Model for Chronic Kidney Disease Diagnosis. *IEEE/ACM Trans. Comput. Biol. Bioinform.* **2019**, 1. [CrossRef]
39. Rady, E.-H.A.; Anwar, A.S. Prediction of kidney disease stages using data mining algorithms. *Inform. Med. Unlocked* **2019**, *15*, 100178. [CrossRef]
40. Gupta, D.; Khare, S.; Aggarwal, A. A method to predict diagnostic codes for chronic diseases using machine learning techniques. In Proceedings of the 2016 International Conference on Computing, Communication and Automation (ICCCA), Greater Noida, India, 29–30 April 2016; pp. 281–287. [CrossRef]
41. Khan, B.; Naseem, R.; Muhammad, F.; Abbas, G.; Kim, S. An Empirical Evaluation of Machine Learning Techniques for Chronic Kidney Disease Prophecy. *IEEE Access* **2020**, *8*, 55012–55022. [CrossRef]
42. Raju, N.V.G.; Lakshmi, K.P.; Praharshitha, K.G.; Likhitha, C. Prediction of chronic kidney disease (CKD) using Data Science. In Proceedings of the 2019 International Conference on Intelligent Computing and Control Systems (ICCS), Madurai, India, 15–17 May 2019; pp. 642–647. [CrossRef]
43. Aljaaf, A.J.; Al-Jumeily, D.; Haglan, H.M.; Alloghani, M.; Baker, T.; Hussain, A.J.; Mustafina, J. Early Prediction of Chronic Kidney Disease Using Machine Learning Supported by Predictive Analytics. In Proceedings of the 2018 IEEE Congress on Evolutionary Computation (CEC), Rio de Janeiro, Brazil, 8–13 July 2018; pp. 1–9. [CrossRef]
44. Ebiaredoh-Mienye, S.A.; Esenogho, E.; Swart, T.G. Artificial Neural Network Technique for Improving Prediction of Credit Card Default: A Stacked Sparse Autoencoder Approach. *Int. J. Electr. Comput. Eng. (IJECE)* **2020**. [CrossRef]

6

A Prostate MRI Segmentation Tool Based on Active Contour Models Using a Gradient Vector Flow

Joaquín Rodríguez [1], Gilberto Ochoa-Ruiz [2] and Christian Mata [3,*]

1 Vibot ERL Laboratory, Université de Bourgogne Franche-Comté, IUT Le Creusot, 12 rue de la Fonderie, 71200 Le Creusot, France; Joaquin_Rodriguez@etu.u-bourgogne.fr
2 Tecnologico de Monterrey, School of Engineering and Sciences, Ave. Eugenio Garza Sada 2501, Monterrey, N.L., México 64849, Mexico; gilberto.ochoa@tec.mx
3 Centre for Technological Risk Studies, Universitat Politècnica de Catalunya, 08034 Barcelona, Spain
* Correspondence: christian.mata@upc.edu

Abstract: Medical support systems used to assist in the diagnosis of prostate lesions generally related to prostate segmentation is one of the majors focus of interest in recent literature. The main problem encountered in the diagnosis of a prostate study is the localization of a Regions of Interest (ROI) containing a tumor tissue. In this paper, a new GUI tool based on a semi-automatic prostate segmentation is presented. The main rationale behind this tool and the focus of this article is facilitate the time consuming segmentation process used for annotating images in the clinical practice, enabling the radiologists to use novel and easy to use semi-automatic segmentation techniques instead of manual segmentation. In this work, a detailed specification of the proposed segmentation algorithm using an Active Contour Models (ACM) aided with a Gradient Vector Flow (GVF) component is defined. The purpose is to help the manual segmentation process of the main ROIs of prostate gland zones. Finally, an experimental case of use and a discussion part of the results are presented.

Keywords: Active Contour Models; snake segmentation; GVF; prostate imaging

1. Introduction

Prostate cancer (PCa) remains one of the most commonly diagnosed solid organ tumor types among men. Early diagnosis and an active follow-up can allow improved prognosis and prevent life-threatening conditions. Once the decision of treatment has been taken, having the most complete information for treatment and follow up is crucial. In 2020, there will be approximately 1,806,590 cancer cases diagnosed and 606,520 cancer deaths are projected to occur in the United States. This classification has been reported by the ICD-O, excepting childhood and adolescent cancers, which were classified according to the ICCC [1]. On the other hand, PCa is the third predicted cause of death in EU with 78,800 death in 2020 [2]. This entails a rate estimation of 10.0/100,000 men.

Medical support systems used to assist in the diagnosis of prostate lesions generally focus on prostate segmentation [3–6]. They rely on computerized techniques for prostate cancer detection applied to ultrasound, magnetic resonance and computed tomodensitometric images [7]. For example, Vos et al. [8] used 3D-T2 imaging to define a specific Region of Interest (ROI), which was subsequently used on diffusion- and perfusion-weighted images to extract relevant features. MRI has been established as the best imaging modality for the detection, localization and staging of PCa on account of its high resolution and excellent spontaneous contrast of soft tissues and the possibilities of multi-planar and multi-parametric scanning [9]. Among the techniques used to detect PCa, MRI also allows non-invasive analysis of the anatomy and the metabolism in the entire prostate gland.

Furthermore, many recent works confirm that the combination of several MRI techniques facilitates the evaluation of prostate diagnoses according to the PI-RADS classification, both for radiologists and medical experts [10]. For instance, a thorough evaluation of various prostate cancer studies was presented in [11]; this study highlights that the correct localization of ROI-containing tumor tissue as the most prevalent problem encountered in the diagnosis of a prostate cancer and other related tasks. Traditionally, clinical experts use different software tools to validate the diagnoses and make annotations in several files. This approach is far from being efficient when managing and dealing with abundant medical data. For the reasons stated above, we propose a new software tool to provide support for the time consuming segmentation process used for annotating images in the clinical practice. Additionally, it enables radiologists to make use of novel semi-automatic segmentation techniques instead of the traditional manual segmentation approaches.

The contributions of this paper are two-fold: we introduce a novel prostate cancer segmentation graphical user interface on which several segmentation algorithms can be easily implemented. In order to demonstrate the strengths and the potential applications of the proposed tool, we included several segmentation algorithms with the software:

- We implemented a modified version of the snake-based active contours segmentation (ACS) algorithm presented in [12] to work with prostate images, which we will refer as *Basic ACS*.
- A simplified version of the *Basic ACS* algorithm, referred as *Simplified ACS*, is included with the program, that runs faster, but with less accuracy.
- Finally, we extended the *Basic ACS* model in order to integrate a Gradient Vector Flow (GVF) component to improve the segmentation process, which we will refer as *GVF ACS* in this paper.

The extensions of original algorithm, in tandem with the novel graphical user interface greatly simplify the segmentation process as it enables a boosted semi-automatic interaction with the clinicians who, eventually, can validate the correctness of the ROI generated by the different methods. Finally, a quantitative study to validate the correctness of the generated segmentation compared to the ground truth and the algorithms is provided. It is worth to mention that the developed program serves as an initial version of a tool that we hope, will create a lot of opportunities to contribute with newer algorithms or improvements to the existing ones in the field of prostate segmentation.

The rest of this paper is organized as follows: in Section 2 we introduce the used dataset and we explain the implementation and features of the proposed Graphical User Interface. Then we describe the Basic ACS and the modifications we introduced to make it work in prostate images. Finally, we present details about the Gradient Vector Flow (GVF) model and its implementation into our tool. In Section 3, we include a single experimental case study to demonstrate the advantages of the proposed approach. In Section 4 we discuss the results in the light of the clinical perspective, and in Section 5 we present the conclusions as well as future works.

2. Materials and Methods

In this section we present the source database and the main contributions of the article, namely the proposed GUI for prostate segmentation process and later on, the integration of the Basic ACS model and its extensions using GVF, the GVF ACS model.

2.1. Database and ROIs References

A database with prostate MRI, based on clinical data with tumor and healthy cases was used. The examinations used in our study contained three-dimensional T2-weighted fast spin-echo (TR/TE/ETL: 3600 ms/143 ms/109, slice thickness: 1.25 mm) images acquired with sub-millimetric pixel resolution in an oblique axial plane. Each study comprises a set of 64 slice images. This database was used in previous works [11] and it has been facilitated for testing the software.

The ground truth annotations were performed using the ProstateAnalyzer tool [11], that allows the drawing of an annotation in a given MRI. For this task, experts with more than 10 years of experience on prostate imaging were asked to provide the annotations using the tool. All the dataset and ground truth data are provided from the medical imaging department of the University Hospital of Dijon

(France). The institutional committee on human research approved the study, with a waiver for the requirement for written consent, because MRI and MRSI were included in the workup procedure for all patients referred for brachytherapy or radiotherapy.

The prostate is composed of a peripheral zone (PZ), central zone (CZ), transitional zone (TZ) and an anterior fibromuscular tissue (AFT) depicted in Figure 1. Most cancer lesions occur in the peripheral zone of the gland, fewer occur in the TZ and almost none arise in the CZ. A detailed description of the influence of the prevalence factor risk according the prostate zone is described in [13]. The T2WI modality was chosen because it provides the best depiction of the prostate's zonal anatomy.

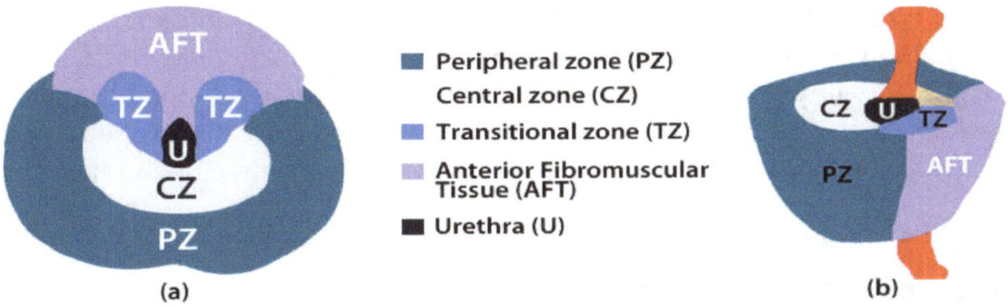

Figure 1. Anatomy of the prostate in (**a**) transversal and (**b**) sagittal planes [11].

The PZ represents up to 70% of a normal prostate gland and around 75% of prostate cancers originate in this zone. The CZ represents about 25% of a normal healthy prostate gland in young adults. Even though the frequency of cancers originating here is much lower, they tend to be of the more aggressive type [14]. An example of a real study case provided by the panel visualization of the prostate tool [11] is depicted in Figure 2. All the overlays are annotated with manual drawings made by radiologists. Each region is represented by different colors (CZ in white and PZ in blue) focusing on a tumor area represented in red (Tum). This example shows the importance of making annotations in regions of interest. In this case, a manual segmentation is validated by experts.

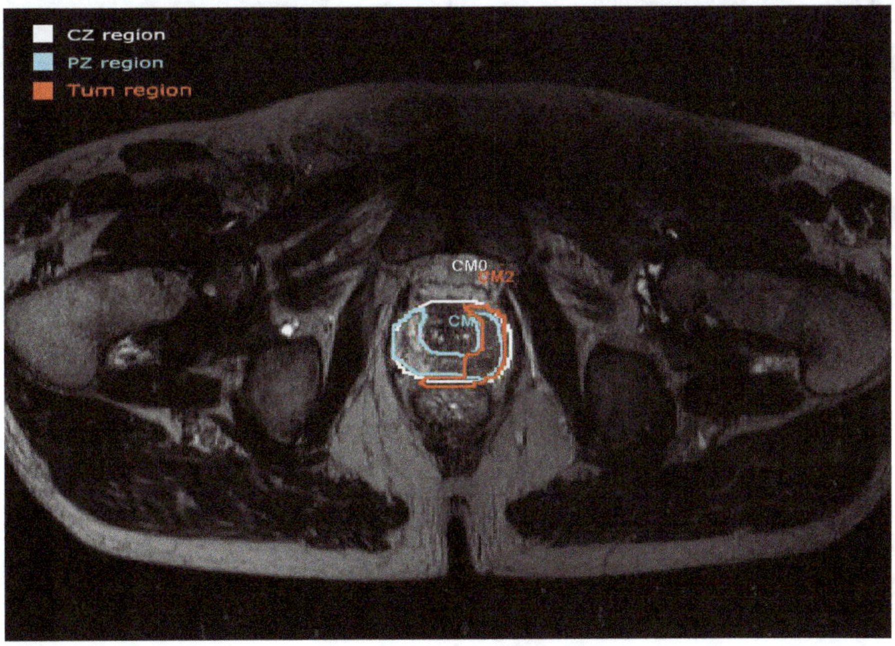

Figure 2. An example of the anatomy (T2WI) panel visualization of the tool developed in [11] with the ROIs annotated by radiologists.

Therefore, one of the main motivations of this work is to develop a new tool focused on improving the results of this initial manual segmentation using Active Contour Models (ACM), facilitating the task of the experts.

In order to attain the above-mentioned goals, we have implemented a novel Graphical User Interface that permits to import, analyze and annotate prostate MR images. The program requires an initial annotation from the user, that does not require to be perfect, and the outcome is an annotation more accurate than the initial one. The modular design of the software allows for integrating segmentation methods as plug-ins or extensions that can be used for testing and clinical purposes. Additionally, this design enables easy performance comparisons between already integrated methods and new methods. In what follows, we will discuss the design of this GUI and subsequently, we will present a study case using three implementations of an ACS model for segmenting the different prostate sections in MR images. It is important to note that this tool and the developed algorithms have not yet been clinically tested and the results presented here represent a proof of concept. However, for the design of the GUI, the expertise and suggestions of clinical experts have been taken into account.

2.2. Implementation of the Graphical User Interface for Prostate Segmentation

In this section, the code organization and the user interface of the program will be explained. The main window of the program is shown in Figure 3. All the code has been developed in Python, using the modules PyQt for the user interface and PyDicom to open the files included in the testing dataset. The code has been organized in modules that do not interact with each other. The integration of all of them has been made in the Main Window class.

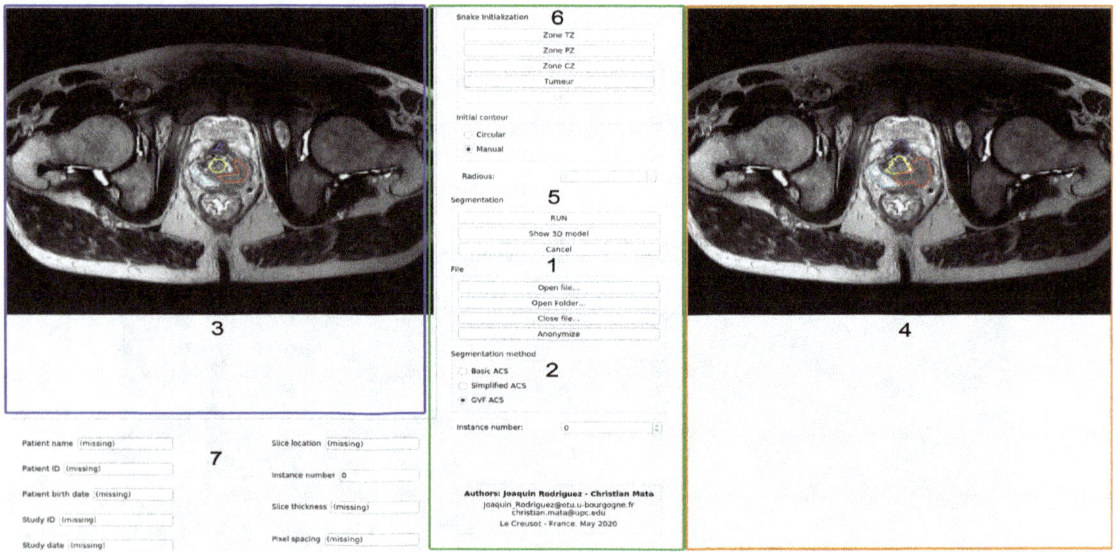

Figure 3. GUI interface of the developed active contour segmentation tool using a prostate MR image.

Each module is placed in folders as follows:

- **DICOM.** This module contains the code that is in charge of handling the Digital Imaging and Communication On Medicine (DICOM) formatted files. It can open either a folder or a single DICOM image. Each file is assumed to contain only one image. The read information will be stored locally on RAM, and after the file or files has/have been opened, a signal will be emitted, and the information can be requested as many times as the user wants.

  The data available to the user includes the images and the patient data fields. This module is also in charge of anonymizing the files and writing them into disc. The functionalities of this module can be accessed through the buttons in the Section 1 of the Figure 3.
- **Image segmentation.** This module stores all the Python code related to the segmentation procedure. The main class in this module is Segmentation-Hub, which is in charge of selecting

the right class for the object that will produce the segmentation, according to the method chosen by the user. The selection of the segmentation method can be done in Section 2 of Figure 3. By implementing the methods in this manner, the actual implementation of the segmentation task is completely transparent for other classes that make use of this module. To select certain segmentation method, only a label that defines the method must be provided.

This module also contains two other files with useful functions:

1. A specific MatLab module which implements some functions that are found in MatLab but not in Python, and their names are the same as in this program.
2. The other file corresponds to a class that finds the ellipse parameters that better fits to a set of points. This code is used for the shape prior of the snake algorithm (Basic ACS) which will be explained in Section 2.3.

- **Image widget.** This module is in charge of showing the image, as well as the initial and the resulting contours from the segmentation. The same module is used for both, left and right images. It also captures the clicks from the user to generate either the circular or the manual initial contour. Both types of initialization will be explained later. The image widget is represented in Sections 3 and 4 of Figure 3.
- **Model 3D widget.** It shows a 3D representation of the output segmentation, based on the Python module Matplotlib. This process is relatively simple as it only replicates the given contour vertically. If the spatial resolution is given in the input DICOM file, the scale of the axis will be given in millimeters. It can be accessed through the button *Show 3D Model* located in Section 5 of Figure 3.
- **Snake init widget.** This widget is in charge of handling all the functionalities of the Snake initialization group, placed at the top of the central control panel of the application.

  Each button will request the main window to ask the user to enter the initial contour in the left image. Once the user has finished, the gathered contours are returned back to this module.

  Afterwards, the corresponding masks for those contours can be generated for the snake algorithm (the mask consists of an image with values of 1 in the interior of the contour, and zeros outside of it). The interface for this module is represented in Section 6 of Figure 3.
- **User data widget.** It is implemented as an efficient and easy to use manner to handle all the user information as an object, and to show it. This class stores all the information related to the patient or the study, retrieved from the DICOM file. It also contains the corresponding widgets that are shown below the left image area, where the gathered information is displayed (see Section 7 of Figure 3).

A block diagram of the proposed tool components is depicted on Figure 4.

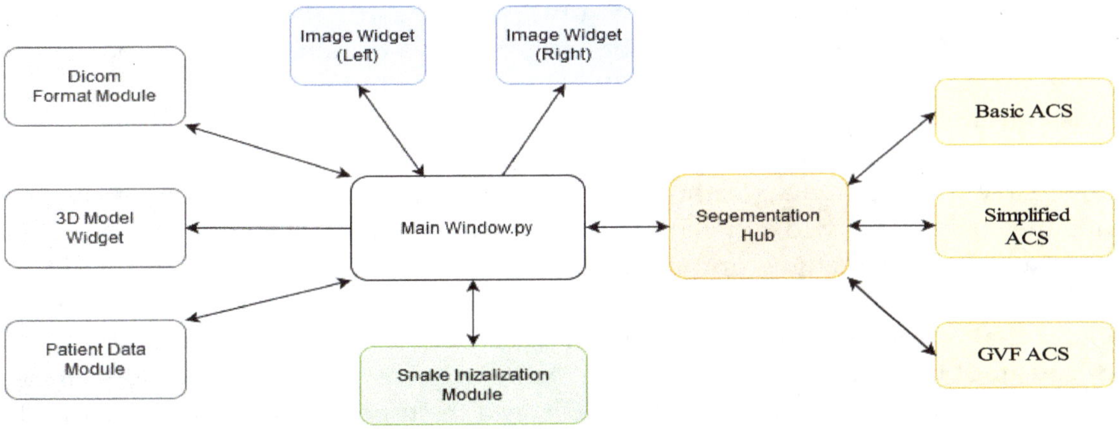

Figure 4. Main software components of the proposed tool. The Segmentation-Hub module can be extended with new modules seamlessly.

Finally, regarding the user interface showed in Figure 3, this program has four well-defined sections:

- **Left panel.** In this area (highlighted in blue), the loaded images are shown, and the user can draw the initial contours of the snake of the different areas of the prostate. Each prostate zone is surrounded with a different color to make it easily distinguishable (see Figure 3)
- **Right panel.** This area (highlighted in orange) shows the loaded images, and the results of the evolution of the selected snake algorithm. Each prostate zone has a pre-defined color, and they match with the colors used for the initial contours (see Section 4 of Figure 3).
- **Bottom area.** The patient information retrieved from the DICOM file is shown (highlighted in blue). Moreover, information related to the spatial resolution and thickness of the gathered slice are included (Section 7 of Figure 3)
- **Central area.** This is the control panel area (highlighted in green). All the functionalities and possible configurations of the program are located in this area. It is represented in the Sections 1, 2, 5 and 6 of Figure 3.

To the best of our knowledge, tools as the proposed in this work, which integrate a Graphical User Interface and semi-automated segmentation algorithms for image annotation do not exist (at least not for prostate MR images). Therefore, a preliminary effort to develop a GUI that includes several active contour model implementations is very important and has driven the development of this work. On the other hand, from the implementation point of view, this program represents an excellent tool to deploy new snake-based algorithms: given that the initial contour and the original image are available in the Segmentation-Hub module, new algorithms can be created using Python, and added as an standalone file to the Image Segmentation folder. This procedure will add another option to the GUI, and the new algorithm's performance and accuracy can be compared with the already existing techniques. This code-base is now available as a GitHub repository to the community [15].

In order to demonstrate how different segmentation methods can be integrated into the proposed tool, we have implemented various versions of an Active Counter Model within the Image Segmentation module of our tool. These methods have been included not only for demonstration purposes, but also to serve as a baseline for future developments in prostate MRI segmentation research (people can improve them, or develop new methods based on them). The proposed Active Contour Model, to be discussed in the following section, also represents a novel contribution, as it has not been previously reported to be used for prostate segmentation purposes.

2.3. Implementation of the Proposed Active Contour Model

The base method implemented is inspired on [12,16]. Both of them are active contours—level-set algorithms. Particularly, the model by Pluempitiwiriyawej et al. [12] was conceived and customized to work with MR images. The general idea of snake algorithms is to modify a curve based on certain forces that push the boundaries of such curve until it reaches the border of the object of interest. A particular feature of this type of segmentation algorithm is that they are unsupervised methods, given that there is not feedback on whether the boundary is following the correct borders or not. Due to this assumption of snake-based methods, an initial contour must be provided, and the closer this initial contour is to the real object, the better the result of the segmentation.

Typically, most snake-based algorithms follow the information about the gradient of the image, which means the curve will try to evolve towards the edges of the object. Nonetheless, if the object does not contain well defined edges, or it has been previously smoothed in order to reduce the noise, this algorithm might fail in following the shape of the object. As a consequence, the outcome will be either a contour that is smaller or larger than the object's boundaries, or in the worst case, the contour will be reduced until it disappears. This is the reason why several researchers developed specific algorithms depending on the type of object to detect, and the type of image to deal with. This is done adding different terms called *priors*. Each constraint added to the algorithm defines a prior, and its corresponding weight will define its contribution to the force.

In this previous work [12], the goal is to segment the shape of the left ventricle of the heart, but since it is aimed to work with MR images, and the priors are similar to the assumptions that can be done for the prostate zones, we considered it as a good starting point for carrying out our experiments and implement the GVF extension to demonstrate its viability in this image modality. The basic assumption of the developed algorithm is that the contour will split the image into two areas, the target object and the background. The evolution of the curve will be driven trying to minimize an energy functional that in this case, it is composed of four components. Each of them will define the priors the final contour must comply with [12]:

1. **Model matching**. it is assumed that the pixel values inside and outside the object follow different statistical models, specified as $M1$ and $M2$, respectively.
2. **Edge information**. the contour must be attracted to certain clues that describe the limits of the object, i.e., the strongest edge values of the image should attract the curve.
3. **Shape prior**. Besides certain possible variations between patients, each prostatic zone has a general shape. This shape information can be thought as a function $C_H(\theta)$, with $\theta = [\theta_1, \theta_2, ..., \theta_n]^T$. The parameters θ_i define a model of the actual shape and size of the requested zone, and depending of how distant is the contour from this estimated shape, this prior will contribute more or less to the snake evolution.
4. **Contour smoothness**: The contour is supposed to not be jagged or too noisy, so this parameter controls that.

Then the functional that defines the energy described above, depending on the contour C, can be expressed as:

$$J(C) = \lambda_1 J_1(C) + \lambda_2 J_2(C) + \lambda_3 J_3(C) + \lambda_4 J_4(C) \tag{1}$$

where λ_i are the weights of each prior included in the energy function. This function will be used to make evolve the contour. It follows that it is possible to transform the information of the contour in a level set function, i.e., the information about the contours can be expressed as a function, where the pixels that belong to the object have certain value (or level), the background ones have another level, and the frontier, which is the contour C, is represented by another level. In the case of this paper, the contour is expressed through the level set function as in Equation (2). As it can be seen, the contour is in the level where the function ϕ is equal to zero. Ω represents the space of the image.

$$C = \{(x, y) \in \Omega : \phi(x, y) = 0\} \tag{2}$$

Then, the energy functional can be expressed as depending on ϕ.

$$J(\phi) = \lambda_1 J_1(\phi) + \lambda_2 J_2(\phi) + \lambda_3 J_3(\phi) + \lambda_4 J_4(\phi) \tag{3}$$

This function ϕ evolves with each iteration (i.e.,time), depending on the direction in which the forces push the contour. In the following sections the particularities of each term will be described.

2.3.1. Region-Based Model Matching—Term $J_1(\phi)$

The aim of this term is to split the image space Ω into two regions that contain homogeneous pixels: the object and the background. Let's call them Ω_1 and Ω_2, respectively. These two regions are separated by the contour C. An homogeneous region implies a region where all the pixels that are contained in it are described by the same stochastic model. The points that belong to the object have intensities $u_1 = \{u_{i,j} : (i, j) \in \Omega_1\}$, and they are described by the model M_1, and the ones that belong to the background have values $u_2 = \{u_{i,j} : (i, j) \in \Omega_2\}$, and they are represented by the model M_2.

The idea of the model is as follows: let's consider the image u_0 to be formed by two regions, of piecewise-constant intensities c_1 and c_2, and that the intensities of the object are represented by

c_1. The boundary of this region is C_0. Then, the pixel values of the image u_0 are c_1 inside C_0, and c_2 outside of it. Given this, it is possible to build the following fitting term:

$$F(C) = F_1(C) + F_2(C) = \int_{inside(C)} |u_0(x,y) - c_1|^2 dxdy + \int_{outside(C)} |u_0(x,y) - c_2|^2 dxdy \tag{4}$$

where C is any variable curve, and c_1 and c_2 are two constants that depend on the contour C. Based on the previous explanation, if $C = C_0$, then $F(C)$ is approximately zero, because each distance between the image value and the constant c_i are approximately zero for each region. If the curve C is outside C_0, then its interior contains parts of the object and parts of the background, while the exterior of C contains only elements of the background. Because of this, $F_1(C) > 0$ and $F_2(C) \approx 0$. In the backwards case, i.e., the contour C is smaller than C_0, the outside contains parts of the object and the background, whilst the inside only contains parts of the object. It follows that $F_1(C) \approx 0$ and $F_2(C) > 0$. Finally, this fitting function can be used to find the boundaries of the object, by minimizing its value such as

$$\underset{C}{inf}\{F_1(C) + F_2(C)\} \approx 0 \approx F_1(C_0) + F_2(C_0) \tag{5}$$

In order to achieve this boundary, the evolution of the curve C is done by moving pixels from the exterior to the interior of the contour, and vice-versa. The first estimation of the energy function for this prior is in Equation (6):

$$J_0(C) = p(u|C, M_1, M_2) \tag{6}$$

where p is the probability density function of the image intensities u, given the contour C, and the models M_1 and M_2. Over these probabilities, it is assumed that each element, object and background, are statistically independent, and they have pdfs p_1 and p_2, respectively. Moreover, the pixel intensities are considered to be independent from each other. With these assumptions, and taking the negative of the logarithm of the pdfs, the Equation (6) becomes Equation (7).

$$J_1(C) = \sum_{(i,j)\in\Omega_1} - \ln(p_1(u_{ij})) + \sum_{(i,j)\in\Omega_2} - \ln(p_2(u_{ij})) \tag{7}$$

Assuming a continuous function, the contour embedded in the zero level-set function ϕ, and considering the Heaviside function in order to create a single integral over all the domain of the image, the Equation (7) can be generalized as shown in Equation (8).

$$J_1(\phi) = \int_{\Omega} - \ln[p_1(u(x,y))]H(\phi(x,y)) - \ln[p_2(u(x,y))](1 - H(\phi(x,y)))dxdy \tag{8}$$

It is assumed that both elements in the image follow a Gaussian distribution, with means m_1 and m_2, and variances σ_1^2 and σ_2^2, which are unknowns, and for each contour C, they will be estimated.

2.3.2. Edge-Based Function—Term $J_2(\phi)$

This term will push the contour towards the edges of the object. The computation of this type of force is done through the edge-map $\Upsilon(x,y)$ generated from the image $u(x,y)$. The most common implementation is the gradient of the smoothed image.

$$\Upsilon(x,y) = -|\nabla G_\sigma * u(x,y)| \tag{9}$$

where G_σ is a Gaussian kernel of parameter σ, ∇ is the gradient operator and $(.) * (.)$ is the convolution operator. Finally, the energy functional, depending on the level set function ϕ, which corresponds to this prior is given by the Equation (10).

$$J_2(\phi) = \int_\Omega \Upsilon(x,y)\delta(\phi(x,y))|\nabla\phi(x,y)|dxdy \tag{10}$$

where $\delta(\phi(x,y))$ will return non-zero values only for the pixels that are on the contour C.

2.3.3. Object Shape Prior—Term $J_3(\phi)$

This term has been introduced in [12] to reinforce an elliptical shape in heart MR images, but it can be changed by any other shape model depending on the specific object to be segmented. The addition of this prior will improve the performance of the general active contour implementation. For instance, if the target to segment has a circle-like shape, then the snake function can be constrained to satisfy an ellipse equation. In that case, the functional corresponding to this energy term can be defined as $J_3(\phi) = \int_C D^2(x,y)ds$ where $D(x,y)$ is the ellipse distance function defined as:

$$D(x,y) = ax^2 + bxy + cy^2 + dx + ey + f \tag{11}$$

The parameters $\theta = [a,b,c,d,e,f]$ are computed in such a way that the cloud of points around the contour C fits with this ellipse equation. This means that the parameters of θ must be computed for each contour C, and they will change the force direction in order to minimize this distance function. Finally, introducing the level set function ϕ, where the contour C is embedded, the shape prior is computed as in Equation (12), when integrating in all the space Ω.

$$J_3(\phi) = \int_\Omega D^2(x,y)\delta(\phi(x,y))|\nabla\phi(x,y)|dxdy \tag{12}$$

2.3.4. Contour Smoothing—Term $J_4(\phi)$

Finally, it is desirable that the generated contour is smooth. This can be achieved if the Euclidean arc length of the contour C is minimized. It follows that the contribution function for this prior is the one represented in Equation (13).

$$J_4(C) = \int_C ds \tag{13}$$

It is worth mentioning that if only this term is included in the functional, the shape of the contour will become a circle, and then it will start shrinking until it eventually disappears. Nonetheless, when all the terms are put together, this situation is avoided, and the effect is to smooth the curve. Again, adding the level set function where the contour is embedded, the final function for J_4 is defined in Equation (14).

$$J_4(\phi) = \int_\Omega \delta(\phi(x,y))|\nabla\phi(x,y)|dxdy \tag{14}$$

The following step is to combine all the functional together, and expand the minimization problem, in such a way the function $\phi(x,y)$, which contains the contour C as its level zero, evolves towards the edge of the object. The entire procedure is well explained in [12], and it consists of three tasks:

1. Define the statistical model constants, in such a way that they comply with the prior that the pixel distribution follows a Gaussian distribution.
2. Estimate the ellipse parameters to obtain the distance functional contribution.
3. Define the contour evolution equation. This can be done by applying the Euler-Lagrange (EL) equation to the functional of the four priors. Then, considering that ϕ is a function of time, the EL equation is equaled to the derivative of ϕ with respect to the time. The resulting function is given in Equation (15).

$$\frac{\partial\phi}{\partial t} = \left[\lambda_1(M_2 - M_1) - \nabla P \frac{\nabla\phi}{||\nabla\phi||} - P\kappa\right]\delta(\phi(x,y)) \tag{15}$$

where M_1, M_2 are the stochastic models of the object and the background, respectively, $\kappa = div\left(\frac{\nabla\phi}{||\nabla\phi||}\right)$ is the curvature of the contour, $\phi(x,y)$ is our level set function, and $P(x,y) = \lambda_2 Y(x,y) + \lambda_3 D^2(x,y) + \lambda_4$ is the potential function.

The different values of λ_1, λ_2, λ_3 and λ_4 will define the contribution of the corresponding energy term, from J_1 to J_4, and the one with the biggest value will enforce its properties over the others. In practice, the parameters setting is done empirically, and there is no rule that defines how to chose them. It depends on the quality and the properties of the input image. One solution is to make the weights to evolve at each iteration to obtain the best results. The general idea of this evolution is that at the beginning, the algorithm should minimize the energy functional trying to cover all the object, pushing the boundaries towards the edges (effect produced by λ_1 and λ_2), and when the algorithm is close to the end, the curve must enforce the shape of the contour and its smoothness (λ_3 and λ_4).

For the particular case of prostate segmentation, several objects with different shapes have to be considered. Therefore, the shape prior cannot be only an ellipse, as it happens in the case of the left ventricle of the heart. Thus for this implementation, the value of λ_3 has been set to zero.

Additionally, through several experiments, we concluded that the contribution produced by the smoothness prior is not noticeable. In fact, it produces small variations in the contour, and the result is that the algorithm takes more time to converge. This is the reason why the value of λ_4 has been set to zero too. Finally, the suggested evolution of the weights is shown in Figure 5.

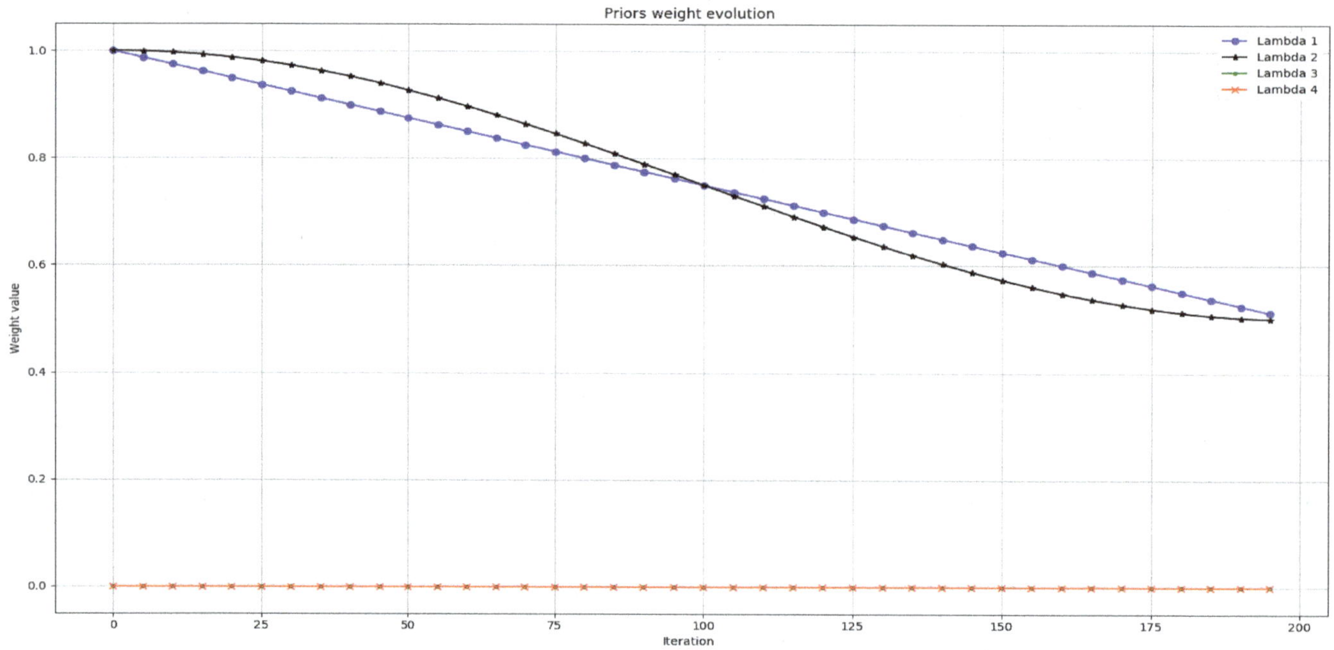

Figure 5. Evolution of λ_i weights for the energy functional.

2.4. Gradient Vector Flow Approach (GVF)

When dealing with snakes algorithms, there are two types of implementations: *Parametric Active Contours (PACs)* or *Geometric Active Contours (GACs)*. They differ in how they define the curve function, since equations formulated for the minimization problem stays almost the same. PACs are based on a parametric curve of a shape represented in Equation (16):

$$C(s) = \{[x(s), y(s)], s \in [0,1]\} \tag{16}$$

with the constraint that it should be closed, i.e., $C(0) = C(1)$. Geometric Active Contours, on the other hand, define the curve to be deformed as embedded in a level-set function, generally as its level zero. This last case is the one implemented and described in Section 2.3. GACs have advantages over PACs, since they are computationally more stable and they are able to change their topology as the function is deformed. Nonetheless, the implemented method is an edge-based method, since it uses the gradient as pushing force, and local intensity information to determine if a pixel belongs to the object or not. Due to this, several problems can appear, such as:

1. If the edges of the object are not well defined, a leaking problem occurs, leading the snake outside of the object's boundaries.
2. If the initial contour is not close to the limits of the object, the gradient will not be able to guide the snake to the edges of the object. If the image is just black and white with one object on it, an initial contour far away from the object will not evolve. On the other hand, if there are other objects around, the snake might be attracted to them, instead of the desired object.
3. Since the snake uses the local pixel information to determine the evolution of the curve, it is sensible to the image noise.

Additionally, the fact of using gradients only, brings another effect related to concavities, that is illustrated in Figure 6.

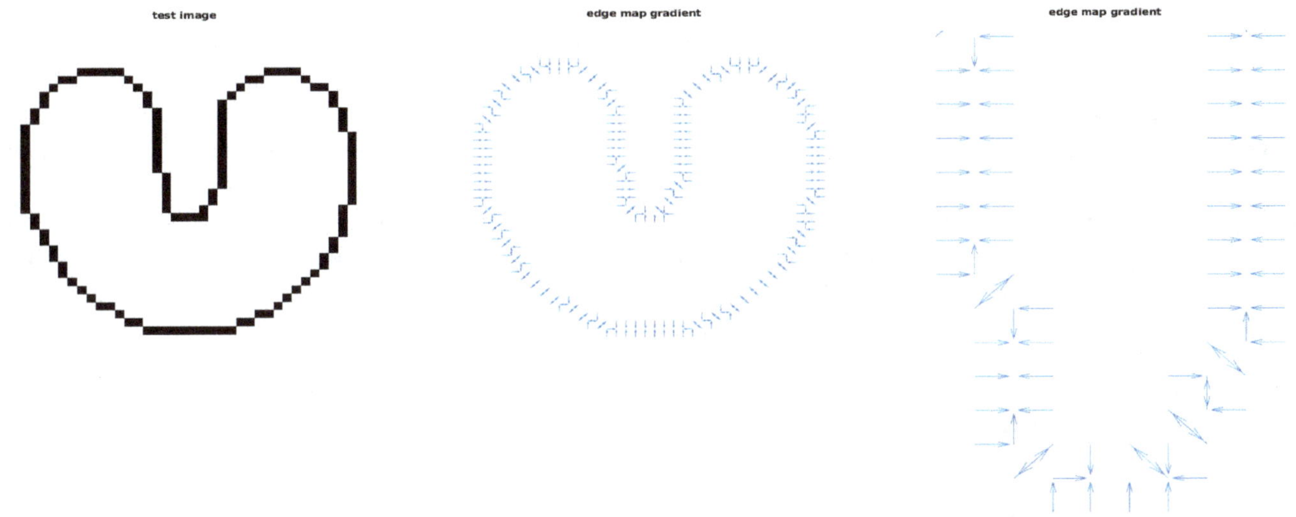

Figure 6. Example of Gradient vector field of a U shape object. (**Left**) Original image. (**Center**) Gradient of the object. (**Right**) Zoom of the vector field in the central concavity of the object.

In this case, a simple object with a narrow concavity, and its corresponding gradient vector field are shown. From it, it is easy to see that:

- In all the space where there the intensities are constant, the gradient is zero. There are gradient vectors only in the borders of the object. This is the main reason why (in an edge-based snake) an initial contour placed far away from the object might not converge to the real object boundaries.
- Narrow concavities start to have horizontal gradient vectors (as it can be seen in the right plot of the Figure 6). As a consequence, the snake will attach to the borders, but it will not address towards the interior of such concavity because the gradient does not have any downwards component.

These last two problems can be solved in the previously explained algorithm with an external force that, not only adds vectors where the gradient is zero, but that also adds a downwards component in the long concavities in such a way that the active contour will be pushed to the interior of this type of areas. This external force is called Gradient Vector Flow (GVF) [17]. Adding this component to the energy described in Section 2.3 will help to not only make the system more robust against initialization effects, but it will improve the outcome by attaching the resulting snake really close to the edges of the object.

The GVF is a dense vector field $\mathbf{v}(x,y) = [u(x,y), v(x,y)]$ derived from the original image, and it is the result of minimizing the energy term defined in Equation (17) [17].

$$\varepsilon = \iint \mu(u_x^2 + u_y^2 + v_x^2 + v_y^2) + |\nabla Y|^2 \, |\mathbf{v} - \nabla Y|^2 \, dxdy \tag{17}$$

where u_x and v_x are the partial derivatives of u and v with respect to the variable x, respectively, u_y and v_y are the partial derivatives of u and v with respect to the variable y, respectively, and $Y(x,y)$ is the edge map of the original image. The parameter μ is a constant that serves as regularization: it adjusts the balance between the first and the second term of the integral, and it should be adjusted based on the noise. The higher the noise, the higher the value of μ. Interpreting the energy term presented in (17), it is possible to see that if the gradient of the edge map is too small, the energy term depends only on the partial derivatives of u and v. On the other hand, if this gradient is large, the integral is dominated by it, and the value of the GVF that minimizes the energy is $\mathbf{v} = Y$, i.e., the gradient vector flow is equal to the gradient of the edge map on those cases. It can be demonstrated that the vector field $\mathbf{v} = (u, v)$ that minimizes (17) is the result of the decoupled pair of differential Equations (18) and (19).

$$\mu\nabla^2 u - (u - Y_x)(Y_x^2 + Y_y^2) = 0 \tag{18}$$

$$\mu\nabla^2 v - (v - Y_y)(Y_x^2 + Y_y^2) = 0 \tag{19}$$

where ∇^2 is the Laplacian operator. Similarly as in Equation (17), it is possible to see that in the regions where the gradient of the edge map is small, the solution of the differential equations for the GVF are the solution of Laplace's equations. Furthermore, this solution is interpolated from the boundaries of the object, and that's the reason why the resulting field, even far away from the object, points to the edges of it. The gradient vector flow of the same image as in Figure 6, is shown in Figure 7. Now, the solution to the Equations (18) and (19) provides vectors in the areas where the gradient is zero, and the vectors in the concavity contains downwards components too.

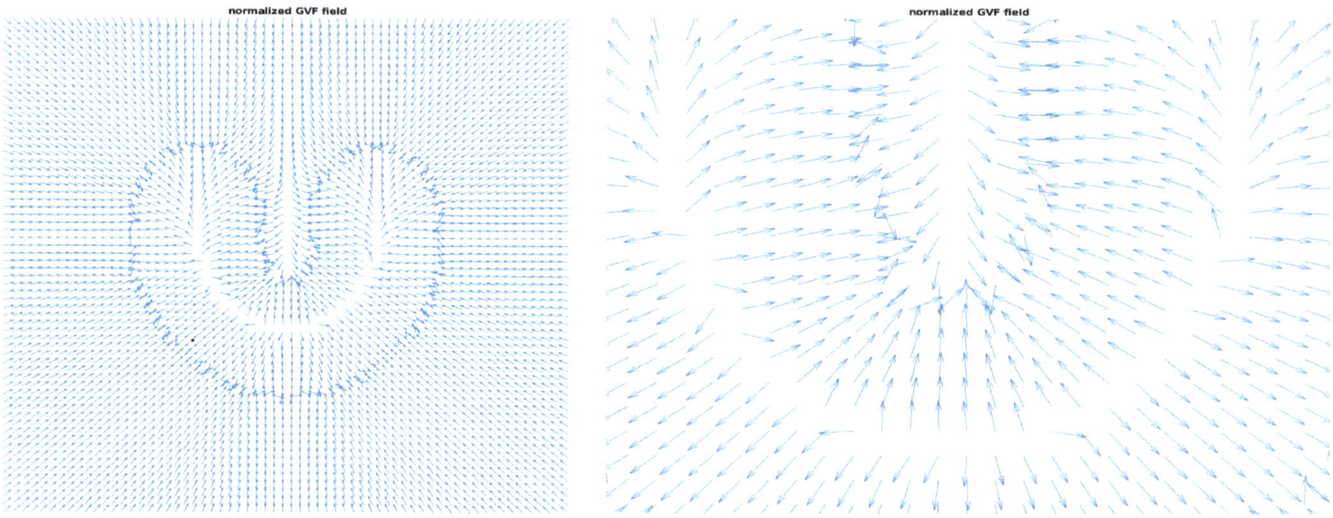

Figure 7. Example of normalized Gradient Vector Flow. (**Left**) GVF vector field for the same image used before. (**Right**) Zoom in the concavity.

Once the GVF has been computed, it is fixed for the entire the image, and what remains is the optimization equation that will guide the deformation of the active contour to the edges of the object, based on this new force. Several researchers have been working on adding gradient vector flow to the traditional snake equations. For the implementation made in Section 2.3, only GACs algorithms can be adapted to be added as an external force to the energy functional defined in the Equation (15), as it has been done in [18,19]. A simplified version of the GVF optimization equation from [19] is used, and defined as:

$$\gamma \frac{\partial \phi}{\partial t} = \left[\alpha \kappa - v . \frac{\nabla \phi}{|\nabla \phi|} \right] |\nabla \phi| \tag{20}$$

The parameter γ regularizes the step size, ϕ is the level-set function, $\kappa = div \left(\frac{\nabla \phi}{|\nabla \phi|} \right)$ is the curvature, **v** is the Gradient Vector Flow vector field, and the parameter α regulates the balance between the two forces. The right hand factor of (20) is added directly to Equation (15), giving Equation (21):

$$\frac{\partial \phi}{\partial t} = \left[\lambda_1 (M_2 - M_1) - \nabla P \frac{\nabla \phi}{||\nabla \phi||} - P\kappa + \beta \left(\left[\alpha \kappa - v . \frac{\nabla \phi}{|\nabla \phi|} \right] |\nabla \phi| \right) \right] \delta(\phi(x, y)) \tag{21}$$

This new segmentation algorithm has been included in the list of options to segment the different prostate zones. After having implemented the *Basic ACS* in Python, the extension with a GVF component is trivial: all the components of this new force are already available in the code except for the vector field **v**. Since this vector field is fixed for a given image, a new class has been created that solves the optimization problem for the GVF. This new piece of code is executed before the main loop of the segmentation algorithm. Since there are no rule for setting both α and γ, we arbitrarily decided to set them to 1. In order to adjust the contribution of this new force, the β factor has been introduced. For the following experiments, this factor has been also set to 1. In the coming sections, the graphical user interface result of the integration of all the modules will be showed. Then, the described algorithms will be tested to show their performance.

3. Experimental Case of Use for Demonstration

In this section a case of use for demonstration is presented. Previously, the proposed GUI has been explained in Section 2.2. A detailed definition of this algorithm and the introduced improvements have been explained in Sections 2.3 and 2.4. The following study case demonstrates how an user can use the proposed tool to manage and segment a real prostate image.

First, the user must load an image in DICOM format. For this application, the snake initialization is required; an example of the initial contours for a study is shown in Figure 8. In the area of the GUI that corresponds to the initialization of the snake, the three first buttons are used for selecting the different zones of the prostate, whereas the fourth one gives the possibility of selecting a tumor.

Located below these buttons, there are two radio buttons, enabling to choose the shape of the initial contour, which can be circular or manual. The first option corresponds to an initial contour with a shape of a circle whose radius can be specified with the spin box located at the end of this area. The possible values are between 1 and 30 pixels. The manual input enables the user to enter a random polygon as initial contour. If selected, the user just has to make a click with the mouse in the vertices of the desired polygon. There are no limits for the amount of points, or the shape of the polygon.

The steps required to initialize the snake for any of the prostate areas are the following:

1. Select the type of contour to enter, circular or manual. In case of circular, enter also the radious.
2. Select an area: TZ, PZ, CZ or Tumour.
3. Create the initial contour for the snake in the left image. If it is a circle, the mouse cursor must be placed in the center of the area of interest, and click with the left button of the mouse. If manual contour has been chosen, the mouse must be placed in the point where the user wishes to start the contour and make click with the left button. Then move the cursor until the next point, make a left click and go to the next point. More than 2 points are required.
4. In manual mode, once the contour is finished, press the "Ok" button. If not, go to step 5.
5. A message box will appear informing if the contour has been correctly added or not.

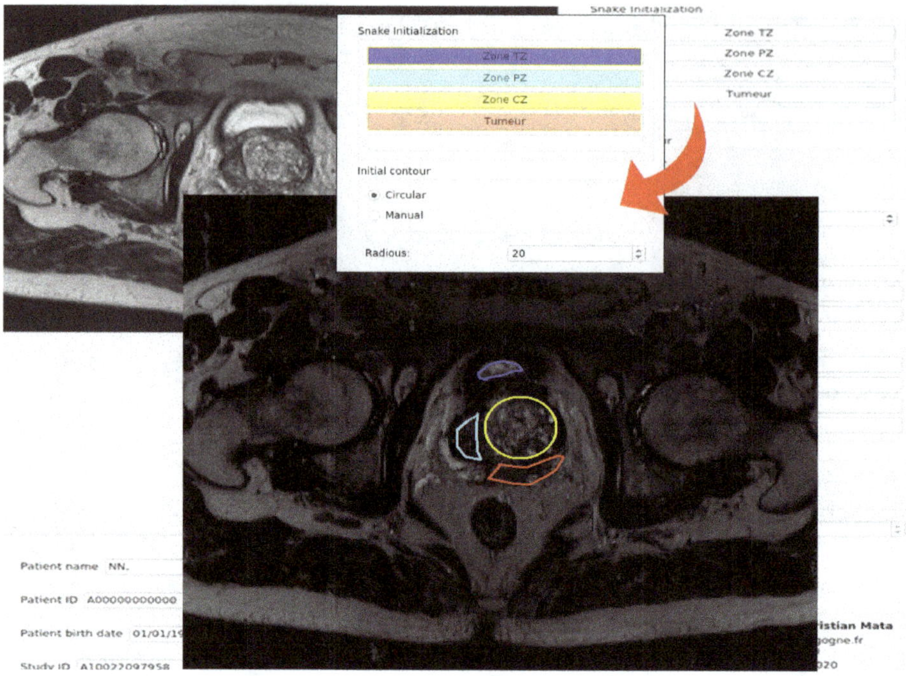

Figure 8. Example of snake initialization for the four zones.

The user can repeat the same procedure for all the zones, or just some of them. In order to differentiate the various selected areas, each initial contour will be drawn with a different color. There are no constraints about the type of contours to use. All the contours can be manual, all of them can be circles or they can be a combination of them.

The following area of the control panel is used for triggering the segmentation. This section is depicted in Figure 9. After an image has been loaded, at least one initial contour has been entered, then the segmentation process will start after pressing the *Run* button. The segmentation method will be triggered as many times as initial contours have been entered, and they will be executed sequentially. During this process, the user can cancel the segmentation at any moment, pressing the *Cancel* button. Once the algorithm had finished, the results will be shown in the right image. Additionally, the color code of the contours is the same for both, left and right images. For instance, the resulting contour of color blue in the right image has as initial contour the blue snake from the left image.

If some results have been produced, then a 3D representation of them can be visualized if the user presses the button *Show 3D model*. This representation consists only of the resulting contours, replicated several times along the Z axis. It is an extra option for users to visualize the main structure of the segmentation in a 3D model. In fact, this option should be improved using better visualization techniques, but it is out of scope of this work for the moment. The amount of repetitions has been set to 50. The axis are represented in real scale, in mm, if the DICOM file contains the information about slice thickness and spatial resolution. If they are not provided, a pop up message will appear reporting the situation, and the X and Y axis will be presented in pixels, and the Z axis will have a size of 10 units. An example of this 3D representation of a result is shown in Figure 10.

Regarding to file management tasks provided to this tool, users can open a DICOM formatted file or a folder that contains several DICOM formatted files. When the *Open file* button is pressed, a pop up window will appear, and it will only allow the user to select a file, not folders. If a file is not in DICOM format, then the program will reject it, and it will not do further actions. If the user wants to open a folder, it should click the *Open folder* button, navigate until the folder it wants, and go into that folder. Without touching any file, users should click the *Choose* button and the system will automatically search for files, and open only the DICOM formatted files. It is important to emphasize that the search system is not recursive. That means, if there are folders inside the selected one, and those folders contain DICOM files, the program will not open them. It will only open the files that are in the current directory.

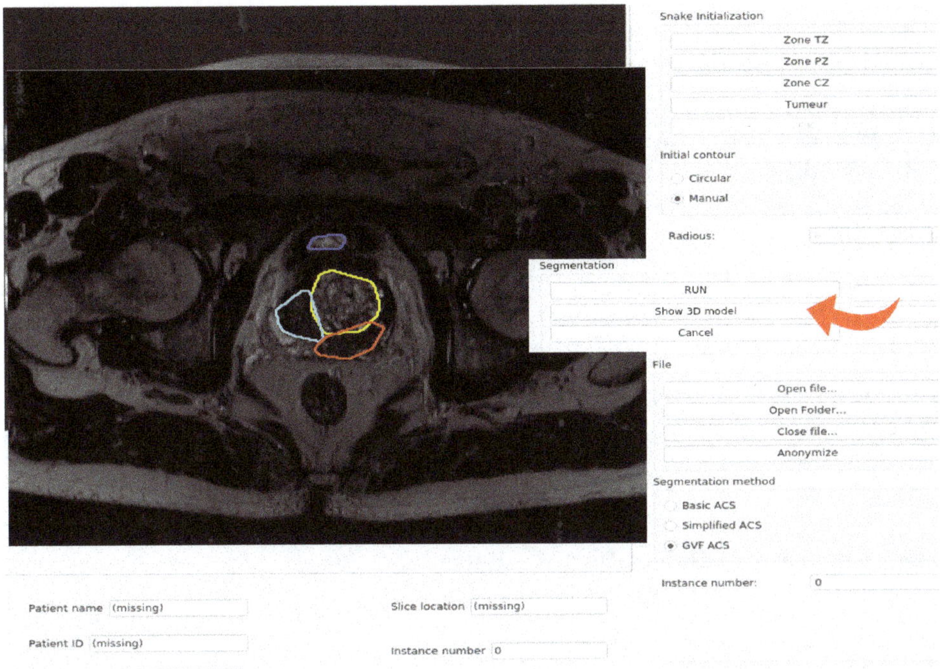

Figure 9. Example of snake results after the snake segmentation.

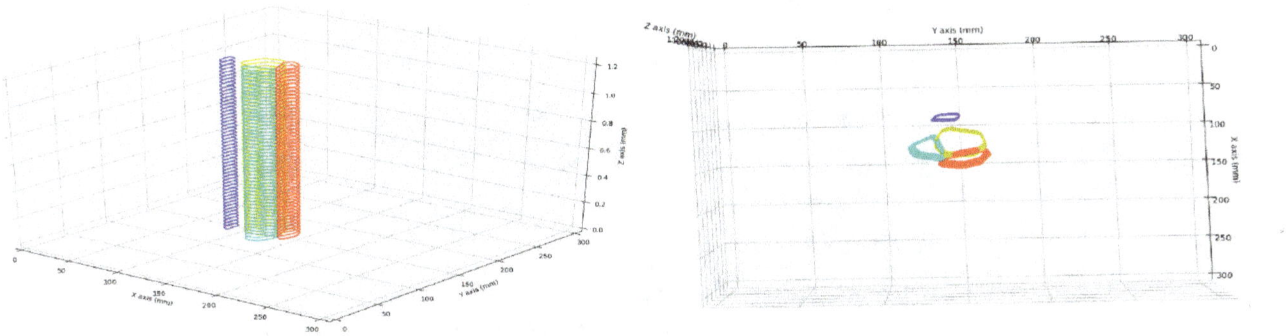

Figure 10. Example of 3D representation of the segmented prostate zones.

As it can be seen in the graphical user interface, there are three types of algorithms: *Basic ACS*, *Simplified ACS* and *GVF ACS*. The first and the second algorithms are based on [12], but the second one does not follow the mathematical approach described in this previous work. On the other hand, *Basic ACS* implements exactly what the paper states, as explained in Section 2.3. Both algorithms have been included so that there is an example in the code of how to add a new algorithm to this code-base. Additionally, the *Simplified ACS* performs a faster than *Basic ACS* but with less accuracy. Nonetheless, in order to produce improvements to the original paper, the *Basic ACS* was required.

Finally, considering that this application is focused on DICOM format and it can be used for radiologists and/or medical experts, it is important to maintain the private information of the patient. For this reason, an anonymization module is integrated in this tool. If the user wants to anonymize the opened file or files, it should click into the *Anonymize* button. If there is a file/files opened, a pop up window will be shown where the user must specify the destination folder of the anonymized files. The name of the output files will be the same as the source files, but the string *_anonymized* will be appended to it. For instance, if the original file is called *Image*00001, the output file will be called *Image*00001*_anonymized*. The fields that are anonymized are: *Patient Name*, *Patient ID* and the

Patient Date of Birth. Those fields are not cleared, but changed by some default data: *Patient Name* is changed by *NN*, *Patient ID* is transformed to *A00000000000*, and the date of birth is changed to 01/01/1970.

We believe that the proposed tool can be beneficial for the research community as it enables to integrate various image management tools thoroughly discussed in previous sections, as well as the capability to segment prostate cancer lesions and other areas as mentioned in the introduction. Even though the application includes the option of segmenting four zones only (CZ, TZ, PZ and Tumor), nothing stops the users of trying to segment other areas of their interest (additional buttons can be appended into the GUI in order to select more areas, or the already existing buttons can be used to segment those areas). These features, as well as the capability to integrate new segmentation models seamlessly make it very appealing for research and teaching purposes in clinical settings. In the former case, it can help in speeding up the creation of datasets for machine learning applications. However, in our experience, doctors are reluctant to use fully automated annotation tools and prefer to use interactive semi-automated tools that enable them to verify and contrast the results with other specialists. In order to test the performance of the proposed tool, we performed one experiment to assess the quality of the segmentation algorithm implemented in this work, which will be detailed in the following section.

4. Discussion of the Segmentation Method Results

In this section, we present a deep analysis of the results of a single segmentation experiment performed using the implemented algorithms, namely the *Basic ACS*, *Simplified ACS* and *GVF ACS* versions of the snake-based models. For all the cases, the initial contours used for all the zones are shown in Figure 11.

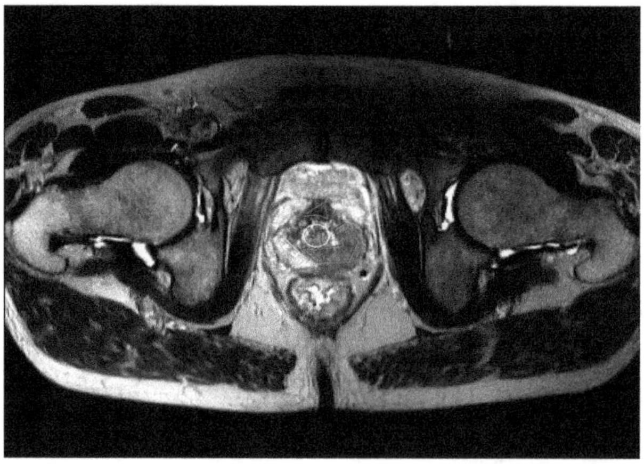

Figure 11. Initialization used for the testing of all the algorithms.

The results for all the algorithms and the ground truth for the selected image are shown in the Figure 12.

From this experiment, it is possible to confirm what it has been said in previous sections. The *Basic ACS* algorithm performs relatively well when there is some gradient information between different areas. In this image, the cyan and the blue contours (corresponding to the PZ and CZ, respectively) are practically attached to the borders; the contour corresponding to the TZ (yellow contour) is almost perfect. Nonetheless, the tumour area invades the TZ area, since the intensities contrast between them is not enough in order to define a good edge.

For the case of *Simplified ACS*, the results are not so satisfactory. This algorithm is uses simplifications of the formulas described in [12]. It has been tested for heart's left ventricle segmentation and it has a good performance in both, quality and speed, but for prostate segmentation, this is not true. Except for the TZ, all the results take part of the other zones, and only when the edge is too strong, the snake seems to be perfectly attached to it.

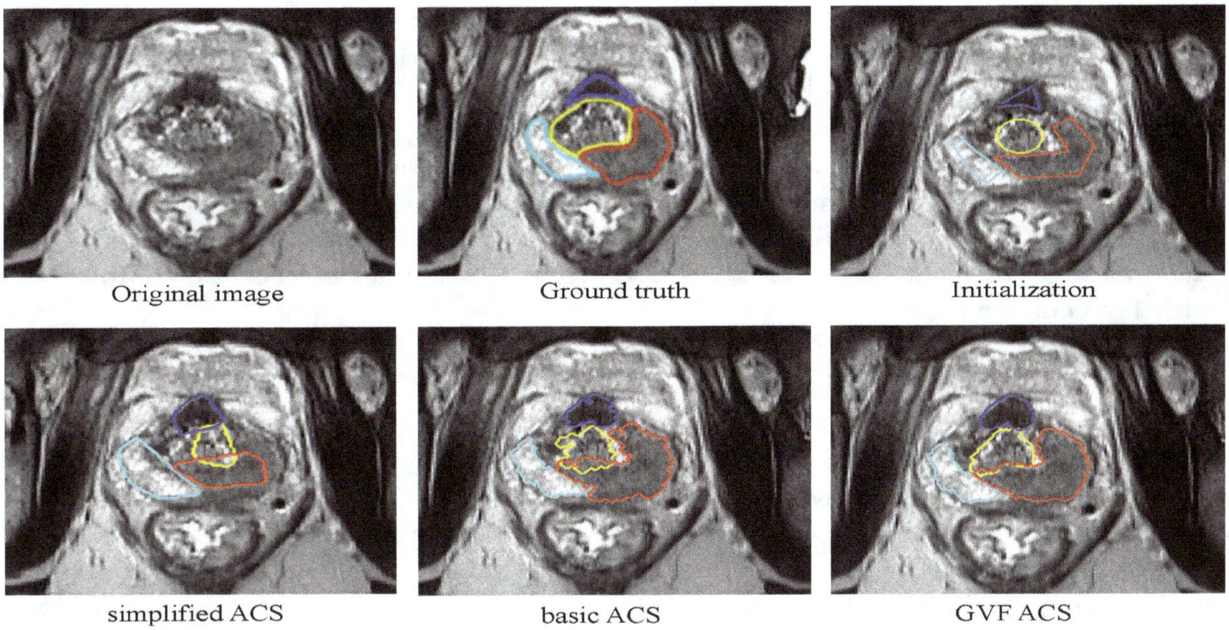

Figure 12. Segmentation results and ground truth for all the algorithms implemented.

Finally, as it is expected, the Gradient Vector Flow implementation overcomes all the problems, and the curves are strongly attached to the borders of each zone. There is only a little overlapping between the tumour and the TZ.

Another point to observe is the smoothness of the results from *Basic ACS* and *GVF ACS*. None of them include either a shape prior or the smoothing factor. This allows the snake to evolve in any shape, which is desired in this case, since there is not a single prior that work for all the prostate zones. Additionally, for the same reason, a generic post-processing that increases the smoothness of the curves is not trivial to implement. This problem is visible mainly in the result given by the *Basic ACS*, where all the contours do not present smooth borders. Nonetheless, the *GVF ACS* generates a result that even without these factors, the outcomes are not so jagged. Once again, the addition of the Gradient Vector Flow component surpasses the results given by the *Basic ACS*.

It is worth mentioning that the initialization (in all the cases) requires to be inside of the object to produce valid results. Since a lot of objects are present in an MR image, a larger contour than the object will produce poor segmentation results. In order to reduce this effect, the image to be segmented is cropped to an square of 150x150 pixels around the center of the initialization contour before starting the segmentation process. As a consequence, not only the influence of other objects over the snake is reduced, but also it reduces the execution time, since less operations are required at each iteration of the algorithm.

In order to measure quantitatively the efficiency of the three model implementations, a contour evaluation of this test was performed. For this evaluation, the Hausdorff distance (HD) and Dice index (DI) metrics for the various segmentation results were compared with a ground truth provided by a specialist. The Hausdorff distance between two finite set of points A and B is defined as follows:

$$HD(A,B) = max(h(A,B), h(B,A)) \tag{22}$$

where $h(A,B)$ is the directed Hausdorff distance defined by:

$$h(A,B) = \max_{a \in A} \min_{b \in B} ||a - b|| \tag{23}$$

where $||.||$ is the Euclidean distance and A and B are the resulting contours of the segmentation.

In computer vision and image processing applications, the largest segmentation errors quantified using the Hausdorff Distance can be a good measure of the usefulness of the segmentation for the intended task. Intuitively, HD is the longest distance one has to travel from a point in one of the two sets to its closest point in the other set. In image segmentation, this metric is computed between boundaries of the estimated and the ground-truth segmentation, which consist of curves in 2D. We computed the Hausdorff distance between the generated segmentation and the ground truth. The methods with the lowest distance are considered to have yielded the best segmentation results.

Another popular metric for image segmentation tasks is based on the Dice coefficient, which is essentially a measure of overlapping between two samples and it is equivalent to the F1 score. This measure ranges from 0 to 1, where a Dice coefficient of 1 denotes perfect and complete overlap. This metric is calculated as:

$$Dice(A, B) = \frac{2\,|A \cap B|}{|A \cup B|} \tag{24}$$

In Table 1, we summarize the results obtained from the performance analysis for the three segmentation methods, using the two above-mentioned metrics. This procedure has been done for each of the prostate's gland zones, which corresponds to the examples of the annotations depicted on Figure 12. The ground truth is used as a reference image to calculate all the measurements. First, according to the initialization image, a comparison of the results between *Simplified ACS*, *Basic ACS* and *GVF ACS* is performed. It can easily be inferred from the table that the *Basic ACS* yields more accurate segmentation results in all the prostate zones than the *Simplified ACS*. Moreover, it can be seen that the *GVF ACS* implementation improves the results in all the cases.

Table 1. Analyses of Hausdorff distance (in mm) and Dice index for the CZ, PZ, TZ and tumour area (TUM).

	Hausdorff Distance			**Dice Index**		
	Simplified ACS	**Basic ACS**	**GVF ACS**	**Simplified ACS**	**Basic ACS**	**GVF ACS**
CZ	11 ± 3	8 ± 1	7 ± 1	0.69 ± 0.20	0.79 ± 0.10	0.79 ± 0.10
PZ	4 ± 2	3 ± 2	2 ± 2	0.88 ± 0.10	0.93 ± 0.10	0.94 ± 0.10
TZ	9 ± 4	7 ± 3	6 ± 3	0.74 ± 0.20	0.73 ± 0.10	0.75 ± 0.10
TUM	5 ± 2	4 ± 2	3 ± 2	0.81 ± 0.10	0.92 ± 0.10	0.93 ± 0.10

The geometry of the CZ zone is considered the most difficult part of the prostate MR image because it is difficult sometimes to demarcate the edges of this area, given that it is surrounded by the other zones; for this reason, it is important to do a good initialization. The results for the PZ are good in all the cases, especially when GVF is used. Moreover, the results on the TZ area are good for all the algorithms considered in this study. Finally, the results for the tumor area indicate that the best segmentation is obtained using *GVF ACS* methods.

Finally, in order to assess the performance of the various studied segmentation methods, a time analysis has been performed. As in Table 1, the analysis has been divided by zones and by algorithm. Then, the execution time of the segmentation algorithm has been assessed for each zone, using the same initialization as in Figure 11. For this test, a computer with a microprocessor i7-8650U @ 1.90 GHz, 16 gb of RAM and running Linux 4.15.0-64 has been used. The execution times are depicted in Table 2. All the measurements has been done in milliseconds. Both *Simplified ACS* and *Basic ACS* run at maximum 200 iterations, and the *GVF ACS* runs at maximum 80 iterations. Both Tables 1 and 2 confirm what it has been said about the *Simplified ACS* algorithm. It is the least accurate, but it runs faster than the other ones. On the other hand, even though the *GVF ACS* runs less iterations than the *Basic ACS*, their running time are similar. This is due to the *GVF ACS* algorithm computes the same code, plus the additional ones in order to get the Gradient Vector Flow contribution. Nonetheless, for this work, this execution time could have been reduced if the equations related to the shape prior and the smoothness would have been removed. Only the weights have been set to zero for those priors. This code has not been erased so that other developers can prove other parameters values, and try to find other combination of weights to make this program work with either, other image modalities, or other organs to be studied.

Table 2. Execution time (in ms) for each segmentation algorithm, and for each prostate zone.

	CZ	PZ	TZ	TUM
Simplified ACS	605.79	231.69	317.19	616.93
Basic ACS	1054.97	574.30	819.18	1108.16
GVF ACS	641.66	644.95	725.72	1058.67

These results show that a good segmentation can be obtained in a reasonably time, which is important for both clinical and machine learning applications. As it is expected, one result is not representative of the quality of these algorithms. An analysis of a larger population must be done in order to have a real measure of quantitative error of our implementations. The work we introduced here is to present the tool, the algorithms implemented and how to use them. As future work, we plan to perform a more comprehensive study encompassing other methods known to have good results to contrast results as well as other regions of interest within the prostate. This will enable us to assess the validity of the proposed segmentation approach in other setting, and to get feedback from a larger pool of specialists. Other avenues of research pertain the validation of the proposed tool, as well as of the segmentation algorithm in a larger pool o prostate MRI images, as well as with a wider number of clinicians. We also plan to integrate other segmentation methods into the proposed GUI tool to carry out a more comprehensive quantitative comparison and to investigate its diagnostic differentiation with other prostate diseases such as BPH, chronic or acute prostatitis.

5. Conclusions

In this paper we described the implementation of a snake-based segmentation algorithm, based on an Active Contours Models (ACM), which has been integrated into a GUI based application. We focused our research in a method originally conceived for segmenting the shape of the heart's left ventricle. A modification of this specific prior has yielded very good results in the context of prostate cancer segmentation: the snake models tries to evolve and to adjust to the boundaries of the proposed zones. The problem with this implementation is that the performance of this previous model highly depends on the quality of the input image, as it uses the pixel intensities and the edges of the object in order to determine the correct curve evolution. As it can be expected, if the boundaries are not well defined, or if the intensities of different sections have similar values, then either the model will not be able to assess the difference, preventing the algorithm of evolving, or it will cause the snake to overlap with other elements in the image. This scenario can be observed in Figure 12, where the red contour overlaps with the area that corresponds to the TZ.

Furthermore, in order to get that segmentation, several shapes for the initial contours had been tested to obtain the best results, which might be very different from one run of the algorithm to another. This entails that the implemented snake-based algorithms are very sensitive to the initialization conditions. This type of problems have fostered researches in image analysis and computer vision to find novel ways of constraining the shape of the force that pushes the objects' boundaries in the right direction. Doing so, the segmentation algorithm becomes robust against to initialization conditions and less sensitive to the quality of the image.

Regarding the performance of both implementations, the *Simplified ACS* and *Basic ACS*, their behaviour are not the same. Since *Basic ACS* includes all the weights and all the functions described by the original document, the boundaries of the final segmentation tends to be closer to the real boundaries of the object to segment than in the case of *Simplified ACS*. Nonetheless, both of them fail in the task of finding the boundaries when the image intensities between two contiguous areas are not noticeably different, like in the case of the tumor and the central zone in Figure 12. This problem has been partially overcame when using the Gradient Vector Flow external force.

Further improvements to this algorithm will thus be directed towards implementing other types of Gradient Vector Flow energy optimization algorithms, or exploring how to include shape priors for each zone of the prostate separately. These modifications would help to create a segmentation that does not go too far from where the real object is. Additionally, no pre-processing nor post-processing functions have been included. Adding pre-processing operations might help to remove the noise that addresses the snake towards the wrong directions, and post-processing of the resulting contour will help to make it smoother, and closer to the real boundaries of the object.

Moreover, since the DICOM files can contain different image modalities, and each modality has its particularities, a profiles section can be added to the program. Each profile will contain a set of parameters (priors weights, GVF weight, regularization constants, and iterations) specific for each algorithm. These profiles will be chosen in a way that they will produce the best segmentation results for the selected image modality, increasing the scope of application of the program.

Other avenues of research pertain the validation of the proposed tool, as well as of the segmentation algorithm in a larger pool o prostate MRI images, as well as with a wider number of clinicians. We also plan to integrate other segmentation methods into the proposed GUI tool to carry out a more comprehensive quantitative comparison and to investigate its diagnostic differentiation with other prostate diseases such as BPH, chronic or acute prostatitis

Author Contributions: Conceptualization, C.M. and J.R.; methodology, all authors.; software, J.R.; validation, C.M., G.O.-R.; resources , C.M and G.O.-R.; data curation, C.M.; writing—original draft preparation, J.R. and C.M.; writing—review and editing, all authors; visualization, all authors; supervision, C.M., G.O.-R. All authors have read and agreed to the published version of the manuscript.

Abbreviations

The following abbreviations are used in this manuscript:

PCa	Prostate Cancer
ICD-O	International Classification of Diseases for Oncology
ICCC	International Classification of Childhood Cancer
EU	European Union
MRI	Magnetic Resonance Imaging
ROI	Region of Interest
T2WI	T2-Weighted Imaging
DWI	Diffusion Weighted Imaging
DCE	Perfusion based on the Dynamic Contrast Enhancement
MRS	Magnetic Resonance Spectroscopy
PI-RADS	Prostate Imaging-Reporting and Data System
CZ	Central Zone
PZ	Peripheral Zone
TZ	Transition Zone
AFT	Anterior Fibromuscular Tissue
Tum	Tumor lession
ACM	Active Contour Models
GVF	Gradient Vector Flow
DICOM	Digital Imaging and Communication On Medicine
HD	Hausdorff distance
DI	Dice Index

References

1. Siegel, R.L.; Miller, K.D.; Jemal, A. An Enhanced Contextual Fire Detection Algorithm for MODIS. *CA Cancer J. Clin.* **2020**, *70*, 7–30. [CrossRef] [PubMed]
2. Carioli, G.; Bertuccio, P.; Boffetta, P.; Levi, F.; La Vecchia, C.; Negri, E.; Malvezzi, M. European cancer mortality predictions for the year 2020 with a focus on prostate cancer. *Ann. Oncol.* **2020**, *31*, 650–658. [CrossRef] [PubMed]
3. Shah, V.; Turkbey, B.; Mani, H.; Pang, Y.; Pohida, T.; Merino, M.J.; Pinto, P.A.; Choyke, P.L.; Bernardo, M. Decision support system for localizing prostate cancer based on multiparametric magnetic resonance imaging. *Med. Phys.* **2012**, *39*, 4093–4103. [CrossRef] [PubMed]
4. Dickinson, L.; Ahmed, H.U.; Allen, C.; Barentsz, J.O.; Carey, B.; Futterer, J.J.; Heijmink, S.W.; Hoskin, P.J.; Kirkham, A.; Padhani, A.R.; et al. Magnetic resonance imaging for the detection, localisation, and characterisation of prostate cancer: Recommendations from a European consensus meeting. *Eur. J. Neurol.* **2011**, *59*, 477–494. [CrossRef] [PubMed]
5. Fradet, V.; Kurhanewicz, J.; Cowan, J.E.; Karl, A.; Coakley, F.V.; Shinohara, K.; Carroll, P.R. Prostate cancer managed with active surveillance: Role of anatomic MR imaging and MR spectroscopic imaging. *Radiographics* **2010**, *256*, 176–183. [CrossRef] [PubMed]
6. Ghose, S.; Oliver, A.; Mitra, J.; Martí, R.; Lladó, X.; Freixenet, J.; Meriaudeau, F.; Sidibé, D.; Vilanova, J.C.; Comet, J. A supervised learning framework of statistical shape and probability priors for automatic prostate segmentation in ultrasound images. *Med. Image Anal.* **2013**, *17*, 587–600. [CrossRef] [PubMed]
7. Ghose, S.; Oliver, O.; Martí, J.; Lladó, X.; Vilanova, J.; Freixenet, J. A survey of prostate segmentation methodologies in ultrasound, magnetic resonance and computed tomography images. *Comput. Methods Programs Biomed.* **2012**, *108*, 262–287. [CrossRef] [PubMed]
8. Vos, P.C.; Hambrock, T.; Barenstz, J.O.; Huisman, H.J. Computer-assisted analysis of peripheral zone prostate lesions using T2-weighted and dynamic contrast enhanced T1-weighted MRI. *Phys. Med. Biol.* **2010**, *55*, 1719–1734. [CrossRef] [PubMed]
9. Chen, M.; Dang, H.; Wang, J.; Zhou, C.; Li, S.; Wang, W. Prostate cancer detection: Comparison of t2-weighted imaging, diffusion-weighted imaging, proton magnetic resonance spectroscopic imaging, and the three techniques combined. *Acta Radiol.* **2008**, *49*, 602–610. [CrossRef] [PubMed]
10. Brancato, V.; Di Costanzo, G.; Basso, L.; Tramontano, L.; Puglia, M.; Ragozzino, A.; Cavaliere, C. Assessment of DCE Utility for PCa Diagnosis Using PI-RADS v2.1: Effects on Diagnostic Accuracy and Reproducibility. *Diagnostics* **2020**, *10*, 164. [CrossRef] [PubMed]
11. Mata, C.; Walker, P.; Oliver, A.; Brunotte, F.; Martí, J.; Lalande, A. Prostateanalyzer: Web-based medical application for the management of prostate cancer using multiparametric mr images. *Inform. Health Soc. Care* **2015**, *87*, 1–21. [CrossRef] [PubMed]
12. Pluempitiwiriyawej, C.; Moura, J.M.; Wu, Y.J.L.; Ho, C. STACS: New active contour scheme for cardiac MR image segmentation. *IEEE Trans. Med. Imaging* **2005**, *24*, 593–603. [CrossRef] [PubMed]
13. De Marzo, A.; Platz, E.; Sutcliffe, S.; Xu, J.; Grönberg, H.; Drake, C.; Nakay, Y. Inflammation in prostate carcinogenesis. *Nat. Rev. Cancer* **2007**, *7*, 256–269. [CrossRef] [PubMed]
14. Verma, S.; Rajesh, A. A clinically relevant approach to imaging prostate cancer: Review. *Am. J. Roentgenol.* **2011**, *196*, S1–S10. [CrossRef] [PubMed]
15. Rodríguez, J.; Ochoa-Ruíz, G.; Mata, C. Prostate-MRI-segmentation-App. GitHub Repos. 2020. Available online: https://github.com/joako1991/Prostate-MRI-segmentation-App (accessed on 2 September 2020).
16. Chan, T.F.; Vese, L.A. Active contours without edges. *IEEE Trans. Image Process.* **2001**, *10*, 266–277. [CrossRef] [PubMed]
17. Xu, C.; Prince, J.L. Snakes, shapes, and gradient vector flow. *IEEE Trans. Image Process.* **1998**, *7*, 359–369. [CrossRef] [PubMed]
18. Paragios, N.; Mellina-Gottardo, O.; Ramesh, V. Gradient vector flow fast geometric active contours. *IEEE Trans. Pattern Anal. Mach. Intell.* **2004**, *26*, 402–407. [CrossRef] [PubMed]
19. Xu, C.; Yezzi, A.; Prince, J.L. On the relationship between parametric and geometric active contours. In Proceedings of the Conference Record of the Thirty-Fourth Asilomar Conference on Signals, Systems and Computers (Cat. No.00CH37154), Pacific Grove, CA, USA, 29 October–1 November 2000; Volume 1, pp. 483–489. [CrossRef]

7

Two-Stage Monitoring of Patients in Intensive Care Unit for Sepsis Prediction Using Non-Overfitted Machine Learning Models

Vytautas Abromavičius, Darius Plonis *, Deividas Tarasevičius and Artūras Serackis

Department of Electronic Systems, Vilnius Gediminas Technical University, Naugarduko str. 41, 03227 Vilnius, Lithuania; vgtu@vgtu.lt or vytautas.abromavicius@vgtu.lt (V.A.); deividas.tarasevicius@vgtu.lt (D.T.); arturas.serackis@vgtu.lt (A.S.)

* Correspondence: darius.plonis@vgtu.lt

Abstract: The presented research faces the problem of early detection of sepsis for patients in the Intensive Care Unit. The PhysioNet/Computing in Cardiology Challenge 2019 facilitated the development of automated, open-source algorithms for the early detection of sepsis from clinical data. A labeled clinical records dataset for training and verification of the algorithms was provided by the challenge organizers. However, a relatively small number of records with sepsis, supported by Sepsis-3 clinical criteria, led to highly unbalanced dataset (only 2% records with sepsis label). A high number of unbalanced data records is a great challenge for machine learning model training and is not suitable for training classical classifiers. To address these issues, a method taking into the account the amount of time the patients spent in the intensive care unit (ICU) was proposed. The proposed method uses two separate ensemble models, one trained on patient records under 56 h in the ICU, and another for patients who stayed longer than 56 h. A solution including feature selection and weighting based training on imbalanced data was proposed in this paper. In addition, several performance metrics were investigated. Results show, that for successful prediction, a particular model having few or more predictors based on the length of stay in the Intensive Care Unit should be applied.

Keywords: early detection; sepsis; evaluation metrics; machine learning; medical informatics; feature extraction; physionet challenge

1. Introduction

Sepsis is a syndrome of physiological, pathological, and biochemical abnormalities induced by infection [1]. The conservative estimates indicate that sepsis is a leading cause of mortality and critical illness worldwide [2,3]. World Health Organization concerned that sepsis continues to cause approximately six million deaths worldwide every year, most of which are preventable [4]. In their study, the Department of Health in Ireland reported that survival from sepsis-induced hypotension is over 75% if it is recognized promptly, but that every delay by an hour causes that figure to fall by over 7%, implying that the mortality increases by about 30%.

In this paper, we present our solution for the early detection of sepsis by joining the PhysioNet/Computing in Cardiology Challenge 2019 [5]. Here, a detailed explanation of the Challenge data, participant evaluation metrics, and primary results are provided, and therefore, we will not explain it in this paper. However, a few important findings we should share in this paper in order to better explain the motivation to construct our algorithm in a particular way.

According to the requirements of the Challenge, our open-source algorithm works on clinical data provided on a real-time basis by giving a positive or negative prediction of sepsis for every single hour.

The algorithm predicts sepsis development for the patient using a pre-trained mathematical model. Therefore, not only the appropriate model should be used but also the training should be performed in the right way.

Data used in the competition was collected from intensive care unit (ICU) patients in three separate hospital systems. However, data from two hospital systems only were publicly available for training (40,336 patients in total). Another set of records (24,819 patients in total), obtained from all three different hospital systems was hidden and used for official scoring only by challenges organizers. Such separation of the data prevented participants from over-fitting their models. Taking into account that the trained model may learn not only dependencies in the clinical records but also hospital system-related behavior, for our approach, we have tested different data selection strategies for training. Models trained on hospital system A data we tested on data from hospital system B and vice versa.

The most challenging issue in the available data records was a high number of unbalanced records. Only 2932 septic patients were included in the dataset, together with 37,404 non-septic patients. From the perspective of mathematical model training, the data balance is much worse. Since the sepsis prediction had to be made on an hourly basis, 6 h in advance to the onset time of sepsis, specified according to Sepsis-3 clinical criteria, a number of non-sepsis examples we also took from the septic patient early records. After such reorganization of training data, only 2% from 1,484,384 [1,424,171] events (16,933 from 752,946 [739,663] in set A and 10,557 from 73,438 [684,508] in set B) had to be classified as an early prediction of sepsis.

The imbalance of the data can be treated in different ways. Nemati et al. successfully used random subsampling to train deep cancer subtype classifier [6]. Vicar et al. used special cost function—Generalized Dice Loss [7]. Sweetly et al. created 54 datasets using the same sepsis data and different non-sepsis data records [8]. He et al. have applied a random subsampling to this Challenge data [9]. Although the rank of their solution was quite high in the Challenge, the model was highly overfitted on hospital systems A and B when comparing to the model performance on hidden hospital system C data. An interesting approach was proposed by Li et al., where they decided to divide data into three stages (1–9, 10–49 and above 50 h stay in ICU) [10].

Dealing with missing values is another decision to be taken and it also may have an influence to the selected model training and overall performance. Forward-fill method [8,11–15]. Singh at al. found in their study, that mean imputation model gave worst results [16]. Other authors successfully used mean calculation over whole dataset [15,17].

Our proposed algorithm was scored on a censored data set, dedicated for scoring and using utility function that rewards early predictions and penalizes late predictions as well as false alarms.

2. Materials and Methods

In this section, we address the challenges regarding the problem of early sepsis detection and propose a methodology to overcome them. A labeled clinical records dataset for training and verification of the algorithms was provided by the PhysioNet/Computing in Cardiology Challenge 2019 organizers [5].

2.1. The Data

Data contained records of 40,336 ICU patients with up to 40 clinical variables divided into two datasets, based on hospital systems A and B. For each patient, the data were recorded at every hour during the stay in ICU. The records were labeled (on an hourly basis) according to Sepsis-3 clinical criteria. A total of 1,407,716 h of data was collected and labeled. Data labels included vital signs, laboratory values, and demographic values of the patients. Eight vital signs were a heart rate (HR), pulse oximetry (O2sat), temperature (Temp), systolic blood pressure (SBP), mean arterial pressure (MAP), diastolic blood pressure (DBP), respiration rate (Resp) and end-tidal carbon dioxide (EtCO2). A total of 26 laboratory values were included in the dataset. Demographic values include age, gender, hospital identifiers, the time between hospital and ICU admission (Hosp), and ICU length of stay (ICULOS). Data were labeled as positive 12 h before and 3 h after the onset time of sepsis. Positive labels of sepsis were found in 2932 of the 40,336 records, which is 7.27% of the data. Labels consisting of positive (sepsis) labels were found in 27,916 rows, which is only 1.98% of all data.

Investigation of the data showed large numbers of missing values. The percentage of missing rows of vital signs is shown in Figure 1. Missing values of vital signs make about 10% of the data, with the exception of Temp (66% missing data) and EtCO2 (100% and 92% missing data, for dataset A and dataset B, respectively). Therefore, EtCO2 was not used as a feature for the model. The percentage of missing rows of laboratory measurements is shown in Figure 2. Missing data of laboratory values makes from 78% to 100% for all values. We did not use laboratory values to develop our model.

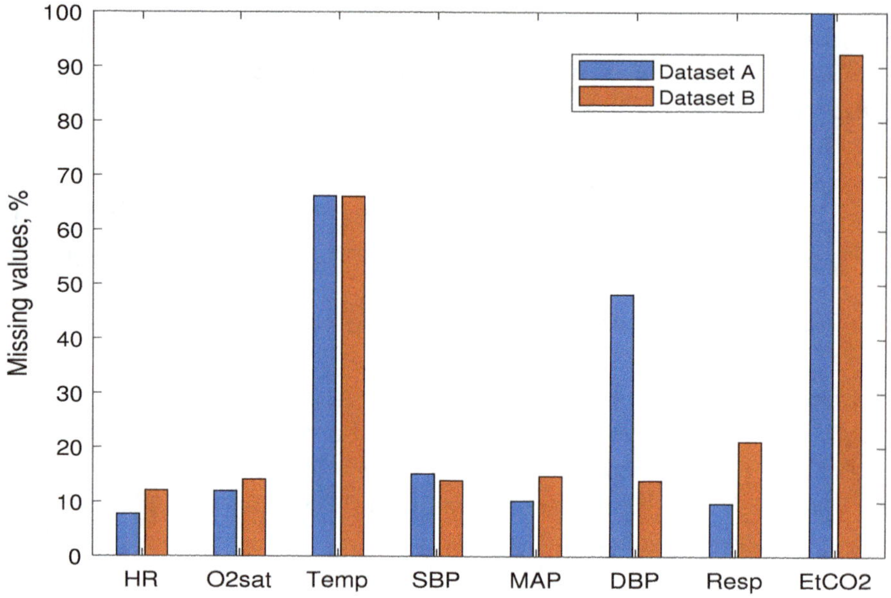

Figure 1. Missing vital values in the data.

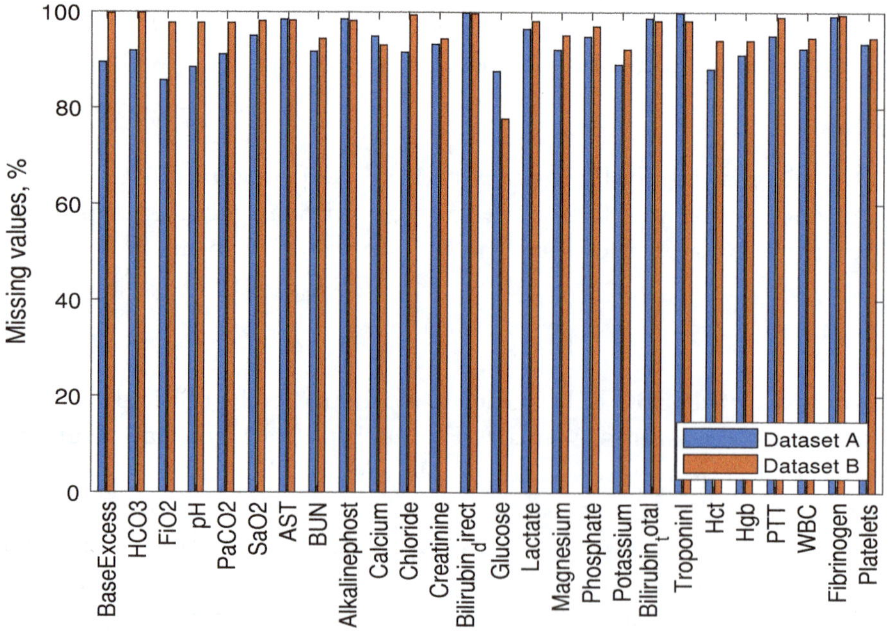

Figure 2. Missing laboratory values in the data.

Average values of vitals are shown in Table 1. Measured SBP, MAP and DBP values are higher in dataset B. Also, the measured HR is slightly lower in dataset B. Having two datasets collected in separate hospitals allowed us to develop models that are robust to measurement errors rising from the specificity of electronic medical record systems. Thus, the nature of data increases the difficulty of predicting sepsis. During the development of the model, we had to take into account the high unbalance of positive and negative cases, large amounts of missing values, and the fact that data was recorded using two different measurement systems.

Table 1. Average values of vitals and their standard error.

Measures	Dataset A	Dataset B
HR	84.6 ± 0.100	83.1 ± 0.106
O2sat	97.2 ± 0.016	97.1 ± 0.014
Temp	36.9 ± 0.004	36.8 ± 0.004
SBP	120.3 ± 0.115	126.4 ± 0.132
MAP	78.5 ± 0.076	86.7 ± 0.091
DBP	60.2 ± 0.070	66.6 ± 0.076
Resp	18.6 ± 0.026	18.5 ± 0.022
EtCO2	NaN	33.1 ± 0.072

2.2. Feature Extraction

A solution proposed in this paper to the early sepsis prediction problem employs information of the ICU length of stay, hospitalization time, age, and seven vital signs—HR, O2sat, Temp, SBP, MAP, DBP, and Resp. We did not use EtCO2 for feature extraction due to a large number of missing values.

We have calculated the mean, standard deviation, and the max-min difference for the vital sign data. We took those values from the whole duration of the record. Additionally, we have considered some other measures for our approach, such as kurtosis, entropy, and the standard error. However, after further analysis, we decided to discard these features. Kurtosis can only be calculated for four or more variables, not including the missing values. Additionally, kurtosis is not a representative statistic estimate for sample sizes less than 200 [18]. The entropy value is proportional to the sample size. In the problem we have investigated in this paper, the sample size changes each hour of the patient stay and can be reduced with missing values for some patients [19]. Therefore, in this case, the entropy just represents a number of samples used for its calculation. Thus, it is unlikely that entropy can carry useful information for the model training. The standard error is calculated by a division by the sample size, and it is inversely proportional to the sample size. Therefore, results can lead to a reduction of standard error for larger data sample sizes, which in its order increases unwanted load model training [20].

After our theoretical investigation, we have calculated 21 features for each hour. Missing values of the data were removed when calculating features. In some cases, features could not be calculated due to a small set of available data (e.g., during the first few hours of ICU stay, or due to a large number of missing values). In such cases, we set the value of the feature to '-1'. Finally, we have assembled a feature set of 24 features for model training: 21 calculated featured from vital signs and three demographic values (Hosp, age, ICULOS). Obtained data had different measurement units, measurement errors, and scales. Therefore, we have applied data standardization to have zero mean and standard deviation '1'. The sample mean and sample standard deviation were used the same for each patient, obtained from all sample data of both datasets containing 40,336 patients in total.

2.3. Data Balancing

The data from the experiment were strongly unbalanced, as discussed in Section 2.1. The balancing of the data can be performed using various oversampling or subsampling techniques that change the data in the dataset before the model is trained. In our investigation, we followed the alternative approach by setting different weights for the individual data points according to their class.

During our investigation of possible data balancing approaches, we surveyed various sampling methods, also used in the Challenge by other authors. The challengers applied undersampling, subsampling methods and some oversampling. The immensity of the imbalance problem is very great; the ratio of the labels is 1:50. Additionally, clinical data is very contextual. Oversampling methods haven't shown good results in the Challenge. Undersampling methods possibly removed valuable information of non-septic patients. Most of the subsampling methods overtrained showed high Utility scores on known datasets and poor scores on hidden datasets. The variability of the clinical (ICU) data is very high. Non-septic cases have various other conditions and unknown prescribed medications. We think that adjustment of classification cost is a more robust and effective way to address this issue of data imbalance. The highest rank in the 2019 Challenge was received by a solution, where the classification cost was calculated using Utility function value differences between correct and incorrect classification [13]. In our solution, we used simple weighting and investigated the behavior of the model training with differently selected weighs.

We have weighed the positive and negative predictions in accordance with the duration before or after the onset time of sepsis. Positive values, with various weights, make only 1.98% of the data. For this reason, the investigated models were trained with uneven classification costs. We have addressed the data balance issue by utilizing and modifying the classification cost function:

$$loss = -\sum_{i=1}^{N} c_i \left| t_i - y_i \right|, \tag{1}$$

where N is the number of observations, t_i is the target output for observation i, y_i is the predicted value for observation i, and c_i is the classification cost for the observation i.

To investigate the influence of the selected weight on the model's behavior during training, we trained our models using different classification costs. A misclassified non-septic observations were weighted by 1 (c_1), and a misclassified septic observation weighted selecting different c_2 (1, 10, 20, 30, 100). Classification cost was selected based on the amount of "unbalance". As it was expected, since the positive values make only 1.98% of the data, the most effective value should be found when the classification cost c_2 is between 20 and 30. Models with c_2 parameter lower than 20 tend to predict most of the data as non-septic, while models with higher c_2 tend to predict all data as septic.

2.4. Model Training

In our investigation, we have used models based on Decision trees, naive Gaussian Bayes, Support Vector Machines (SVM), and Ensemble learners. All models were trained using stratified 5-fold cross validation. Decision trees based models were important in this stage of the problem solution. The Decision tree models give insights about the relevance of selected features. However, they tend to overfit the data [21]. Less over-fitting can be expected when using Ensemble learner models [22]. We have trained the ensemble learning-based models using hyperparameter optimization among Bag, GentleBoost, LogitBoost, AdaBoost, and RUSBoost methods. Hyperparameter tuning was performed for the number of decision tree splits, number of learners used in the model, learning rate, number of features in the ensemble. The number of decision tree splits search scaled in the range from 1 to 500. Many branches tend to overfit the data, while simpler trees can be more robust, which is especially important for the clinical data. The number of learners used in the search was from 10 to 100. A high number of learners can produce higher accuracy but can be time-consuming to train. We changed the learning rate in the ranged from 0.0001 to 1, and the number of features in ensemble hyperparameter tuning scaled from 1 to 24.

Gaussian naive Bayes based models are known for their simplicity, high bias, and low overfit. Typically good results using Naive Bayes are achieved using low variance data. These models are not recommended for high variance data [23]. Models trained using SVM tends to overfit data less. However, they are not very successful in problems with a high number of missing values in data [24].

We have trained each model separately using features estimated on an hourly basis in random order. In order to avoid over-fitting and increase robustness, we have trained the models on records taken from a single hospital system (dataset A) and tested on records from another hospital (dataset B, hidden during the training). We trained models on the dataset A using 5-fold cross-validation. Using our selected approach, only half of the available data was used for training. However, as it was shown in the results of the challenge [5], proposed solutions to the problem performed well on known datasets, even if scoring was done on a hidden part of the same set, and performed marginally worse on new hospital system C, hidden from challenge contestants. Additionally, the advantage of this approach to train and evaluate models is supported by Biglarbeigi [25].

Based on the results of the trained models and insights into the data, we proposed a method that takes into account the amount of time the patients have already spent in the ICU. The first model used AdaBoost ensemble method with a decision tree to evaluate features of patients extracted during the first 56 h (11,146 sepsis labels and 654,866 non-sepsis labels; it makes approximate imbalance ratio of 1:59). The second model is applied for patients with ICULOS time greater than 56 (5990 sepsis labels and 118,213 non-sepsis labels; it makes an approximate imbalance ratio of 1:20). The second model was developed using the discriminant subspace-based ensemble method. The method generates decision trees using pseudorandomly selected feature components. Decisions of the trees are then combined by averaging the estimates. As this method is based on decision trees, it is fast to train and easy to interpret [26]. Both models were using features described in Section 2.2. Additionally, our proposed model was trained on both datasets, 75% of the data used for training. This allowed us to investigate how much model overtrains on known hospital systems.

2.5. Model Scoring

Models, proposed in this paper for Sepsis prediction, were evaluated using several different metrics. Traditional scoring metrics, such as the area under the receiver operating characteristics (AUROC), the area under the precision-recall curve (AUPRC), accuracy, F-measure, and Matthews correlation coefficient (MCC) were used. Additionally, investigated models were scored using a specific scoring function developed by the authors of the dataset, called Utility score. Performance of the investigated models was based on the Utility score metric. Additionally, using different scoring metrics allowed us a better comparison of investigated models. AUPRC is recommended for imbalanced data over the AUROC measure [27,28]. F-measure is a harmonic mean of precision and recall [29]. Lately, MCC measure was shown to be more advantageous over F-measure in the binary classification of imbalanced data [30].

The utility score metric was proposed by the authors of the dataset for the 2019 physionet Challenge [5]. This metric was recently proposed. The utility score metric reward algorithms that facilitate early sepsis detection and treatment. Additionally, it addresses the problem of infrequent events and sequential prediction tasks. It is designed to capture the clinical utility of early sepsis detection by weighting early and late predictions. Moreover, decision threshold metrics (AUROC and AUPRC) have problems evaluating unbalanced datasets. Additionally, other challengers evaluated their models using the Utility score, therefore, it is easier to compare the results. However, the experimental results showed that Utility score correlates with two traditional metrics F-measure and MCC.

Utility score—a specifically designed scoring function rewards algorithms for early predictions and penalizes them for late or missed predictions and false alarms. Scoring was conducted by predicting each hourly label for each patient. Each positive label had a defined score depending on correct prediction time to sepsis. Scoring function awarded models for correct prediction at most 12 h before and 3 h after the onset time of sepsis. Scoring function penalized models who predicted septic state 12 h before onset time of sepsis and slightly penalized models with false-positive predictions.

True negative predictions were not penalized or rewarded by the function. Best Utility score the most optimal model could achieve would be 1. Thus, a better model would have higher Utility score. A more detailed scoring description can be found in the original paper. The utility score was a reference metric. Using it, we evaluated the performance of our investigated models. AUROC, AUPRC, accuracy, F-measure, and MCC scores were used to gain insight into the models (e.g., if they correlate with any other parameter of the experiment, such as classification cost, feature reduction, model configuration, or Utility score).

Our investigated and proposed models were compared with five challengers who received the highest Utility score on hidden test C. Additionally, a result of three baseline models was generated. Baseline models were scored using all positive, all negative and random performance to clearly show the unbalance of the data and the difficulty of the challenge.

3. Results

As it was noted in Section 2.4, decision trees, naive Gaussian Bayes, SVM and ensemble learners were investigated in our experiment. Various parameters of the models were adjusted. Additionally, the effect of classification cost and feature reduction was investigated. The performance of developed models was evaluated using Utility score as a reference metric. To complement, several other metrics, such as AUROC, AUPRC, accuracy, F-measure, and MCC were calculated to compare investigated models. Models were trained using dataset A, and scored using dataset B. Results of the experiment are given in Table 2. Models, based on decision trees, are labeled from 1 to 14. Models, based on the Naive Bayes algorithm, are labeled from 21 to 25. SVM based models are labeled from 31 to 34. Models from 41 to 44 were using an optimizable ensemble method for searching the best model for the problem.

The random guess of the sepsis with an accuracy of 50% showed −0.529 Utility score and 0.125 AUROC. By labeling all cases as positive, the Utility score was reduced to −1.059 and AUROC was 0, F-measure—0.029. Labeling all cases as negative increased the Utility score to 0, AUROC was 0.5 and F-measure—0. AUROC was generally expected to be equal or above 0.5 when the dataset is balanced. In Table 2, the third row indicates the AUROC value of a random performance, having an accuracy of 50%). The AUROC value in such a case is 0.125 (for balanced datasets it would be 0.5). It is a direct insight into the importance of the problem.

Based on the results of the Physionet challenge 2019 on the hidden dataset, several of the highest Utility scores were from 0.017 to 0.193. The highest Utility score (0.193) was achieved by Hong et al. using deep recurrent reinforcement learners [31]. Murugesan et al. applied XGBoost algorithm and achieved 0.182 Utility score on hidden test set [32]. Our proposed method was developed based on the results of further described investigations and results. The proposed method predicted 3753 true positive, 707,606 true negative, 7027 false positive and 43,309 false negative observations of dataset B. The precision of the method was 34.82%, recall—7.98%. Our proposed method achieved 0.306 AUROC, 0.009 AUPROC, 0.934 accuracy, 0.129 F-measure, 0.142 MCC and 0.245 Utility scores. Additionally, this model was trained on both datasets (70% of the data used for training) achieved 0.276 Utility score.

Decision trees are fast to train and to evaluate. We started our investigation using these models. The baseline score of Model1, with default parameters, gave a Utility score of 0.01. Secondly, a feature reduction using principal component analysis (PCA) was applied. Six features to explain 95% variance was kept. Model2 gave Utility score of 0.004. For Model3, increasing feature set to 14 (out of 24) increased Utility score to 0.0124. Forth model used 14 features and a modified classification cost ratio of 1:10. Model4 obtained Utility score of 0.1236. Further increasing classification (Model5) ratio to 1:100 Utility score decreased to −0.296. Using all available features in the set (24 features) Utility score was slightly improved to −0.242, for Model6. Using 24 features and classification cost 1:10 obtained Utility score was 0.184 for Model7. For Model8 we modified classification cost to 1:20, obtained Utility score was 0.22. Further increasing classification cost to 1:30 (Model9) decreased Utility score to 0.216.

Model10, having a modified classification cost of 1:20, and a reduced feature set to 20 got Utility score decreased to 0.157. Next, we limited the tree split criterion to 50. Model11 achieved Utility score of 0.232. Higher Utility score was achieved by reducing split criterion to 4, it was 0.233 (Model12). Reducing split criterion to 2 for Model13 got a similar Utility score of 0.233. Model14, with a further reduced split criterion to 1, achieved the highest Utility score of 0.242. Only 1 tree branch was used for this model. A feature that was used for this model was ICULOS. Features used for Model12 and Model14 also included ICULOS, and also mean SBP and Resp.

Models labeled from 21 to 25 were based on the Naive Bayes algorithm. Model21 without feature reduction and using classification cost 1:20 achieved Utility score of 0.1334. For Model23, using PCA, the number of features was reduced to 14, achieved Utility score was 0.129. Further reducing the number of features to 6 (95% explained variance using PCA) improved Utility score to 0.150, as shown in Table 2 Model24 row. Adjusting the classification cost led to a reduced score—Model22 and Model25 used a reduced feature set and a modified classification cost of 1:10 and 1:30; they yielded Utility scores of 0.097 and 0.143, respectively. SVM models were computed using the Gaussian kernel function. Results of the SVM models are shown in Table 2, under Model31 to Model34. Model31, using a classification cost ratio of 1:20 and 24 features for training, achieved a 0.151 Utility score. Model32, using 6 features to explain 95% variance, achieved a 0.144 Utility score. Model33 and Model34, using classification costs 1:30 and 1:10, respectively, achieved 0.1294 and 0.1302 Utility scores.

Models labeled from 41 to 44 were trained using ensemble methods, searching between Bag, GentleBoost, LogitBoost, AdaBoost, and RUSBoost methods and other hyperparameters. The classification cost for all investigated models were set to 1:20. Model41 using a full feature set achieved Utility score of 0.082. Reducing the tree split criterion to 10 (Model42) gave an improved Utility score of—0.124. Ensemble model (Model43) using bagged decision trees, having 29 learners, 4 splits and using 24 features achieved a Utility score of 0.173, further reducing split criterion to 1 did not improve the Utility score—0.173. Using principal component analysis (95%) reduced the Utility score to 0.008 (Model44).

High AUROC, AUPRC and accuracy scores using decision tree models were achieved when classification cost was 1:1, for example, 0.492, 0.497, 0.491 AUROC score for Model1, Model2, Model3, respectively. Model12 and Model14 with high Utility scores gave low AUROC (0.313 and 0.309, respectively), AUPRC (0.009, both) and accuracy (0.931 and 0.937, respectively) scores.

High AUROC, AUPRC, and accuracy scores using ensemble learners were achieved using Model41: 0.413, 0.012, and 0.955, respectively. However, this ensemble model achieved low Utility (0.082). In the same manner, low AUROC (0.347), AUPRC (0.01), and accuracy (0.939) scores, and the highest Utility score (0.173) was achieved using Model43. Other investigated models performed similarly, high AUROC, AUPRC and accuracy, and low Utility score; or low AUROC, AUPRC and accuracy, and higher Utility score was observed in all investigated models, namely decision trees, SVM, naive Bayes, and ensemble-based models.

Highest F-measure and MCC scores using decision tree models were achieved for models that showed the highest Utility scores. F-measure score of Model14 was 0.133 (Utility—0.242), score of Model11 was 0.131 (Utility—0.232). MCC score of Model14 was 0.143; the score of Model11 was 0.14. Lowest F-measure and MCC scores were achieved using Model2: F-measure—0.011, MCC—0.018. However, the lowest Utility score (-0.296) using decision tree models was achieved using Model5. F-measure score of Model5 was 0.04, MCC—0.057.

Naive Gaussian Bayes models achieved lowest F-measure (0.062) and MCC (0.085) scores when Model22 (Utility score—0.097) was scored, highest F-measure (0.099) and MCC (0.122) scores using Model24 (Utility score—0.15).

Model32 trained using SVM achieved F-measure (0.108) and MCC (0.104) score, and scored 0.144 using Utility performance metric. However, Model31's Utility score (0.1515) was slightly higher, while F-measure (0.099) and MCC (0.1) score lower. Low F-measure (0.081) and MCC (0.087) scores also showed low Utility scores—0.129, for Model33.

Comparably low F-measure (0.025) and MCC (0.02) scores using ensemble learners were achieved using Model44 (Utility score—0.008). Model43 with a high Utility score (0.173) demonstrated a high F-measure (0.115) and MCC (0.113) scores.

Table 2. Results of the investigated models, baseline scores, and five highest Utility scores on hidden test set from the challenge. Our Investigated models labeled from 1 to 14 were based on decision trees. Models labeled from 21 to 25 were based on naive Bayes algorithm. SVM based models were labeled from 31 to 34. Models labeled from 41 to 44 were using ensemble methods with hyperparameter search. Best performing models, having the highest Utility score, were highlighted.

Model	AUROC	AUPRC	Accuracy	F-Measure	MCC	Utility
All positive	0.000	0.000	0.014	0.029	0.000	−1.059
All negative	0.500	0.014	0.986	0.000	0.000	0.000
Random performance	**0.125**	**0.007**	**0.500**	**0.027**	**0.000**	**−0.529**
Hong et al. [31]	**0.060**	**0.003**	**0.937**	**0.094**	N/A	**0.193**
Murugesan et al. [32]	0.256	0.006	0.962	0.113	N/A	0.182
Narayanaswamy et al. [33]	0.701	0.069	0.881	0.059	N/A	0.062
Alfaras et al. [34]	0.702	0.078	0.877	0.058	N/A	0.055
Deogire [35]	0.586	0.016	0.984	0.048	N/A	0.017
Proposed method	**0.307**	**0.009**	**0.934**	**0.130**	**0.143**	**0.245**
when trained on both datasets	0.291	0.009	0.934	0.140	0.158	0.276
Model1	0.492	0.014	0.984	0.024	0.028	0.010
Model2	**0.497**	**0.014**	**0.985**	0.011	0.018	0.004
Model3	0.491	0.014	0.984	0.028	0.033	0.012
Model4	0.379	0.011	0.945	0.095	0.090	0.124
Model5	0.058	0.003	0.486	0.040	0.057	−0.296
Model6	0.097	0.005	0.562	0.040	0.051	−0.242
Model7	0.357	0.011	0.950	0.126	0.125	0.184
Model8	0.314	0.010	0.930	0.118	0.129	0.220
Model9	0.278	0.009	0.901	0.100	0.119	0.216
Model10	0.321	0.010	0.914	0.091	0.098	0.157
Model11	0.321	0.010	0.940	0.131	0.140	0.232
Model12	0.309	0.009	0.931	0.124	0.136	0.233
Model13	0.309	0.009	0.931	0.124	0.136	0.233
Model14	0.313	0.009	0.937	**0.133**	**0.143**	**0.242**
Model21	0.226	0.008	0.828	0.070	0.092	0.133
Model22	**0.241**	**0.009**	**0.874**	0.062	0.085	0.097
Model23	0.23	0.008	0.831	0.069	0.090	0.129
Model24	0.201	0.006	0.785	**0.099**	**0.122**	**0.150**
Model25	0.202	0.006	0.790	0.092	0.118	0.143
Model31	0.353	0.011	0.935	0.099	0.100	**0.151**
Model32	0.375	0.011	0.949	**0.108**	**0.104**	0.144
Model33	0.320	0.010	0.904	0.081	0.087	0.129
Model34	**0.392**	**0.012**	**0.956**	**0.109**	0.101	0.130
Model41	0.413	0.012	0.955	0.084	0.072	0.082
Model42	0.358	0.011	0.937	0.100	0.099	0.124
Model43	0.347	0.010	0.939	**0.115**	**0.113**	**0.173**
Model44	**0.489**	**0.014**	**0.981**	0.025	0.020	0.008

4. Discussion

The highest Utility score was achieved using our proposed method, which divided patients based on their length of stay and then the appropriate model was applied. Additionally, decision trees with a low number of nodes achieved high Utility scores when ICU length of stay was included as a branch of decision tree. Therefore, we believe that future models should be developed based on ICU-stay time. For example, one model predicting recently hospitalized ICU patients, another would be used if a patient's ICU length of stay reaches a certain length of time. Also, this approach can be implemented using three or more temporal divisions. This finding of our investigation is supported by Lauritsen [36], Vincent [37] and Shimabukuro [38] papers. Each intervention, vital measurement, intravenous therapy, and duration of stay in general increases a chance of infection—a direct cause of sepsis.

Regarding the dataset, other papers tackled this problem and proposed methods, which were trained on both datasets, and officially scored on hidden set C. Dataset C is not available anymore. Therefore, one must find other means to compare the results with the challenge score. Most of the challengers performed well on known hospital systems, obtaining Utility scores of about 0.4. However, Utility scores for the hidden hospital systems were low [5]. One author suggested evaluating the proposed methodology using one dataset and testing it on another [25]. Our achieved Utility score was for the known dataset, but the hidden percentage of data was 0.276 when trained on 75% of the records. This shows that our proposed model is robust to overtrain.

We assume that the Utility score can be improved a little by finding better value for classification cost, where a true positive prediction reward would be multiplied somewhere between 20 and 30. However, this would fit the data and would not solve the general problem of the Challenge. Therefore, we recommend using an arbitrary value between 20 and 30 to increases the robustness of the system.

MCC and F-measure scores gave similar results, which increases and decreases with the Utility score. However, the bounds of MCC are from -1 to 1, while the F-measure is from 0 to 1. The bounds of the Utility score are from -2 to 1. We support the idea of using the Utility score as a metric for this dataset. Moreover, we showed that the MCC and F-measure are effective metrics for this problem, while other traditional metrics AUROC, AURRC and Accuracy are misleading for a highly unbalanced dataset. Additionally, due to the nature of the Utility score, results can be difficult to interpret, as Roussel et al. pointed out in their work [39].

Investigated decision trees achieved Utility score of 0.242, AUROC score of 0.313, and MCC score of 0.143 on hidden set. Models with such results are far from applicable to the clinical setting. Additionally, our investigation showed that increasing AUROC and accuracy usually leads to decreased Utility, F-measure, and MCC scores. Moreover, accuracy is high for all investigated models. Accuracy can be miss-leading when interpreting models, results for this kind of highly unbalanced data, and a large number of negatives [22]. When developing methods for this kind of problem, one needs to be careful; the accuracy of 98.2% can be achieved just by guessing all rows as negative. We showed that balancing data reduces AUROC, accuracy scores and improves F-measure, MCC, and Utility scores.

There are many models to experiment with, for example, k-Nearest Neighbor (kNN) and Long Short-Term Memory (LSTM) models were not tested in our work. LSTM models are more difficult to configure to use them effectively. Additionally, LSTM tends to overfit the data. Moreover, even if one successfully tackles the overfitting problem, there is still another downside, which is more important in the current state of the early sepsis prediction problem. The developed model may be hard to interpret and would not reveal much insight into data [40]. The clustering of unbalanced data (including Sepsis-related records) may give promising results for sepsis prediction. However, kNN overfits data with large variances [41]. On the other hand, a trained kNN model having 1000 or 2000 clusters to represent the data can be expected to be robust. In general, we believe results using these models can be promising, and we encourage future works exploring LSTM and kNN model capabilities.

It is notable that investigated models do not differ significantly in Utility score if a number of features is reduced. This shows that some features are not useful for the model. On the other hand, our proposed features were relatively simple. We believe that more advanced features are needed to solve the early detection of the sepsis problem. Using advanced features should improve the score. However, feature engineering is a difficult, time-consuming process, which also requires understanding the nature of the data. In this paper, we provide many insights into the nature of the data, different scoring metrics, advantages of various models, and feature combinations.

We believe that the results of our investigation presented in this paper will benefit the fundamental need of early sepsis prediction and will answer some basic questions about the limits of early detection. Our results should benefit the search for advanced combinations of features, ease the use of machine learning tools. With meaningful insights peer researchers can apply advanced feature engineering techniques and develop more sophisticated and robust models in order to reach reliable results. Reaching better results is available through the use of combined models and handcrafted features [42], thus, further contributing to this field. The main challenges of this problem, as we revealed, are—the highly unbalanced dataset, the high number of missing data, simple features calculated using vitals does not have enough predictive power, proposed solutions are prone to overtrain. Adjusting the classification cost function helps to address the latter problem. In addition, the insights and conclusions of our experiment may benefit not only machine learning specialists, researchers, but also ICU personnel and scientists in the medical field.

5. Conclusions

In this study, we provide a comparison of several alternative methods for early sepsis prediction. The performance of the investigated models was based on the Utility score metric. Our selected models and insights show how to deal with unbalanced data and with a large number of missing values.

The results, obtained during an experimental investigation, are based on publicly available data containing 40,336 records with 1,407,716 of rows and 40 dimensions. Results showed:

1. Our proposed method, using two separate ensemble models, based on length of stay in the ICU, performed better than other tested models when using vital and demographic data to calculate simple features.
2. Adjusting classification cost function improves the Utility score of the tested models. Best results, on the investigated dataset, were achieved when the reward of true positive prediction was increased 20 times.
3. Feature ranking, using PCA, applied for our proposed features does not always improve Utility score. Utility score changes, when reducing the number of features based on the investigated model. In some models, such as Naive Gaussian, reducing the number of features improved the Utility score.
4. Performance metrics AUROC, AUPRC, and accuracy are not suitable for this highly unbalanced dataset. Additionally, these metrics do not reflect the Utility score. These metrics can be high for models with low Utility scores. Dealing with the early sepsis prediction problem, one should not apply these performance metrics. On the contrary, F-measure and MCC performance metrics reflect the Utility score.
5. High Utility score was obtained using decision tree models limited to 50 and fewer splits. All investigated decision trees chose ICULOS—ICU length of stay, as an important feature. Additionally, reducing the number of tree splits up to 4, and 1 further increased the Utility score. Utility score of 0.242 was achieved using only ICULOS as a single feature for the decision tree model.

Author Contributions: Conceptualization and methodology, all authors; validation, V.A. and D.T.; Analysis, A.S. and V.A.; writing—original draft preparation, A.S. and V.A.; project administration, A.S.; supervision, D.P.; writing—review and editing, all authors. All authors have read and agreed to the published version of the manuscript.

References

1. Singer, M.; Deutschman, C.S.; Seymour, C.W.; Shankar-Hari, M.; Annane, D.; Bauer, M.; Bellomo, R.; Bernard, G.R.; Chiche, J.D.; Coopersmith, C.M.; et al. The third international consensus definitions for sepsis and septic shock (sepsis-3). *JAMA* **2008**, *10*, 142–149. [CrossRef]
2. Vincent, J.L.; Marshall, J.C.; Ñamendys-Silva, S.A.; François, B.; Martin-Loeches, I.; Lipman, J.; Reinhart, K.; Antonelli, M.; Pickkers, P.; Njimi, H.; et al. Assessment of the worldwide burden of critical illness: The intensive care over nations (icon) audit. *Lancet Respir. Med.* **2014**, *2*, 380–386. [CrossRef]
3. Fleischmann, C.; Scherag, A.; Adhikari, N.K.; Hartog, C.S.; Tsaganos, T.; Schlattmann, P.; Angus, D.C.; Reinhart, K. Assessment of global incidence and mortality of hospital-treated sepsis. current estimates and limitations. *Am. J. Respir. Crit. Care Med.* **2016**, *193*, 259–272. [CrossRef]
4. Reinhart, K.; Daniels, R.; Kissoon, N.; Machado, F.R.; Schachter, R.D.; Finfer, S. Recognizing sepsis as a global health priority—A who resolution. *N. Engl. J. Med.* **2017**, *377*, 414–417. [CrossRef]
5. Reyna, M.A.; Josef, C.S.; Jeter, R.; Shashikumar, S.P.; Westover, M.B.; Nemati, S.; Clifford, G.D.; Sharma, A. Early prediction of sepsis from clinical data: The PhysioNet/Computing in Cardiology Challenge 2019. *Crit. Care Med.* **2020**, *48*, 210–217. [CrossRef]
6. Nemati, S.; Holder, A.; Razmi, F.; Stanley, M.D.; Clifford, G.D.; Buchman, T.G. An Interpretable Machine Learning Model for Accurate Prediction of Sepsis in the ICU. *Crit. Care Med.* **2018**, *46*, 547–553. [CrossRef] [PubMed]
7. Vicar, T.; Hejc, J.; Novotna, P.; Ronzhina, M.; Smisek, R. Sepsis Detection in Sparse Clinical Data Using Long Short-Term Memory Network with Dice Loss. In Proceedings of the 2019 Computing in Cardiology (CinC), Singapore, 8–11 September 2019.
8. Sweely, B.; Park, A.; Winter, L.; Liu, L.; Zhao, X. Time-Padded Random Forest Ensemble to Capture Changes in Physiology Leading to Sepsis Development. In Proceedings of the 2019 Computing in Cardiology (CinC), Singapore, 8–11 September 2019.
9. He, Z.; Chen, X.; Fang, Z.; Yi, W.; Wang, C.; Jiang, L.; Pan, Y. Early Sepsis Prediction Using Ensemble Learning with Features Extracted from LSTM Recurrent Neural Network. In Proceedings of the 2019 Computing in Cardiology (CinC), Singapore, 8–11 September 2019.
10. Li, X.; Kang, Y.; Jia, X.; Wang, J.; Xie, G. TASP: A Time-Phased Model for Sepsis Prediction. In Proceedings of the 2019 Computing in Cardiology (CinC), Singapore, 8–11 September 2019.
11. Nejedly, P.; Plesinger, F.; Viscor, I.; Halamek, J.; Jurak, P. Prediction of Sepsis Using LSTM with Hyperparameter Optimization with a Genetic Algorithm. In Proceedings of the 2019 Computing in Cardiology (CinC), Singapore, 8–11 September 2019.
12. Yang, M.; Wang, X.; Gao, H.; Li, Y.; Liu, X.; Li, J.; Liu, C. Early Prediction of Sepsis Using Multi-Feature Fusion Based XGBoost Learning and Bayesian Optimization. In Proceedings of the 2019 Computing in Cardiology (CinC), Singapore, 8–11 September 2019.
13. Morrill, J.; Kormilitzin, A.; Nevado-Holgado, A.; Swaminathan, S.; Howison, S.; Lyons, T. The Signature-Based Model for Early Detection of Sepsis from Electronic Health Records in the Intensive Care Unit. In Proceedings of the 2019 Computing in Cardiology (CinC), Singapore, 8–11 September 2019.
14. Anda Du, J.; Sadr, N.; de Chazal, P. Automated Prediction of Sepsis Onset Using Gradient Boosted Decision Trees. In Proceedings of the 2019 Computing in Cardiology (CinC), Singapore, 8–11 September 2019.
15. Hammoud, I.; Ramakrishnan, I.; Henry, M. Early Prediction of Sepsis Using Gradient Boosting Decision Trees with Optimal Sample Weighting. In Proceedings of the 2019 Computing in Cardiology (CinC), Singapore, 8–11 September 2019.
16. Singh, J.; Oshiro, K.; Krishnan, R.; Sato, M.; Ohkuma, T.; Kato, N. Utilizing Informative Missingness for Early Prediction of Sepsis. In Proceedings of the 2019 Computing in Cardiology (CinC), Singapore, 8–11 September 2019.
17. Tran, L.; Shahabi, C.; Nguyen, M. Representation Learning for Early Sepsis Prediction. In Proceedings of the 2019 Computing in Cardiology (CinC), Singapore, 8–11 September 2019.

18. DeCarlo, L.T. On the meaning and use of kurtosis. *Psychol. Methods* **1997**, *2*, 292. [CrossRef]
19. Dehmer, M. Information processing in complex networks: Graph entropy and information functionals. *Appl. Math. Comput.* **2008**, *201*, 82–94. [CrossRef]
20. Hamaker, E.L.; Ryan, O. A squared standard error is not a measure of individual differences. *Proc. Natl. Acad. Sci. USA* **2019**, *116*, 6544–6545. [CrossRef]
21. Tanha, J.; van Someren, M.; Afsarmanesh, H. Semi-supervised self-training for decision tree classifiers. *Int. J. Mach. Learn. Cybern.* **2017**, *8*, 355–370. [CrossRef]
22. Hu, B.; Wang, J.; Zhu, Y.; Yang, T. Dynamic Deep Forest: An Ensemble Classification Method for Network Intrusion Detection. *Electronics* **2019**, *8*, 968. [CrossRef]
23. Chen, Y.; Lu, L.; Yu, X.; Li, X. Adaptive Method for Packet Loss Types in IoT: An Naive Bayes Distinguisher. *Electronics* **2019**, *8*, 134. [CrossRef]
24. Gu, B.; Quan, X.; Gu, Y.; Sheng, V.S.; Zheng, G.S. Chunk incremental learning for cost-sensitive hinge loss support vector machine. *Pattern Recognit.* **2018**, *83*, 196–208. [CrossRef]
25. Biglarbeigi, P.; McLaughlin, D.; Rjoob, K.; Abdullah, A.; McCallan, N.; Jasinska-Piadlo, A.; Bond, R.; Finlay, D.; Ng, K.Y.; Kennedy, A.; et al. Early Prediction of Sepsis Considering Early Warning Scoring Systems. In Proceedings of the 2019 Computing in Cardiology (CinC), Singapore, 8–11 September 2019.
26. Ho, T.K. The random subspace method for constructing decision forests. *IEEE Trans. Pattern Anal. Mach. Intell.* **1998**, *20*, 832–844.
27. Boyd, K.; Eng, K.H.; Page, C.D. Area under the precision-recall curve: Point estimates and confidence intervals. In *Joint European Conference on Machine Learning and Knowledge Discovery in Databases*; Springer: Berlin/Heidelberg, Germany, 2013.
28. Saito, T.; Rehmsmeier, M. The precision-recall plot is more informative than the ROC plot when evaluating binary classifiers on imbalanced datasets. *PLoS ONE* **2015**, *10*, e0118432. [CrossRef] [PubMed]
29. Rousseau, R. The F-measure for research priority. *J. Data Inf. Sci.* **2018**, *3*, 1–18. [CrossRef]
30. Chicco, D.; Jurman, G. The advantages of the Matthews correlation coefficient (MCC) over F1 score and accuracy in binary classification evaluation. *BMC Genom.* **2020**, *21*, 6. [CrossRef]
31. Hong, S.; Shang, J.; Wu, M.; Zhou, Y.; Sun, Y.; Chou, Y.H.; Song, M.; Li, H. Early Sepsis Prediction with Deep Recurrent Reinforcement Learning. *Physionet Chall.* **2019**. Available online: https://docs.google.com/spreadsheets/d/1PPQY0SdguwCx_CxbR1BYlkh0dwpINlhEFxejc10xwgM/edit?fbclid=IwAR3psdL1QQ_PxlukPT89fE-v0ZVFgLdax11mrAeQwkdCO9WXeEKFfn8ek2o#gid=0 (accessed on 5 May 2020).
32. Murugesan, I.; Murugesan, K.; Balasubramanian, L.; Arumugam, M. Interpretation of Artificial Intelligence Algorithms in the Prediction of Sepsis. In Proceedings of the 2019 Computing in Cardiology (CinC), Singapore, 8–11 September 2019.
33. Narayanaswamy, L.; Garg, D.; Narra, B.; Narayanswamy, R. Machine Learning Algorithmic and System Level Considerations for Early Prediction of Sepsis. In Proceedings of the 2019 Computing in Cardiology (CinC), Singapore, 8–11 September 2019.
34. Alfaras, M.; Varandas, R.; Gamboa, H. Ring-Topology Echo State Networks for ICU Sepsis Classification. In Proceedings of the 2019 Computing in Cardiology (CinC), Singapore, 8–11 September 2019.
35. Deogire, A. A Low Dimensional Algorithm for Detection of Sepsis From Electronic Medical Record Data. In Proceedings of the 2019 Computing in Cardiology (CinC), Singapore, 8–11 September 2019.
36. Lauritsen, S.M.; Kalør, M.E.; Kongsgaard, E.L.; Lauritsen, K.M.; Jørgensen, M.J.; Lange, J.; Thiesson, B. Early detection of sepsis utilizing deep learning on electronic health record event sequences. *Early Detect. Sepsis Util. Deep Learn. Electron. Health Rec. Event Seq.* **2020**, *104*, 101820. [CrossRef]
37. Vincent, J.L. The clinical challenge of sepsis identification and monitoring. *PLoS Med.* **2016**, *13*, e1002022. [CrossRef]
38. Shimabukuro, D.W.; Barton, C.W.; Feldman, M.D.; Mataraso, S.J.; Das, R. Effect of a machine learning-based severe sepsis prediction algorithm on patient survival and hospital length of stay: A randomised clinical trial. *BMJ Open Respir. Res.* **2017**, *4*, e000234. [CrossRef] [PubMed]
39. Roussel, B.; Behar, J.; Oster, J. A Recurrent Neural Network for the Prediction of Vital Sign Evolution and Sepsis in ICU. In Proceedings of the 2019 Computing in Cardiology (CinC), Singapore, 8–11 September 2019.
40. Wan, R.; Mei, S.; Wang, J.; Liu, M.; Yang, F. Multivariate temporal convolutional network: A deep neural networks approach for multivariate time series forecasting. *Electronics* **2019**, *8*, 876. [CrossRef]

41. Mullick, S.S.; Datta, S.; Das, S. Daptive Learning-Based *k*-Nearest Neighbor Classifiers With Resilience to Class Imbalance. *IEEE Trans. Neural Networks Learn. Syst.* **2018**, *29*, 5713–5725.
42. Sawada, Y.; Sato, Y.; Nakada, T.; Yamaguchi, S.; Ujimoto, K.; Hayashi, N. Improvement in Classification Performance Based on Target Vector Modification for All-Transfer Deep Learning. *Appl. Sci.* **2019**, *9*, 128. [CrossRef]

8

Medical Assistant Mobile Application for Diabetes Control by Simulating a Compartmental Model

Martín Hernández-Ordoñez [1,*], Marco Aurelio Nuño-Maganda [2], Carlos Adrián Calles-Arriaga [2], Abelardo Rodríguez-León [3,*], Guillermo Efren Ovando-Chacon [1,*], Rolando Salazar-Hernández [4], Omar Montaño-Rivas [5] and José Margarito Canseco-Cortinas [2]

1 Department of Metal-Mechanics, México National Technological/I.T. Campus, Veracruz 91860, Mexico
2 Intelligent Systems Department, Polytechnic University of Victoria, Tamaulipas 87138, Mexico; mnunom@upv.edu.mx (M.A.N.-M.); ccallesa@upv.edu.mx (C.A.C.-A.); 1229002@upv.edu.mx (J.M.C.-C.)
3 Department of Systems and Computing, México National Technological/I.T. Campus, Veracruz 91860, Mexico
4 Facultad de Comercio, Administración y Ciencias Sociales, Universidad Autónoma de Tamaulipas, Tamaulipas 87000, Mexico; rsalazar@uat.edu.mx
5 Academy of Information Technologies, Polytechnic University of San Luis Potosí, San Luis 78369, Mexico; omar.montano@upslp.edu.mx
* Correspondence: martin.ho@veracruz.tecnm.mx (M.H.-O.); abelardo.rl@veracruz.tecnm.mx (A.R.-L.); guillermo.oc@veracruz.tecnm.mx (G.E.O.-C.)

Featured Application: Mobile application for iterative simulation of a diabetic model.

Abstract: This paper presents an educational mobile assistant application for type 1 diabetes patients. The proposed application is based on four mathematical models that describe the glucose-insulin-glucagon dynamics using a compartmental model, with additional equations to reproduce aerobic exercise, gastric glucose absorption by the gut, and subcutaneous insulin absorption. The medical assistant was implemented in Java and deployed and validated on several smartphones with Android OS. Multiple daily doses can be simulated to perform intensive insulin therapy. As a result, the proposed application shows the influence of exercise periods, food intakes, and insulin treatments on the glucose concentrations. Four parameter variations are studied, and their corresponding glucose concentration plots are obtained, which show agreement with simulators of the state of the art. The developed application is focused on type-1 diabetes, but this can be extended to consider type-2 diabetes by modifying the current mathematical models.

Keywords: mathematical models; Iterative simulation; compartmental model; diabetes control; mobile assistant

---

1. Introduction

In recent years, obesity and overweight have become a severe problem for human health. In 2014 more than 1.9 billion adults aged 18 and older were overweight globally, from which over 600 million were obese. The data indicated that 39% of these adults were overweight and 13% were obese [1]. Body mass index (BMI) provides the most useful population-level measure of overweight and obesity as it is the same for both sexes and all ages of adults. Patients with higher BMI are at greater risk for having diabetes. In 2014, more than 422 million people had diabetes in the world, with a global prevalence of 8.5% among adults over 18 years old. Diabetes is a leading cause of blindness, kidney failure, heart attacks, stroke and lower limb amputation. In 2012, an estimated 1.5 million deaths were directly caused by diabetes, and another 2.2 million deaths were attributable to high blood glucose [2]. Diabetes was promoted from 21st place in 1990 to the 14th in 2010 in the list of death causes worldwide [3], and recently, to the 6th place in 2016 [4].

In Mexico, about 72.5% of adults from 18 years and over, 36.3% of teenagers, and 33.2% of children were overweight or obese in 2016. Diabetes statistics are not too optimistic; Mexico is in sixth place in countries with more diabetes, just behind China, India, US, Brazil and Russia [5]. Recent statistics show that 9.17% of adults from 18 years (about 6.4 million people) have diabetes [6]. Type 2 diabetes has become the leading cause of death in Mexico. The disease claims nearly 80,000 lives each year, and forecasters say the health problem is expected to get worse in the decades to come [7].

On the other hand, smartphones have been accessible to more people due to the high worldwide market growth rate. In 2016, around 1.5 billion smartphones were sold worldwide [8]; by the end of 2016, more than 3.2 billion individuals worldwide used the Internet regularly, accounting for nearly 45% of the world's population; about 2.5 billion people access the web via mobile phone [9], which represents novel opportunities for designing applications running on smartphones, accessible to large population groups. Specifically, healthcare and disease management have benefited with applications such as fitness tracking, drug dose calculators, information apps, tutorials, surveys, diaries, and other tools created to help empower users to put more emphasis on their health care. Some benefits of using smartphones with Internet connectivity consists of the possibility of sharing data with family, friends, classmates, colleges, collaborators but especially with professionals who can guide the user and give feedback regarding treatment to be followed.

This paper is structured as follows. In Section 2, a concise review of the state of the art is given. A description of the models used in the developed application is provided in Section 3. In Section 4, the results and discussion are described. Finally, in Section 5, the conclusion is presented where final recalls are established, and future work is outlined.

2. State of the Art

2.1. PC or Web Simulators for Glucose Concentration Levels

In recent years, an effort to implement glucose levels simulators has been made. One standard option for implementing simulators are PCs or Laptops. PCs have as their main advantage the inherent high computational power for performing simulations. In addition, there has been a trend to replace PCs with much more compact devices, such as smartphones, but most simulators for glucose concentration are PC-based. Another implementation option consists of Web systems, allowing for a broad range of devices to access such simulation systems. Web-based simulators have an advantage: many platforms can access the simulator compared to a particular PC implementation. Web-based simulators have as main disadvantage the requirement of Internet connectivity, making the simulator difficult to access in places with connectivity problems.

In [10], the AIDA diabetes simulator is presented, and extensive evaluation about this simulator has been reported in [11]. Recently, new types of rapid-acting insulins have been added to the AIDA diabetes simulator [12]. AIDA's mathematical model was created to simulate glucose tolerance; however, its use is not based on daily periods.

In [13], the REACTION project is presented. This project consists of a set of healthcare services oriented to diabetic patients and caregivers through a cloud-based application focusing on management and therapy services. The REACTION project is a management system created for the implementation of logistics related to medical personnel. The dosage management algorithm is based on basic rules, and it is not a pharmacological-dynamic behavioral study of insulin. In other words, it is a mathematical model with experimental parameters.

In [14], GLUCOSIM is proposed as a desktop application designed to do virtual experiments to show the effects of food intake changes and insulin therapy on glucose levels. A more detailed version of this system is reported in [15], where a Web-based solution was included. It is important to mention that GLUCOSIM is a tool designed to study, train and analyze the external effects that modify glucose concentration. It uses three mathematical models to consider all the mentioned effects; however, it does not describe periods of exercise or other modeled effects.

In [16], a system is proposed based on the combination of Compartmental Models (CMs) and artificial Neural Networks (NNs). Data from a Type 1 diabetes patient, which contains information about measured blood glucose levels, insulin intake, and food intake description, along with the corresponding time, were used as input to the model. The proposed strategy was not adequately validated. Furthermore, no performance criteria were mentioned to assess the results objectively.

The literature review indicates that early studies of compartmental modelling of glucose/insulin interactions were proposed since the 1980s in [17–19]. On the other hand, recently, different research groups have reported important works related with the implementations of compartmental models to develop glucose level simulators, for example, in [20,21] are presented a glucose forecasting algorithm based on a compartmental composite model of glucose-insulin dynamics. In [22] is developed a dynamic model for type 1 diabetic patient that focuses on blood glucose regulation. A first model for insulin adsorption in infusion sets using a minimal lumped two-compartment modelling approach is reported in [23]. A review of the key role of the UVA/Padova simulator is presented in [24], which has tested the use of new molecules for better glucose control.

2.2. Mobile Applications for Diabetes Management

The universe of mobile applications for diabetes care is enormous. A first step consists in determining the utility of apps. One standard classification includes exercise and fitness apps, med adherence, weight management, blood glucose trackers, support, healthcare professional apps, and educational simulators. There is extensive availability of applications related to any of the previously mentioned apps, but few efforts are related to educational simulators for smartphones.

One interesting branch of smartphone applications for health care is the simulators. In this paper, we are specifically interested in creating a smartphone-based simulator of glucose-insulin metabolism. In recent years, there have been advances in creating models that can replicate the behavior of parts (or entire) of human organisms and their corresponding implementation as a computer simulation. A smartphone-based simulation can be useful for patients with recently diagnosed diabetes to help them estimate the insulin doses and food intake, but also for patients at risk of developing diabetes or without diabetes, for contributing to raising awareness of the benefits of changing their food consumption and exercise habits. In [25], a review of several diabetes simulators is presented, but the applications reported in that paper is out of the scope of this work, since there is an interest in providing a realistic simulation of blood glucose levels.

There are several reviews of applications for diabetes management. In [26], a set of critical factors to be considered when designing diabetes management applications are explored. These factors come from patient demographics, technology costs, platform varieties, and ease of use. They also categorize the applications in the following classes: blood glucose logging, nutrition databases, carbohydrate tracking, tracking physical activity and weight, data-sharing and social support, and short messages and reminders. An important point to consider is that the FDA does not approve most applications. In [27], several commercial applications for diabetes management available on the Apple App Store and articles published in relevant databases are reviewed. The reviewed applications support self-management tasks such as physical exercise, insulin dosage or medication, blood glucose testing, and diet. Other support tasks considered include decision support, notification/alert, tagging of input data, and social media integration. Analysis indicates that application usage is associated with improved attitudes favorable to diabetes self-management. Limitations of the applications include lack of personalized feedback; usability issues, particularly the ease of data entry; and integration with patients and electronic health records. In much more detail, in [28], it is concluded that a critical feature strongly recommended by clinical guidelines—namely, personalized education is not assimilated in current diabetes applications. In [29] a critical assessment was reported of several smartphone apps for calculating insulin dose. The conclusion was that popular apps offering insulin dose calculations carry a risk of incorrect dose recommendations ranging from those that might lead to suboptimal disease control to those with potentially life-threatening consequences. In [30], an analysis of the benefits of smartphone apps for type 2 diabetes mellitus (T2DM) self-management was presented. It can be concluded that more research with valid study designs and longer follow-up is needed to evaluate the impact of health apps for diabetes care and self-management, specifically for T2DM. In [31], both Heuristic and keystroke level modeling (KLM) are used to measure efficiency for each analyzed mobile diabetes management application for patients with Type-1 Diabetes Mellitus.

With recent advances in connectivity technologies, there are some efforts to build tools based on cloud computing [32] or social network support [33,34]. One disadvantage of these tools is that they always require Internet connectivity at all times, which makes them useless in places with connectivity problems. Some applications are targeted to a particular segment of the population, such as pregnant women; one of these applications is reported in [35,36], where a tool to follow patients with gestational diabetes is described. In [37], an application for insulin dose calculation is reported. The authors establish that this application's innovation consists of the incorporation of exercise and alcohol intake to the calculator in addition to carbohydrates intake. In [38], an application created explicitly for controlling an insulin pump taking as real-time input data from a continuous glucose monitor is reported. A closed-loop control system used to automatically manage insulin infusion to maintain the desire range´s glucose level is proposed. To summarize, there is a strong interest from the scientific community in developing applications around the problems associated with diabetes. This article adds to this trend with an emphasis on the exercise model.

3. Models

The idea of creating an artificial model for a glucose-insulin system for several purposes has been widely explored. In [39], a minimal glucose-insulin system is proposed; the model starts with the Bergman model [17] and presents modifications to improve, considering the glucose level´s description in the subcutaneous layer and a meal disturbance term. The developed application uses four mathematical models related to them, following the different dynamics that they describe:

1. Glucose-Insulin Model: Sorensen in [40] proposed it. This model comprises 19 nonlinear differential equations, which include significant metabolic effects related to glucose regulation. The model was obtained through a compartmental technique, where the pancreas compartment is omitted to consider a type 1 diabetic patient. Recently, this glucose-insulin model was extended to consider exercise periods [41].
2. Subcutaneous Insulin model: Berger and Rodbard [42] obtained it. This model describes the subcutaneous insulin uptake pattern after an insulin injection. The model considers interactions between components after subcutaneous injections such as insulin absorption and elimination in plasma insulin, active insulin, glucose utilization, plasma glucose, and glucose input. The model is based on a set of differential equations. Variations in plasma insulin concentration (I) can be estimated by Equation (1).

$$\frac{dI}{dt} = \frac{I_{abs}}{V_i} - k_e \cdot I \tag{1}$$

where I_{abs} represents the rate of insulin absorption, V_i is the volume of insulin distribution, and k_e is the first-order rate constant of insulin elimination. The absorption of insulin can be calculated as follows:

$$I_{abs} = \frac{st^2 T_{50}^s D}{t\left(T_{50}^s + t^s\right)^2} \tag{2}$$

where s is a parameter associated with the insulin absorption pattern, t represents the time of the injection, T_{50} is when the dose (D) is absorbed in an amount of 50%.

3. To estimate steady-state conditions, insulin profile (I_{ss}) using the superposition principle is computed assuming three days as follows:

$$I_{ss}(t) = \mathrm{I}(t) + I(t+24) + I(t+48) \tag{3}$$

$$I_{a,ss}(t) = \mathrm{I}_a(t) + I_a(t+24) + I_a(t+48) \tag{4}$$

where I_a is the build-up and the deactivation of the insulin pump.

4. Meal Intake model: this model was proposed in 1992 by Lehmann and Deutsch [43]. It describes the gastric glucose absorption into the bloodstream by a meal intake represented by its carbohydrates content. According to this model, glucose utilization G_{out} (G) at plasma insulin concentration is:

$$G_{out}(G) = \frac{V_{max}G}{k_m + G} \tag{5}$$

G represents the glucose concentration, V_{max} maximal glucose utilization for reference insulin concentration, and K_m is glucose concentration for the half-maximal response. V_{max} depends on insulin; mathematically, this is

$$V_{max}(I_{ss}) = \frac{G_{out}(I_{ss})(K_m + G_x)}{G_x} \tag{6}$$

where I_{ss} is plasma insulin concentration equivalent to steady-state insulin, and G_x is the reference glucose value. Glucose utilization for any combination of plasma glucose and insulin levels is given by

$$G_{out}(G, I_{ss}) = \frac{G(c \cdot I_{ss} + d)(K_m + G_x)}{G_x(K_m + G)} \tag{7}$$

where c is insulin sensitivity, and d represents insulin-independent glucose utilization. The insulin absorption dynamics for regular, NPH, lente, ultralente formulations were characterized in [42] just by changing some specific parameters in the general model. Recently, in [44], the Lispro insulin formulation was also characterized by the model in [42].

5. The exercise model was considered from [41]. The liver's glycogen reservoir (GLY) can be calculated as shown in Equation (8).

$$\frac{dGLY(t)}{dt} = -\varnothing\left(PVO_2^{max}(t), GLY(t)\right) + \Psi(G_{abs}(t) + GLY(t)) \tag{8}$$

$$\varnothing\left(PVO_2^{max}, GLY\right) = \begin{cases} \varsigma\left(PVO_2^{max}\right) & \text{if} \quad 0 < GLY \le GLY_{max} \\ 0 & \text{if} \quad GLY \ge 0 \end{cases} \tag{9}$$

$$\Psi(G_{abs}, GLY) = \begin{cases} G_{abs} & \text{if} \quad GLY < GLY_{max} \\ 0 & \text{if} \quad GLY > GLY_{max} \end{cases} \tag{10}$$

$$\varsigma\left(PVO_2^{max}\right) = 0.006\left(PVO_2^{max}\right)^2 + 1.226PVO_2^{max} - 10.1958\ \text{mg/min} \tag{11}$$

where φ is the net glycogenolysis rate, Ψ represents the absorptive period, ζ is the glucose uptake due to exercise intensity, and $PVO_2{}^{max}$ is the percentage of the maximum oxygen consumption rate.

In Figure 1, the block diagram of the diabetic patient utilized in this work is shown. There are four subsystems, each one corresponds to a previously described model, and their interactions are shown as solid arrows. The dotted lines delimit the mathematical models proposed in the literature, which describe different but comparable physiological phenomena because they have the same scale.

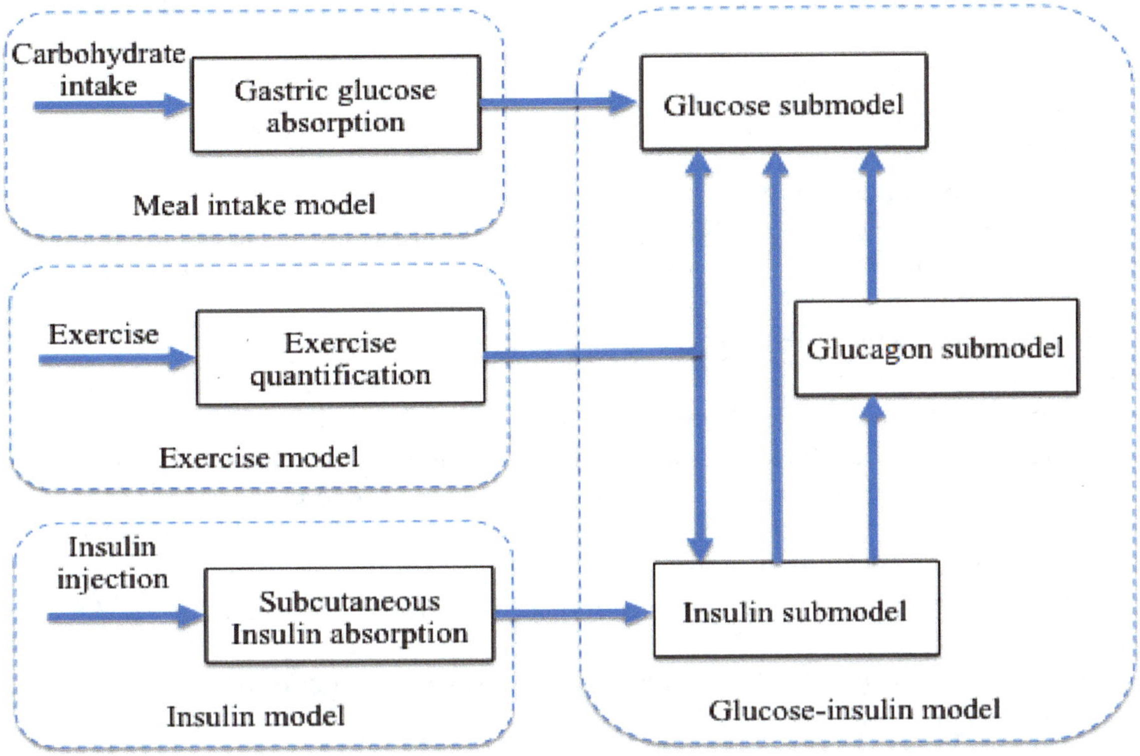

Figure 1. The diabetic patient model utilized for the implementation of simulations reported in this work.

4. Results and Discussion

4.1. *Mobile Application for Educational Similar*

4.1.1. Hardware and Software Tools

The proposed education simulator was developed based on the models described in the last section. The models were implemented in Java using Android Studio IDE with Android Studio SDK and Java SE Development Kit; besides, Android MPChart Library is used for showing results of the glucose level simulation in a plot [45].

The proposed application was validated on devices with several versions of Android. Table 1, shows the list of devices and its specifications used for testing the proposed application.

Table 1. Devices utilized for testing the proposed application.

Device	Processor	RAM	Android Version
Galaxy S2	Dual-core 1.2 GHz Cortex-A9	1 GB	4.1
Galaxy S4	Dual-core 1.7 GHz Krait 300	1.5 GB	5.0.1
Polaroid Tab	Dual-core 1.0 GHz Broadcom 21663	1 GB	4.2.2
Galaxy Tab 10.1	Quad-core 2.3 GHz Krait 400	3 GB	5.1.1
LG G3 Stylus	Quad-core 1.3 GHz Cortex-A7	1 GB	5.0.2

4.1.2. System Architecture

In Figure 2, the architecture of the proposed application is shown. The architecture takes as an input the following data:

1. Meal parameters: these parameters are related to carbohydrate intake (in grams) and the day´s carbohydrate intake schedule.

2. Insulin dose parameters: these parameters are related to the type (fast or slow actions) and the dose of insulin (in units).
3. Exercise parameters: these parameters are related to the quantity and intensity of exercise.
4. Simulation configuration: these parameters are related to the simulation's duration and the type of plot to be generated.
5. The architecture contains the following blocks:
6. Simulation variables container: this block stores data required to be accessed and shared by all model blocks. It contains three profiles: meal dosing, insulin dosing, and exercise quantification.
7. Meal model block: this block takes as input the meal profile and generates as output the glucose obtained according to the carbohydrate intake grams.
8. Insulin model block: this block takes as input the insulin dosing profile and generates as output the quantity and duration of insulin in the blood flow.
9. Exercise model block: this block takes as input the exercise dosing profile and generates as output the blood redistribution volume according to the quantity of exercise.
10. Simulation loop block: this block updates each model block with required data from others and controls the simulation's start and end.
11. Plot generation module: this block generates data from the simulation to be used for generating a plot.
12. Plot visualization module: this block takes as input the vector generated by the plot generation module and displays the plot.

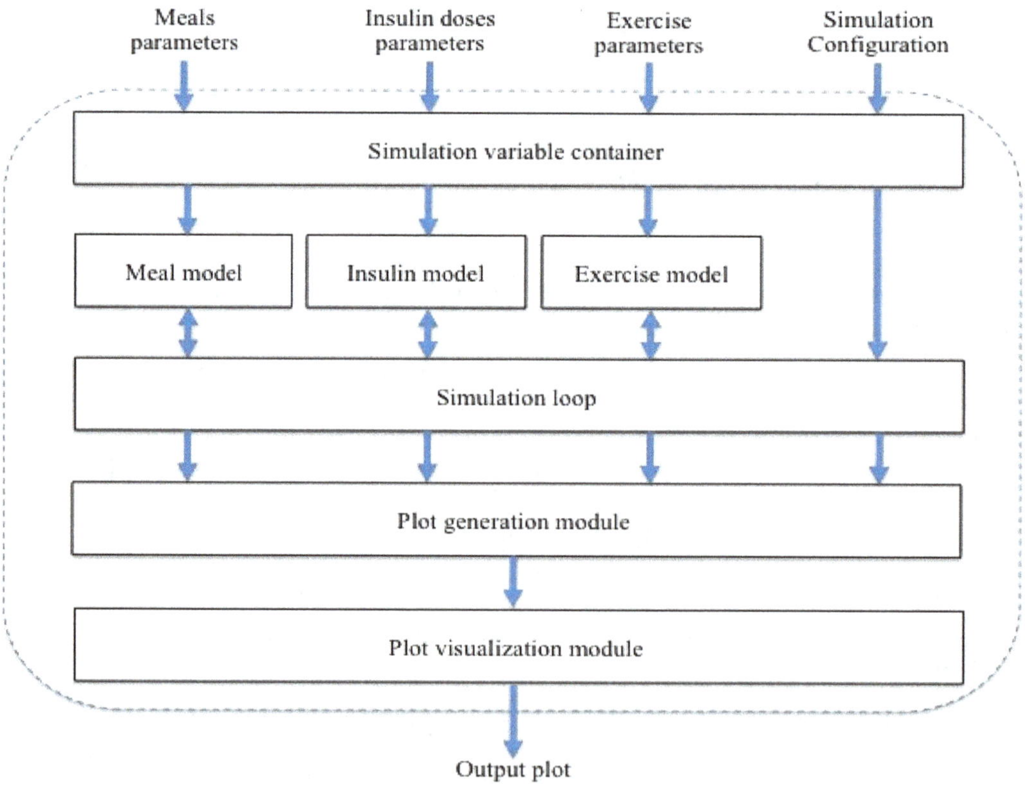

Figure 2. The system architecture.

Finally, the architecture generates as the output the plot with the information according to the user's input.

4.1.3. User Interface

In Figure 3a, a welcome screen of the proposed application is shown. The proposed application's main objective is the generation of a plot of the blood glucose concentration based on the parameters defined in the previous section. For user commodity and better distribution application's controls, a tabbed document interface (TDI) was conceived as the main container for hosting all the needed user controls required to set the simulation parameters and show the results. Specifically, for the Android SDK environment, a tab host container was utilized. This control enables the integration of plenty of components in a single form. The proposed application contains four tabs: the first three tabs allow the user to define the parameters of meal, insulin, and exercise models, and the last one is designed to generate simulation data and show the blood glucose concentration in a plot.

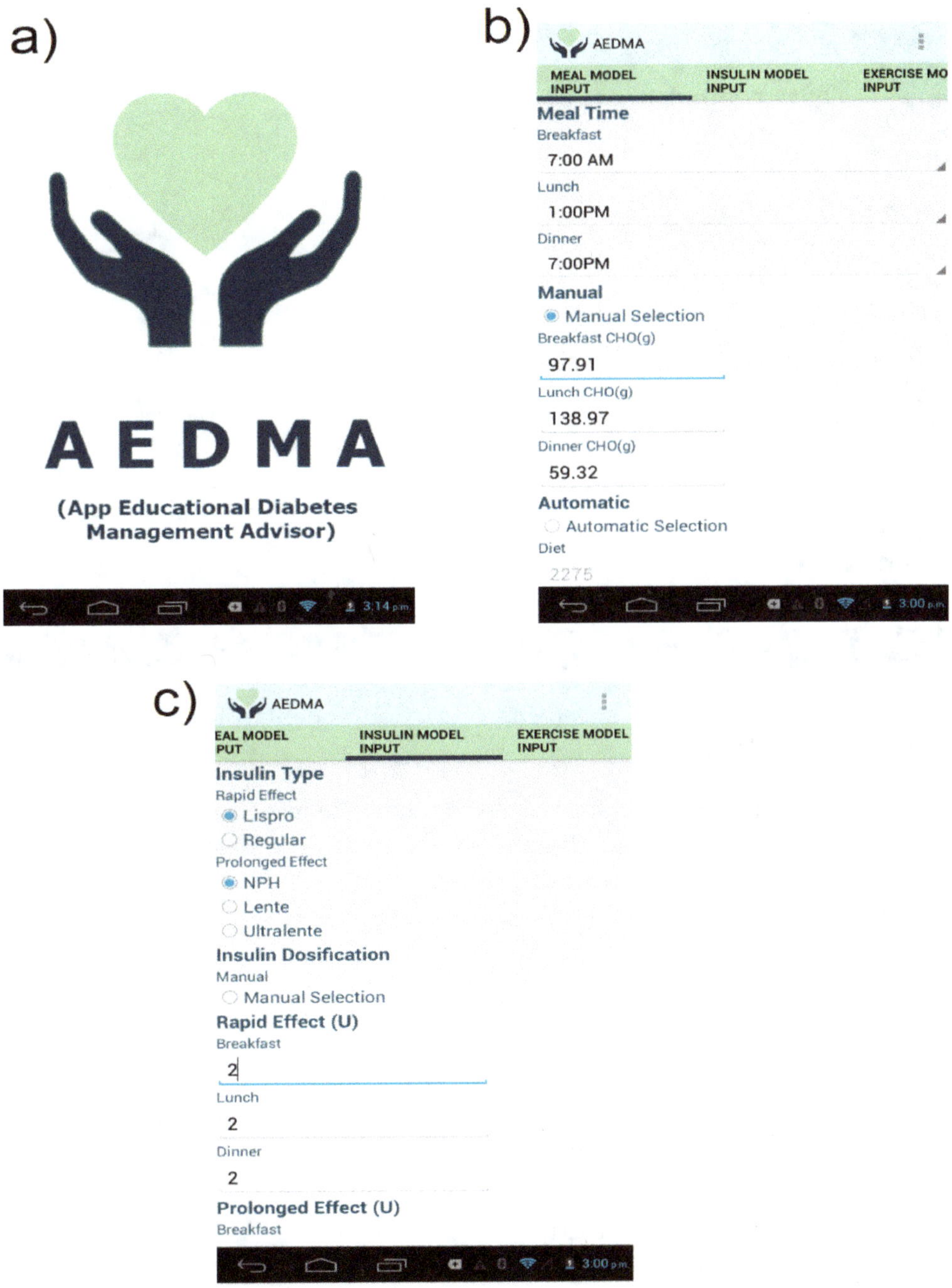

Figure 3. Screens of the proposed AEDMA app. (**a**) Main screen of the proposed applications. (**b**) Components of the meal model input Table. (**c**) Components of the insulin model tab.

In Figure 3b, the tab for the meal model parameters is shown. This tab contains interface controls where users can define each meal's time and its estimated carbohydrate contents (in grams). The estimated carbohydrate contents also can be automatically calculated based on a default estimation of calories for a day, or user can input the total calories, and the application estimates the carbohydrate content in grams based on the given calories.

In Figure 3c, the tab for the insulin model is shown. This tab contains interface controls that define the type of insulin and the unit to be dosed in each meal, for both the rapid and prolonged effect.

In Figure 4a, the tab for the exercise model is shown. This tab contains interface controls where the user defines the intensity, duration, start time, and exercise routine.

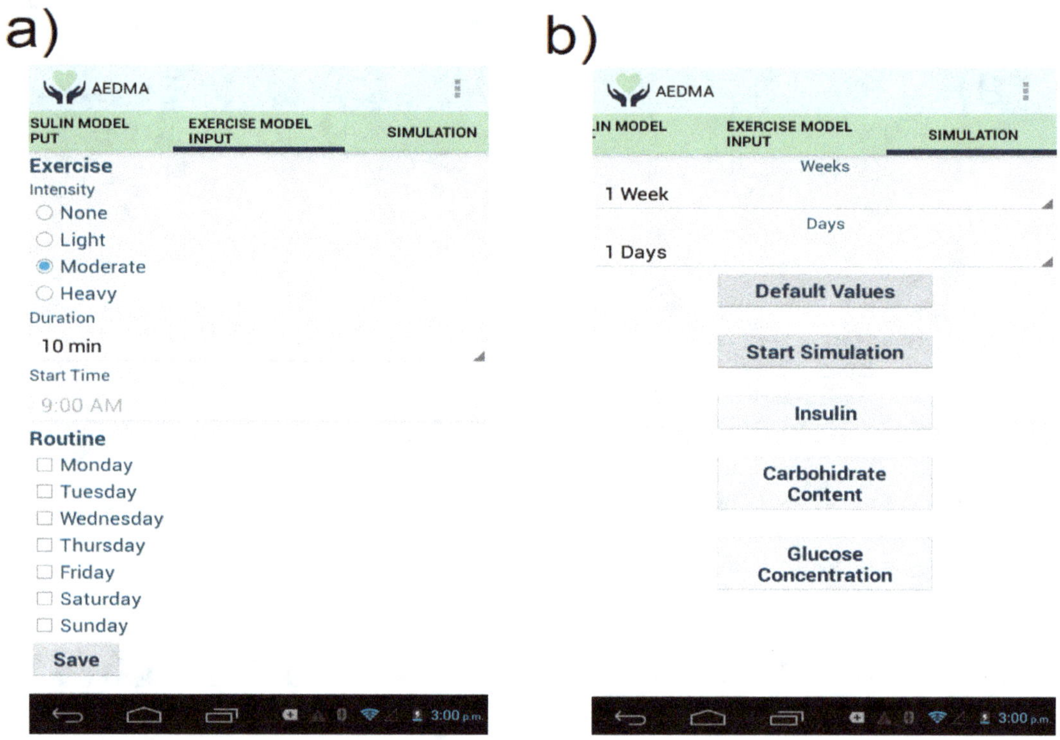

Figure 4. The last two configuration screens. (**a**) Components of the exercise model Table. (**b**) Components of the simulations tab.

In Figure 4b, the tab for simulation is shown. In this tab, the user defines the time of the simulation in weeks and days. It is also possible to set all variables to their default values, start simulation, shown insulin, carbohydrate, or glucose concentration plots.

In Table 2, the application's default values are listed, but the user can syntonize this to get a better understanding of the model behavior.

Table 2. Default parameter values for the proposed application.

Meal Model	
Breakfast time	7:00 AM
Lunch time	1:00 PM
Dinner time	7:00 PM
Breakfast CHO (g)	97.91
Lunch CHO (g)	138.97
Dinner CHO (g)	59.32

Table 2. *Cont.*

Insulin Model	
Rapid effect insulin type	Lispro
Prolonged effect insulin Type	NPH
Rapid effect insulin units at breakfast	2
Rapid effect insulin units at lunch	2
Rapid effect insulin units at dinner	2
Prolonged effect insulin units at breakfast	3
Prolonged effect insulin units at dinner	3
Exercise Model	
Intensity	Light
Duration	10 min
Start time	9:00 AM
Routine	Monday checked

4.2. Reported Experiments

In Table 3, the parameters utilized for validating the meal and insulin models are shown. The abbreviations in the column names are experiment number (Exp), carbohydrate grams in breakfast (B-CHO), carbohydrate grams in lunch (L-CHO), carbohydrate grams in dinner (D-CHO), insulin units at breakfast (B-u), insulin units at lunch (L-u), insulin units at dinner (D-u). In the first experiment, the default values for carbohydrate and insulin units are used. In the second experiment, carbohydrate grams are reduced to half, but the insulin units are left at their default values. In the third experiment, default values for carbohydrate grams are used, but the insulin dose is doubled, and in the last experiment, carbohydrate grams are reduced to half, and the insulin dose is doubled.

Table 3. Selected parameters set of four experiments.

Exp	Meal			Insulin Dossification						
	Carbohydrate Grams Intake			Rapid Effect				Prolongated Effect		
	B-CHO	L-CHO	D-CHO	Type	B-u	L-u	D-u	Type	B-u	D-u
1	97.91	138.97	59.32	Lispro	2	2	2	NPH	3	3
2	49.85	69.48	29.66	Lispro	2	2	2	NPH	3	3
3	97.91	138.97	59.32	Lispro	4	4	4	NPH	6	6
4	49.85	69.48	29.66	Lispro	4	4	4	NPH	6	6

Figure 5 shows a glucose concentration plot for a 5-day simulation for each experiment reported in Table 3. In Figure 5a, the maximum glucose peak is close to 195 mg/dL every day of the reported simulation. In contrast, in Figure 5b, the maximum glucose peak surpasses 175 mg/dL due to the reduction of carbohydrate intake. In Figure 5c, the same carbohydrate intake is used, but both prolonged and rapid insulin doses are doubled. It can be shown that glucose levels are lower when compared with the plot of experiment 1, and in Figure 5d, also the carbohydrate intake is reduced to half to validate both meal and insulin models. In both experiments (3 and 4), it can be shown for its corresponding plots that even a risk of hyperglycemia is present due to the high insulin dose.

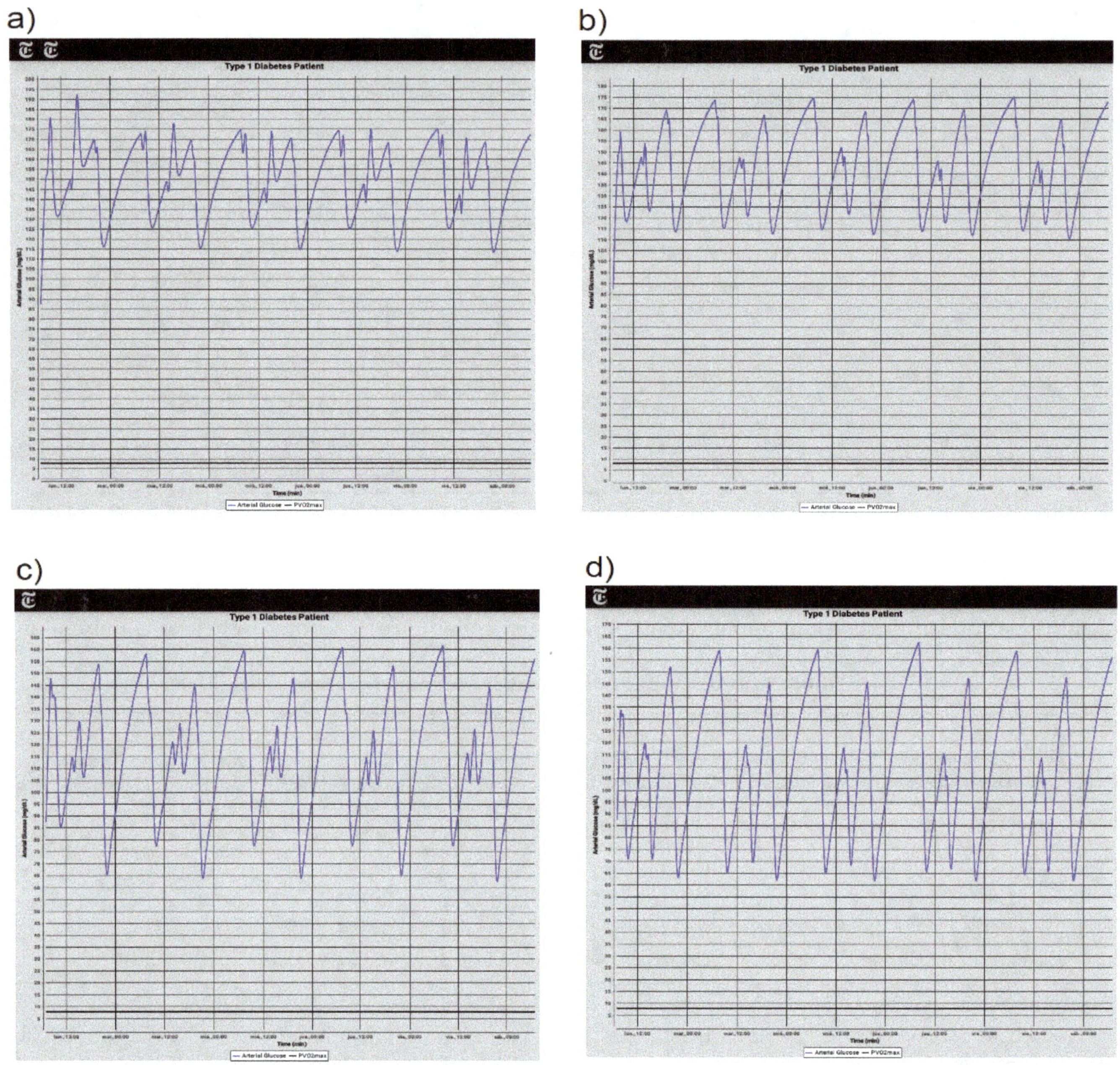

Figure 5. Comparison of blood glucose plots generated by AEDMA application for several values of carbohydrate grams and insulin units. (**a**) Experiment 1. (**b**) Experiment 2. (**c**) Experiment 3. (**d**) Experiment 4.

In Figure 6, a validation of the exercise models through the corresponding simulation plots are shown. In order to obtain the reported plots, the used exercise intensities are light, moderate, and heavy, and the exercise durations are 10, 30, and 90 min. The default values for grams of carbohydrate intake and insulin doses are used. In Figure 6a, the simulation using 10 min of light exercise is shown. The value of the glucose peaks after exercise (at 9:00 AM) is close to 185 mg/dL, but using 30 min of light exercise, this is under 180 mg/dL (Figure 6b), and when using 90 min of light exercise, the glucose peaks is close to 175 mg/dL (Figure 6c). Similar behavior is shown when using the same duration but with moderate exercise (Figure 6d–f). The value of the glucose peaks after exercise (at 9:00 AM) is close to 175 mg/dL, and it is low when compared with the same peak obtained when using light exercise (180 mg/dL). Finally, this behavior remains when using heavy exercise (Figure 6g–i). For comparing exercise intensities, it can be shown from plots that the glucose peaks after 10 min exercise are: close to

185 mg/dL for light exercise, over 175 mg/dL for moderate exercise, and below 170 mg/dL for heavy exercise. Similar results are obtained for 30 and 90 min of exercise duration. In general, there are many applications, however, long-term prediction of glucose still remains a challenge [20]. In this work, an app has been developed capable of predicting the behavior of glucose levels for several days (see Figure 5) or during a day with different exercise regimes (see Figure 6).

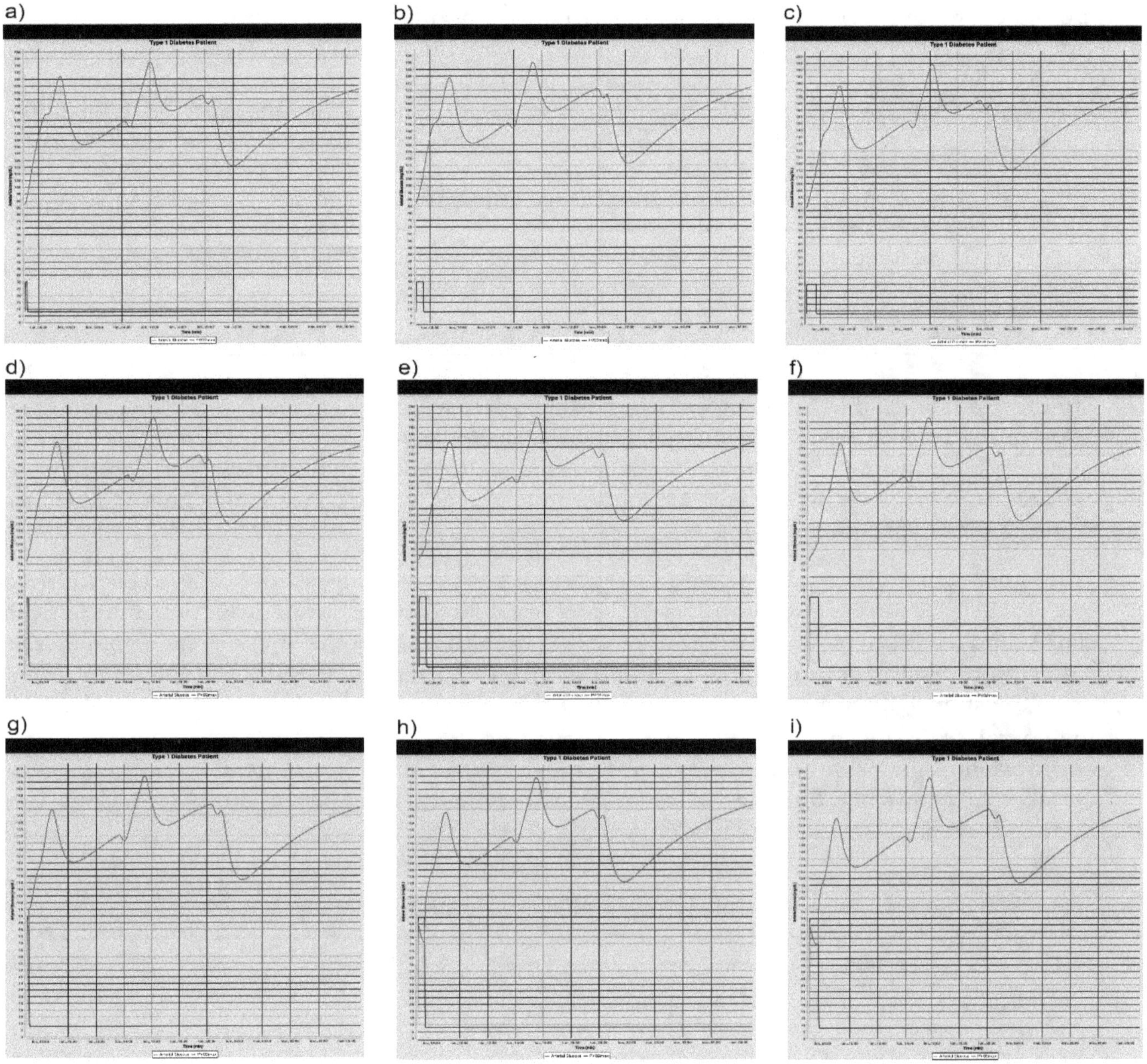

Figure 6. Comparison of blood glucose plots generated by AEDMA application for several exercise intensities using experiment 1 settings. (**a**) Light exercise—10 min. (**b**) Light exercise—30 min. (**c**) Light exercise—90 min. (**d**) Moderate exercise—10 min. (**e**) Moderate exercise—30 min. (**f**) Moderate exercise—90 min. (**g**) Heavy exercise—10 min. (**h**) Heavy exercise—30 min. (**i**) Heavy exercise—90 min.

Until now, the complete software of the presented application has not been compared with other applications since our priority is to focus on the diet and physical activity of the Mexican population with diabetes. There are many applications, but with European or United States standards. However, each submodel has been compared and validated separately by its respective authors. It is important to point out that the current version of the application presented in this work is an extension of a previous compartmental model that takes into account exercise periods. This model was developed by the main author, who validated and compared its results with experimental data [41]. So far, we have performed a prototype test on 26 young adults and execution times comparison for different devices.

4.3. Qualitative Study

For validating the AEDMA, we perform a prototype test using a questionnaire to evaluate the main points of the proposed system. We applied a questionnaire to 26 young adults (age 15–25). This application is focused mainly on this user group, which is highly familiar with tablet or smartphone devices, and they are regular users of mobile apps. We restrict the participants of the prototype test to have an android device because we designed AEDMA specifically for this mobile OS. In Table 4, relevant information about the distribution of the testing subjects is shown.

Table 4. Relevant data of testing subjects.

Gender		Age		Previous Knowledge of Mobiles Apps for Diabetes Treatment	
Male	Female	15–19	20–25	Yes	No
76.9%	23.1%	38.5%	61.5%	15.4%	84.6%

After testing the ADEMA by at least 1 h in the participant's device, they were asked to answer a questionnaire that contains 10 questions related to the key aspects of the AEDMA. Each question has 5 options, rated from NO, Rather NO, Do not know, Rather YES, and YES. The questions and the percentage of responses for each option are summarized in Table 5. From the obtained responses, we can summarize the following remarks:

1. From questions 1, 3, 4, and 5, a preliminary conclusion about important points to be improved to the AEDMA can be guessed. These points are related to improving the user interface, the clarity, and legibility of presented glucose level graphs, and the ease of use of the app. Question 8 gives a general panorama showing that the mobile app in its current state can be improved. From question 9, the variability of glucose levels is adequate from the user's perspective.
2. In general, from questions 2 and 7, we can conclude that the AEDMA is useful and to give an appropriate impression to the test user, to reuse the application if a next version is released. Question 10 allows highlighting the importance of giving users an important role to involve them in the design of these types of apps.

Table 5. Results of the questionnaire for the test group.

Question	1 (No)%	2 (Rather No)%	3 (Do Not Know)%	4 (Rather Yes)%	5 (Yes)%
(1) Are the user interface controls adequate to the type of data required by the app?	15.4%	15.4%	15.4%	38.5%	15.4%
(2) Is the application useful?	23.1%	0%	0%	0%	76.9%
(3) Are the generated graphs easy to understand?	7.7%	0%	23.1%	46.2%	23.1%
(4) Do the application's user interface controls allow to manage the application in an ease way?	0%	7.7%	7.7%	46.2%	38.5%
(5) How difficult has been the use of the app?	15.4%	38.5%	30.8%	15.4%	0%
(6) Does the application motivate to study more in depth the phenomena?	0%	0%	15.4%	46.2%	38.5%
(7) Will you reuse the app?	0%	7.7%	7.7%	15.4%	69.2%
(8) Do you consider that current app can be improved?	7.7%	0%	0%	23.1%	69.2%
(9) Do you consider appropriate the functionality of the application for learning the glucose levels variability?	0%	0%	7.7%	38.5%	53.8%
(10) Do you consider the mobile application are sufficient to assess whether in the future you would like to participate in similar experiences with mobile apps?	0%	0%	23.1%	38.5%	38.5%

4.4. Execution Time Comparison

We obtain a measurement of the time required to conclude the simulation using several parameters for each application's deployment device. Table 6 shows the obtained measurements for each device. We compute each measurement using only one thread environment because a multithread environment was not conceived in the original application. We choose the following simulation times: 4 days, one week, two weeks, and three weeks. A Polaroid tablet device obtained the biggest execution time, while a Galaxy Tab 10.1 device obtained the shortest one. The rows in Table 6 start from the slower to the higher simulation time. The mobile devices used for the application's deployment were not recent models, because even when some of them were featured as high-end devices when released, they are old devices and, with recent advances in mobile technology, many of them can be featured as low or middle-end devices when compared with the existing technology available at the time of writing this paper.

Table 6. Time to complete computation of glucose concentration plots (in seconds) using several simulation time durations.

Device	Simulation Time Duration			
	4 Days	1 Week	2 Weeks	3 Weeks
Polaroid Tab	12.30	13.53	16.24	21.11
Galaxy S2	9.53	10.97	13.16	18.16
Galaxy S4	6.53	7.64	9.17	12.84
LG G3 Stylus	5.53	6.59	7.90	11.30
Galaxy Tab 10.1	5.53	6.70	8.04	11.73

5. Conclusions

In this paper, an application for diabetes education is proposed. The proposed application was designed to provide a software tool to help support therapy in patients with diabetes, seeking to improve the quality of life. The simulation is fixed, but an interactive simulation functionality can be added to provide a richer user experience. The software is based on four mathematical models originally designed as a desktop computer program. An exercise option in the interface helps patients to schedule their routines and to estimate in advance its impact on blood glucose. This app could also be developed for Apples' iOS products. Besides, this app could potentially be implemented as a smartwatch app. The most important conclusions are:

1. The App includes glucose regulation associated with metabolism and the application of an insulin injection.
2. The App is capable of taking into account the effects of food intake and physical activity.
3. The developed application can simulate the behavior of glucose levels for long periods.
4. The App is capable of considering three types of physical activity: light, moderate and heavy.
5. The developed application is focused on type-1 diabetes, but this can be extended to consider type-2 diabetes.
6. As a future improvement, the application should be modified to split the simulation processing into smaller operations running on multiple threads. This could be beneficial in devices with more than one core.

Author Contributions: Conceptualization, M.H.-O., M.A.N.-M.; Formal Analysis, C.A.C.-A., A.R.-L.; Investigation, M.A.N.-M., G.E.O.-C., J.M.C.-C.; Methodology, M.H.-O., C.A.C.-A., G.E.O.-C., R.S.-H., O.M.-R.; Project Administration, M.H.-O., R.S.-H.; Software, M.H.-O., G.E.O.-C., J.M.C.-C., O.M.-R.; Supervision, M.H.-O., M.A.N.-M., A.R.-L., O.M.-R.; Validation, A.R.-L., R.S.-H., J.M.C.-C.; Visualization, A.R.-L., J.M.C.-C., O.M.-R.; Writing Original Draft, M.H.-O., M.A.N.-M., C.A.C.-A., G.E.O.-C.; Writing Review and Editing, M.A.N.-M., C.A.C.-A., R.S.-H. All authors have read and agreed to the published version of the manuscript.

Acknowledgments: The present project was partially funded by the National Council of Science and Technology of México (CONACYT) through a scholarship (no. 337087) granted to José Margarito Canseco-Cortinas. The authors are grateful for the support provided by TNM-ITV, CONACYT and PRODEP.

References

1. World Health Organization. *Obesity and Overweight Fact Sheet*; WHO: Geneva, Switzerland, 2016.
2. World Health Organization. *Diabetes Fact Sheet*; WHO: Geneva, Switzerland, 2016.
3. Institute for Health Metrics and Evaluation. *The Global Burden of Disease: Generating Evidence, Guiding Policy*; IHME: Washington, DC, USA, 2013.
4. World Health Organization. *The Top 10 Causes of Death*; WHO: Geneva, Switzerland, 2017.
5. International Diabetes Federation. *IDF Diabetes Atlas*, 7th ed.; International Diabetes Federation: Brussels, Belgium, 2015.
6. Levy, T.S.; Nasu, L.C.; Dommarco, J.R.; Ávila, M.H. *Informe Final de Resultados, Encuesta Nacional de Salud y Nutrición de Medio Camino 2016*; Instituto Nacional de Salud Pública INSP: Mexico City, Mexico, 2016.
7. Institute for Health Metrics and Evaluation (IHME). Country Profile Mexico. Mexico, 2017. Available online: http://www.healthdata.org/ (accessed on 7 October 2018).
8. Statista Inc. Global Smartphone Sales to End Users 2007–2016. Available online: https://www.statista.com/statistics/263437/global-smartphone-sales-to-end-users-since-2007/ (accessed on 12 October 2018).
9. eMarketer. Worldwide Internet and Mobile Users: eMarketer's Updated Estimates and Forecast for 2015–2020. 2016. Available online: https://www.emarketer.com/Report/Worldwide-Internet-Mobile-Users-eMarketersUpdated-Estimates-Forecast-20152020/2001897#moreReport (accessed on 25 September 2018).
10. Lehmann, E. Preliminary experience with the Internet release of AIDA—An interactive educational diabetes simulator. *Comput. Methods Programs Biomed.* **1998**, *56*, 109–132. [CrossRef]
11. Hernandez-Ordonez, M.; Montano, O.; Campos-Delgado, D.U.; Palacios, E. Development of an Educational Simulator and Graphical User Interface for Diabetic Patients. In Proceedings of the 2007 4th International Conference on Electrical and Electronics Engineering, Mexico City, Mexico, 5–7 September 2007; pp. 82–85. [CrossRef]
12. Lehmann, E.D.; Tarín, C.; Bondia, J.; Teufel, E.; Deutsch, T. Development of AIDA v4.3b Diabetes Simulator: Technical Upgrade to Support Incorporation of Lispro, Aspart, and Glargine Insulin Analogues. *J. Electr. Comput. Eng.* **2011**, *2011*, 427196. [CrossRef]
13. Thestrup, J.; Gergely, T.; Beck, P. Exploring new care models in diabetes management and therapy with a wireless mobile eHealth platform. In *Wireless Mobile Communication and Healthcare: Second International ICST Conference, MobiHealth 2011, Kos Island, Greece, 5–7 October 2011*; Revised Selected Papers; Nikita, K.S., Lin, J.C., Fotiadis, D.I., Arredondo Waldmeyer, M.T., Eds.; Springer: Berlin/Heidelberg, Germany, 2012; pp. 203–210.
14. Erzen, F.C.; Birol, G.; Cinar, A. Glucosim: A simulator for education on the dynamics of diabetes mellitus. In Proceedings of the 23rd Annual International Conference of the IEEE Engineering in Medicine and Biology Society, Istambul, Turkey, 25–28 October 2001; Volume 4, pp. 3163–3166. [CrossRef]
15. Agar, B.U.; Eren, M.; Cinar, A. Glucosim: Educational software for virtual experiments with patients with type 1 diabetes. In Proceedings of the 2005 IEEE Engineering in Medicine and Biology 27th Annual Conference, Shanghai, China, 17–18 January 2006; pp. 845–848. [CrossRef]
16. Mougiakakou, S.G.; Prountzou, K.; Nikita, K.S. A Real Time Simulation Model of Glucose-Insulin Metabolism for Type 1 Diabetes Patients. In Proceedings of the 2005 IEEE Engineering in Medicine and Biology 27th Annual Conference, Shanghai, China, 17–18 January 2005; pp. 298–301. [CrossRef]
17. Bergman, R.N.; Phillips, L.S.; Cobelli, C. Physiologic evaluation of factors controlling glucose tolerance in man: Measurement of insulin sensitivity and beta-cell glucose sensitivity from the response to intravenous glucose. *J. Clin. Investig.* **1981**, *68*, 1456–1467. [CrossRef] [PubMed]
18. Cobelli, C.; Caumo, A.; Omenetto, M.; Sacca, L. Minimal model SG overestimation and SI underestimation: Improved accuracy by a Bayesian two-compartment model. *Am. J. Physiol.* **1999**, *277*, E481–E488.

19. Hovorka, R.; Shojaee-Moradie, F.; Carroll, P.V.; Chassin, L.J.; Gowrie, I.J.; Jackson, N.C.; Tudor, R.S.; Umpleby, A.M.; Jones, R.H. Partitioning glucose distribution/trans-port, disposal, and endogenous production during IVGTT. *Am. J. Physiol.* **2002**, *282*, E992–E1007.
20. Liu, C.; Vehí, J.; Avari, P.; Reddy, M.; Oliver, N.; Georgiou, P.; Herrero, P. Long-Term Glucose Forecasting Using a Physiological Model and Deconvolution of the Continuous Glucose Monitoring Signal. *Sensors* **2019**, *19*, 4338. [CrossRef]
21. Liu, C.; Avari, P.; Leal, Y.; Wos, M.; Sivasithamparam, K.; Georgiou, P.; Reddy, M.; Fernández-Real, J.M.; Martin, C.; Fernández-Balsells, M.; et al. A Modular Safety System for an Insulin Dose Recommender: A Feasibility Study. *J. Diabetes Sci. Technol.* **2019**, *14*, 87–96. [CrossRef]
22. Sangeetha, S.; Sreepradha, C.; Sobana, S.; Bidisha, P.; Panda, R.C. Modeling and Control of the Glucose-Insulin-Glucagon System in Type I Diabetis Mellitus. *ChemBioEng Rev.* **2020**, *3*, 89–100. [CrossRef]
23. Knopp, J.L.; Hardy, A.R.; Vergeer, S.; Chase, J.G. Modelling insulin adsorption in intravenous infusion sets in the intensive care unit. *IFAC J. Syst. Control* **2019**, *8*, 100042. [CrossRef]
24. Visentin, R.; Schiavon, M.; Basu, R.; Basu, A.; Man, C.D.; Cobelli, C. Physiological models for artificial pancreas development. In *The Artificial Pancreas: Current Situation and Future Directions*, 1st ed.; Sánchez-Peña, R.S., Cherñavvsky, D.R., Eds.; Academic Press: Cambridge, MA, USA, 2019; Volume 1, pp. 123–152.
25. Maas, A.H.; van der Molen, P.; van de Vijver, R.; Chen, W.; van Pul, C.; Cottaar, E.J.; van Riel, N.A.; Hilbers, P.A.; Haak, H.R. Concept Development of the Eindhoven Diabetes Education Simulator Project. *Games Health J.* **2016**, *5*, 120–127. [CrossRef]
26. Ristau, R.A.; Yang, J.; White, J.R. Evaluation and Evolution of Diabetes Mobile Applications: Key Factors for Health Care Professionals Seeking to Guide Patients. *Diabetes Spectr.* **2013**, *26*, 211–215. Available online: http://spectrum.diabetesjournals.org/content/26/4/211.full.pdf (accessed on 17 September 2018). [CrossRef]
27. El-Gayar, O.; Timsina, P.; Nawar, N.; Eid, W. Mobile Applications for Diabetes Self-Management: Status and Potential. *J. Diabetes Sci. Technol.* **2013**, *7*, 247–262. [CrossRef] [PubMed]
28. Chomutare, T.; Fernandez-Luque, L.; Arsand, E.; Hartvigsen, G. Features of mobile diabetes applications: Review of the literature and analysis of current applications compared against evidence-based guidelines. *J. Med Internet Res.* **2011**, *13*, e65. [CrossRef] [PubMed]
29. Huckvale, K.; Adomaviciute, S.; Prieto, J.T.; Leow, M.K.S.; Car, J. Smartphone apps for calculating insulin dose: A systematic assessment. *BMC Med.* **2015**, *13*, 106. [CrossRef] [PubMed]
30. Cui, M.; Wu, X.; Mao, J.; Wang, X.; Nie, M. T2DM Self-Management via Smartphone Applications: A Systematic Review and Meta-Analysis. *PLoS ONE* **2016**, *11*, e0166718. [CrossRef] [PubMed]
31. Garcia, E.; Martin, C.; Garcia, A.; Harrison, R.; Flood, D. Systematic Analysis of Mobile Diabetes Management Applications on Different Platforms. In Proceedings of the 7th Conference on Workgroup Human-Computer Interaction and Usability Engineering of the Austrian Computer Society: Information Quality in e-Health, Graz, Austria, 25–26 November 2011; Springer: Berlin/Heidelberg, Germany, 2011. USAB'11. pp. 379–396.
32. Baskaran, V.; Prescod, F.; Dong, L. A Smartphone-Based Cloud Computing Tool for Managing Type 1 Diabetes in Ontarians. *Can. J. Diabetes* **2015**, *39*, 200–203. [CrossRef]
33. Chomutare, T.; Tatara, N.; Arsand, E.; Hartvigsen, G. Designing a diabetes mobile application with social network support. In *Studies in Health Technology and Informatics*; IOS Press: Clifton, NJ, USA, 2013.
34. Nguyen, H.D.; Jiang, X.; Poo, D.C.C. Designing a Social Mobile Platform for Diabetes Self-management: A Theory-Driven Perspective. In *Social Computing and Social Media: 7th International Conference, SCSM 2015, Held as Part of HCI International 2015, Los Angeles, CA, USA, 2–7 August 2015, Proceedings*; Meiselwitz, G., Ed.; Springer International Publishing: Cham, Switzerland, 2015; pp. 67–77.
35. Garnweidner-Holme, L.M.; Borgen, I.; Garitano, I.; Noll, J.; Lukasse, M. Designing and Developing a Mobile Smartphone Application for Women with Gestational Diabetes Mellitus Followed-Up at Diabetes Outpatient Clinics in Norway. *Healthcare* **2015**, *3*, 310–323. [CrossRef]
36. Borgen, I.; Garnweidner-Holme, L.M.; Jacobsen, A.F.; Bjerkan, K.; Fayyad, S.; Joranger, P.; Lilleengen, A.M.; Mosdøl, A.; Noll, J.; Småstuen, M.C.; et al. Smartphone application for women with gestational diabetes mellitus: A study protocol for a multicentre randomised controlled trial. *BMJ Open* **2017**, *7*, e013117. Available online: http://bmjopen.bmj.com/content/7/3/e013117.full.pdf (accessed on 12 December 2018). [CrossRef]
37. Lloyd, B.; Groat, D.; Cook, C.; Kaufman, D.; Grando, A. IDECIDE: A mobile application for insulin dosing using an evidence based equation to account for patient preferences. In *Studies in Health Technology and Informatics*; IOS Press: Clifton, NJ, USA, 2015; Volume 216, pp. 93–97. [CrossRef]

38. Keith-Hynes, P.; Mize, B.; Robert, A.; Place, J. The Diabetes Assistant: A Smartphone-Based System for Real-Time Control of Blood Glucose. *Electronics* **2014**, *3*, 609–623. [CrossRef]
39. González, A.A.; Voos, H.; Darouach, M. Glucose-Insulin System Based on Minimal Model: A Realistic Approach. In Proceedings of the 2015 17th UKSIM-AMSS International Conference on Modelling and Simulation, Cambridge, UK, 25–27 March 2015; IEEE Computer Society: Washington, DC, USA, 2015. UKSIM '15. pp. 55–60. [CrossRef]
40. Sorensen, J.T. A Physiologic Model of Glucose Metabolism in Man and Its Use to Design and Assess Improved Insulin Therapies for Diabetes. Ph.D. Thesis, Massachusetts Institute of Technology. Dept. of Chemical Engineering, Berkeley, CA, USA, 1985.
41. Hernández-Ordoñez, M.; Campos-Delgado, D. An extension to the compartmental model of type 1 diabetic patients to reproduce exercise periods with glycogen depletion and replenishment. *J. Biomech.* **2008**, *41*, 744–752. [CrossRef]
42. Berger, M.; Rodbard, D. Computer simulation of plasma insulin and glucose dynamics after subcutaneous insulin injection. *Diabetes Care* **1989**, *12*, 725–736. [CrossRef] [PubMed]
43. Lehmann, E.; Deutsch, T. A physiological model of glucose-insulin interaction in type 1 diabetes mellitus. *J. Biomed. Eng.* **1992**, *14*, 235–242. [CrossRef]
44. Wilinska, M.E.; Chassin, L.J.; Schaller, H.C.; Schaupp, L.; Pieber, T.R.; Hovorka, R. Insulin kinetics in type-1 diabetes: Continuous and bolus delivery of rapid acting insulin. *IEEE Trans. Biomed. Eng.* **2005**, *52*, 3–12. [CrossRef] [PubMed]
45. Jahoda, P. MPAndroidChart. 2016. Available online: https://github.com/PhilJay/MPAndroidChart (accessed on 15 November 2018).

9

Intelligent Fog-Enabled Smart Healthcare System for Wearable Physiological Parameter Detection

Muhammad Ijaz [1,2], Gang Li [1,2], Huiquan Wang [3], Ahmed M. El-Sherbeeny [4], Yussif Moro Awelisah [1,2], Ling Lin [1,2,*], Anis Koubaa [5,6] and Alam Noor [5,*]

1 State Key Laboratory of Precision Measurement Technology and Instrument, Tianjin University, Tianjin 300072, China; ijazm09@gmail.com (M.I.); ligang59@tju.edu.cn (G.L.); yussif@tju.edu.cn (Y.M.A.)
2 China and Tianjin Key Laboratory of Biomedical Detecting Techniques and Instruments, Tianjin University, Tianjin 300072, China
3 School of life sciences, Tiangong University, Tianjin 300387, China; huiquan@tiangong.edu.cn
4 Industrial Engineering Department, College of Engineering, King Saud University, PO Box 800, Riyadh 11421, Saudi Arabia; aelsherbeeny@ksu.edu.sa
5 Robotics and Internet-of-Things Lab, Prince Sultan University, Riyadh 11586, Saudi Arabia; akoubaa@psu.edu.sa
6 CISTER, INESC-TEC, ISEP, Polytechnic Institute of Porto, 4249-015 Porto, Portugal
* Correspondence: linling@tju.edu.cn (L.L.); eng.alamnoor@gmail.com (A.N.)

Abstract: Wearable technology plays a key role in smart healthcare applications. Detection and analysis of the physiological data from wearable devices is an essential process in smart healthcare. Physiological data analysis is performed in fog computing to abridge the excess latency introduced by cloud computing. However, the latency for the emergency health status and overloading in fog environment becomes key challenges for smart healthcare. This paper resolves these problems by presenting a novel tri-fog health architecture for physiological parameter detection. The overall system is built upon three layers as wearable layer, intelligent fog layer, and cloud layer. In the first layer, data from the wearable of patients are subjected to fault detection at personal data assistant (PDA). To eliminate fault data, we present the rapid kernel principal component analysis (RK-PCA) algorithm. Then, the faultless data is validated, whether it is duplicate or not, by the data on-looker node in the second layer. To remove data redundancy, we propose a new fuzzy assisted objective optimization by ratio analysis (FaMOORA) algorithm. To timely predict the user's health status, we enable the two-level health hidden Markov model (2L-2HMM) that finds the user's health status from temporal variations in data collected from wearable devices. Finally, the user's health status is detected in the fog layer with the assist of a hybrid machine learning algorithm, namely SpikQ-Net, based on the three major categories of attributes such as behavioral, biomedical, and environment. Upon the user's health status, the immediate action is taken by both cloud and fog layers. To ensure lower response time and timely service, we also present an optimal health off procedure with the aid of the multi-objective spotted hyena optimization (MoSHO) algorithm. The health off method allows offloading between overloaded and underloaded fog nodes. The proposed tri-fog health model is validated by a thorough simulation performed in the iFogSim tool. It shows better achievements in latency (reduced up to 3 ms), execution time (reduced up to 1.7 ms), detection accuracy (improved up to 97%), and system stability (improved up to 96%).

Keywords: Tri-Fog Health System; fault data elimination; health status prediction; health status detection; health off

1. Introduction

In recent times, smart healthcare becomes an emerging application of the internet of things (IoT). A smart healthcare system consists of wearable sensors used to monitor the specific health status of the users or patients [1,2]. Most importantly, wearable technology has become a vital part of not only remote patient monitoring but also for user health monitoring regularly. The introduction of wearable devices minimizes the frequent involvement of doctors in health monitoring. It also assists in the early detection of diseases, drug research, smart hospital development, and safety provisioning [3,4]. Two major technologies have to be investigated to develop a smart healthcare system. Firstly, through biomedical sensors like temperature, motion, blood pressure, and how the wearable devices are appended on the user's body to acquire, their health status is studied [5]. Secondly, the useful fog computing technology that enables real-time and delay minimized health services [6,7] should be examined. As a result of the fog enabled healthcare system, the data acquired from the wearable devices are analyzed by the fog layer, which further minimizes the latency for healthcare services.

In the wearable based physiological monitoring, fault data detection from biosensors is one of the main issues [8]. Analyzing the fault data sensed by the wearable leads to inaccurate decision making. As the health data must be more reliable, the adaptive neuro-fuzzy inference system (ANFIS) is presented to diagnose health data [9]. A distributed similarity test has been introduced to detect the sensor data fault [10]. Based on the sensor reading variations, the sensor fault is detected. Thus, in a smart healthcare system, fault data diagnosis and elimination are the first and foremost process. In recent times, deep learning is addressed as one of the effective solutions for classification and prediction problems [11,12]. Deep learning algorithms are capable of handling and analyzing the massive amount of data without minimum prediction errors [13,14]. When it comes to fog-enabled smart healthcare, the faultless data need to be analyzed by the fog nodes. In most fog-based smart healthcare systems, a deep learning approach is incorporated to detect the abnormalities in the user's health status [15,16]. The deep learning approaches analyze the user's physiological data aggregated from the wearable devices. The multi-classifier system works based on data fused from different kinds of wearable sensors [17]. Both data fusion and multi-classifier methods offer better performance. A transfer learning model is proposed to detect Parkinson's disease from the wearable data [18].

In conventional healthcare systems, the data are analyzed in the cloud layer, which means the latency is high. Thus, fog computing becomes an essential part of the smart healthcare system [19]. Although the smart healthcare system has potentiality worked in many applications; still, the fault data detection has not yet been addressed. Firstly, while all works focus on the data analysis in the fog layer, the major issue of fog computing (i.e., fog overloading) is not yet concentrated for the healthcare environment. With the increase in users or patients in the healthcare system, there are relatively increasing concerns about the overloading issue [20]. Secondly, most research works utilized only biosensors or body sensors or wearable data to monitor the user's health status. However, environmental factors are also equally important to detect the user's health status accurately [21]. Environmental data like environment temperature, noise level, pollution level have a direct impact on the user's health data generated by wearable devices [22]. Both of the issues, including fog offloading and environmental data analysis, are not thoroughly analyzed in the prior research works from the perspective of healthcare systems. Apart from these issues, another challenge is that the duplicate data processing in fog or cloud layer leads to unnecessary resource consumption [23]. For example, the sensors report the data for each fraction of seconds. But the temperature data may be the same for a while. Thus, redundant data elimination will speed up the analysis process and also preserve the resources of fog and cloud computing.

1.1. Motivation and Inspiration

This research work is motivated by the existing problems in the smart healthcare system, such as high latency for emergency health status, fault and duplicate data analysis, and fog overloading. The brief summarization on research issues in our smart healthcare is provided here:

- Latency—High latency is introduced due to data processing in the cloud layer. In general, healthcare services need on-time data transmission. Latency in healthcare applications directly affects the patient's or user's health.
- Fault Data—Most wearable or biosensors are deployed in the open or mobile (on the human) environment. It makes the sensors to generate erroneous data. Analyzing the inaccurate data ultimately leads to incorrect prediction.
- Low Accuracy—Health status prediction accuracy is down due to improper algorithms and attributes. All research works considered only wearable sensor data, which are unable to provide accurate results. However, environmental data are also crucial for accurate prediction. As the wearable data consists of duplicate data, it also affects the data processing accuracy.
- Fog Overloading—One of the best solutions for minimizing latency is to use fog computing. However, when more users are connected in the same region, the fog will become overloaded. This overloading problem is the major research issue in smart healthcare.

These research issues motivate us to design a novel smart healthcare system. This paper concentrates on all these aspects to design an efficient smart healthcare system. For those, we formulate the following research objectives:

- Design a family healthcare system by using wearable for monitoring physiological parameters.
- Accurately predict the user state through physiological parameters.
- Minimize latency and detect the user state promptly.

To achieve these objectives, we designed a novel tripartite fog-enabled healthcare (Tri-FogHealth) architecture to monitor the health status of users through wearable physiological parameters. Apart from this, we made the following contributions in Tri-FogHealth architecture:

- Erroneous data from the wearable is diagnosed by using a rapid kernel principal component analysis (RK-PCA) algorithm. The RK-PCA algorithm is incorporated in a personal data assistant (PDA) (i.e.,) the faulty data is detected and eliminated in the wearable layer.
- From the faultless data, the data deduplication process is carried by the data on-looker node. To detect and eliminate duplicate data, we present a fuzzy assisted objective optimization by ratio analysis (FaMOORA) algorithm. If no duplicate data is found, then the fog node predicts the user's health status through temporal features using the two-level health hidden Markov model (2L-2HMM). The 2L-2HMM appends the severity level of the user's health status and provides apt action for severe cases.
- To prevent the fog layer from overloading the issue, we enable the health off procedure. The health of works upon two states. In the first stage, the offloading decision is made based on two rules. Then, an optimal node is selected for offloading by using the multi-objective spotted hyena optimization (MoSHO) algorithm.
- Then, the user's current health status is detected in the cloud layer based on behavioral, biomedical, and environmental attributes. All these attributes are fed into the spiking quantum neural network (SpikQ-Net) that accurately classifies the user's health status into normal action required, no action required, and immediate action required classes.

1.2. Paper Layout

The rest of this paper is organized as follows: Section 2 surveys existing research works held on smart healthcare systems. In Section 3, we highlight the problem statement and the background of the problems considered in this work. Section 4 clearly explains the overall proposed work with all algorithms. In Section 5, we describe the experimentation detail of the proposed work with experimental setup and comparative analysis. Section 6 concludes the overall contributions of this work.

2. Related Work

In this section, we present existing important research works proposed in the smart healthcare system.

2.1. Research Works on Cloud-Based Smart Healthcare System

A smart healthcare system is designed to monitor elderly peoples and optimal access control [24]. For providing access control, the Pearson correlation coefficient (PCC) algorithm is presented with the Manhattan distance measure. Firstly, algorithms work in parallel to identify older people. Then, the PCA algorithm is applied to reduce the dimensionality reduction for the collected elderly data. Lately, the normalization cross-correlation (NCC) algorithm is utilized for final results. However, the PCA and NCC algorithms are insufficient to process the large amount of data collected from elderly peoples. In a smart healthcare system designed with multiple heterogeneous wearable sensors [25], the proposed approach uses an analytical hierarchy process (AHP) with the VIseKriterijumska Optimizacija I Kompromisno Resenje (VIKOR) method to make a proper decision on hospital selection based on two steps. Firstly, the data from the wearable device was collected and analyzed. Then, the hospital is selected by considering the user's health status and multiple criteria. In this work, the processing algorithm is only applied to determine the optimal hospital; however, a more intelligent mechanism will make decisions based on the health data.

For reliable medical monitoring, fault data detection was performed by the threshold tuning method [26]. The medical data is collected from wearable devices. As it could be corrupted from the environmental factors and sensor faults, the fault detection using Bayesian neural network was performed initially. Although fault data detection improves data reliability, health status monitoring performance is still inefficient. The Bayesian neural network increases the complexity of the personal devices of the patient.

As a result, a statistical approach was presented for patient monitoring [27]. The vital signs are acquired from the wearable, and the data is processed to predict the patient's health status. First, gaussian process (GP) models are built for interpretive signs with varying complexity. For this purpose, the covariance kernels and the fixed parameters are utilized. Then, the Bayesian model is proposed to find the health status of the user based on two main hypotheses, such as (i) use of patient-specific model and (ii) use of optimal hyperparameter values. Here, the selection of hyperparameters increases the complexity of the system.

A new cloud digital twins (CloudDTH) framework was introduced for smart healthcare monitoring [28]. The concept of digital twins is integrated multi-physics, multi-scale and probabilistic simulation of a system. In CloudDTH, a virtual object is created for all users in the cloud environment. The virtual object data was used for modelling, simulating, and evaluating the user data. From the analysis of the virtual object, the healthcare status of the user was predicted. In general, digital twins are hard to deploy and manage. In addition, to create a digital twin for each user is not scalable.

To further enhance the prediction accuracy, a complement naïve Bayesian (CNB) classifier was deployed in the cloud environment to classify the user's health data [29]. Firstly, the medical data was acquired from the wearable and biosensors. Before classification, the preprocessing mechanism was applied to handle the noisy data. The CNB classifier uses double learning processes to improve classification accuracy. First, the naïve Bayes classifier was trained with the dataset. Then, the classifier was tested by using the same dataset. It is known as double learning. Here the misclassified data was used for original test data classification.

2.2. Research Works on Fog-Enabled Healthcare System

The concept of edge computing is introduced to mitigate latency in healthcare applications [30]. The proposed system computed the criticality measure index (CMI) from the gathered wearable data. Then the alert message was triggered in emergencies. Here, the CMI value is calculated for each data without considering temporal and environmental data. It tends to inaccurate health status prediction.

The fog computing-based gateway design explores a geo-distributed intermediary layer of intelligence [31]. This layer was introduced between the sensors and the cloud. In the fog enabled healthcare systems, the fog node takes the responsibility of the sensors such as severity detection. The highlight is that the use of the fog layer in the e-healthcare system improves energy efficiency, scalability, and reliability problems and also supports user mobility. Therefore, fog computing plays a pivotal role in e-healthcare applications.

However, the data analysis accuracy is low since there no intelligence algorithm is applied to the collected health data. Therefore, a smart treatment for personalized healthcare (STPH) model was presented with edge computing [32]. The STPH model provides the optimal treatment solution to minimize the cost of the intelligent agent. This approach uses an intelligent agent (IA), which assists in constructing a personalized treatment plan. Furthermore, the edge servers were introduced to help the cloud server in the data processing. Here the treatment plan is optimally selected for emergencies. However, optimal treatment plan selection without detecting the user's current health status results in low accuracy.

An edge of thins (EoT) driven ambient assisted living framework was proposed for e-healthcare applications [33]. This framework uses a hybrid classifier to predict the health status of the user. The hybrid classifier is made up of the hybrid ambient assisted living with naïve bayes classifier and the firefly algorithm (HAAL-NBFA). The firefly algorithm is employed to select the optimal features for classification. Upon optimal features chosen by the firefly algorithm, the naïve Bayes classifier detects the state of the user. Before the imbalanced dataset is balanced by the synthetic minority over-sampling technique (SMOTE), the naïve Bayes classifier has less accuracy due to the class dependencies. This work fails when the incoming data has faulty reading.

A HealthFog framework was developed to monitor the heart diseases in the IoT environment to minimize the latency and response time for personalized healthcare [34]. The HealthFog integrates the ensemble deep learning algorithm with edge computing. Further, the fog-enabled framework is defined as FogBus, which efficiently detects the health status of heart patients. At the same time, real-time medical data is collected from the sensors of the wearable. The FogBus is designed using the broker node, the worker node, and the cloud data center. The same data is analyzed in different worker nodes, and the results are ensemble for final classification. Here the deep learning model is trained in each worker node of each fog node; this increases the time consumption.

As fog overloading increases the latency for the emergency data, an ubiquitous cloud edge enabled healthcare (UbeHealth) system was aimed to improve the quality of service (QoS) in the healthcare system [35]. The healthcare data was processed in both the cloudlet and network layer. In the cloudlet layer, the deep learning-based data prediction approach was applied, and in the network layer, data classification by deep learning approach was proposed. Both deep learning approaches use a recurrent neural network (RNN) for classification. In the cloudlet layer, the flow clustering and analysis (FCA) process was employed with the density-based spatial clustring of application with noise (DBSCAN) clustering algorithm. Consequently, using two deep learning algorithms increases the time consumption.

2.3. Research Works on Fog Offloading

Load balancing in fog-based healthcare applications was focused on improving service quality [36]. The fog computing resources were consolidated in this work to balance the load among foglets. Only critical resources were redirected to cloud computing, and the rest requests were scheduled to fog nodes locally. Although this work utilizes fog nodes to prevent overloading, a random selection of fog nodes leads to that the fog nodes to become overloaded.

Multiple agents are deployed in the smart healthcare system to maintain load balancing among fog nodes [37]. The primary aim of the multi-agent fog computing model was to serve critical tasks within the given time. For this, optimal scheduling was enabled by the multiple agents to access the fog resources. Here, the most suitable fog node was selected based on resource availability information. However, numerous criteria are required to process critical and emergency tasks.

A novel four-tier fog architecture was presented to balance load among fog nodes [38]. A dual fuzzy logic algorithm classified the tasks received from the IoT devices to assign priority levels for the tasks. Then the tasks were scheduled based on an artificial neural network. Herein, the single objective is considered for fog node selection, where the energy utility is inefficient.

An energy-efficient offloading strategy was presented for IoT applications [39]. The objective was to achieve better QoS and energy efficiency. For this, a firefly algorithm based offloading scheme was proposed. The firefly algorithm uses a weighted-sum method to determine fitness function. The firefly algorithm is inefficient in local search as it is not suitable for optimal fog node selection.

Comment on Literature: In Table 1, we summarize the literature works with limitations. The analyzes show a massive research gap that needed to be addressed while designing a smart healthcare system.

Table 1. Summarization of literature survey.

Category	Presented Works	Research Issues
Cloud-Smart Healthcare	• PCC and NCC [24] • AHP-VIKOR Model [25] • Fault Monitoring [26] • Statistical Approach [27] • CloudDTH [28] • CNB-Cloud [29]	• Health status detection time is high • Unable to process a large amount of data • Involvement of inefficient algorithms
Fog-Smart Healthcare	• CMI-Fog [30] • Fog-Gateway [31] • STPH [32] • EoT-Hybrid Classifier [33] • HealthFog [34] • UbeHealth [35]	• Low accuracy due to ineffective algorithms • Not able to support a large number of users • High processing time due to the presence of redundant data
Fog Offloading	• Health Load Balancing [36] • Multi-Agent Fog Model [37] • Four-Tier Fog Architecture [38] • QoS Offloading [39]	• Nonoptimal fog selection degrades the offloading performance • single objective is insufficient to select optimum fog node

3. Problem Overview

In this section, we present the problem statement of this work with the background of the problems.

3.1. Overall Problem Statement

In wearable-based smart healthcare, more research works have been presented in the view of a clinical study, and non-clinical home-based health monitoring is concentrated less. The biomedical sensors have been used only for health monitoring, but environmental factors play a pivotal role in healthcare monitoring. Furthermore, fault and duplicate data processing often results in inaccurate outcomes and increases time consumption. Although fog-enabled IoT healthcare systems minimize the latency, this depreciation is not sufficient for emergency events. Because the regional fog node where the number of users is high or the environmental status is worst will become overloaded, it drastically increases the latency for the particular region.

3.2. Background of the Problem

A cognitive dynamics (CDS) concept is presented for smart healthcare and disease diagnosis, along with decision tree-based classification [40]. Here, the decision tree is unstable, i.e., a small change in the data results in a massive change in the structure, which leads to wrong decisions. Further, it is not suitable to handle streaming data like smart healthcare. The overall analysis is performed here in the cloudlet layer, which will increase latency drastically. A structured Gaussian process is proposed for patient-specific physiological monitoring based on its health trajectory [41]. The Gaussian method is a highly parametric approach that considers all parameters known in prior while increasing the complexity. This work finds a single vital sign for determining the health level of the patients.

Furthermore, this work is not suitable to handle mobile users since the cluster formation become complex. Mobile-based physiological sensor system (MoPS) uses a smart shirt and wearable technology [42]. Analysis of the massive data from wearable demands highly efficient algorithms and methodologies. Here the data analysis is performed in a cloud server without using proper algorithms and based on the conventional threshold. It leads to inaccurate classification and also increases the time consumption.

Further, the user status is detected based on the current physiological sign only. But in general, the health status of a user depends upon the time series data. The overall analysis considers a single physiological sign which is insufficient for health status detection.

In a fog-assisted patient health monitoring, Bayesian belief network (BBN) was introduced in the fog layer for health status prediction [43]. In the cloud layer, the temporal information is used to compute the temporal health index (THI) for the patients. In this work, both fog and cloud layers work upon the same attributes (environmental, medical, and behavior). This time consumption increasing makes it not suitable for healthcare monitoring. Processing in the cloud layer increases the latency of emergency events. This work is not appropriate to handle large-scale systems and also unable to support mobile users. However, patients with chronic disease will have mobile nature instead of static. This system is not suitable for real-time analysis. In addition, the BBN classifier is hard to construct and also has low classification accuracy. A hierarchical data fusion method uses the complex event processing (CPE) method for clinical patient monitoring [44]. In each level (sensor, fog, and cloud), data fusion is performed based on a threshold value. All three levels consider biosensor reading only for the patient's health status monitoring. However, environmental factors also play a pivotal role in healthcare monitoring. CPE, which is used in all three levels, uses some pre-defined rules to detect the patient status. However, this is not suitable in the practical scenario since each user has different signs and parameters. Thus, the CPE based analysis is not suitable for real-time analysis. In the fog-cloud smart office healthcare system, the severity index is computed based on environmental, behavior, and posture data [45]. The Bayesian classifier is complex and has less accuracy. Thus, data classification by Bayesian classifiers often results in inaccurate outcomes. The final decision on the user's health status is determined at the cloud layer. It increases the latency considerably for emergency events. Poor load management in the fog layer affects the overall processing ability of the fog layer.

4. Proposed Tri-Fog Health System

In this section, we discuss the proposed tri-fog healthcare system in detail. Each proposed methodology is explained in each subsection.

4.1. System Overview

The proposed tri-foghealth system is designed with three primary layers, such as the wearable layer, the intelligent fog layer, and the cloud layer, as shown in Figure 1. The main intention of the system is to enable remote health monitoring for wellbeing lifestyle. It also supports mobile users. The first layer consists of n users $(u_1, u_2, .; u_n)$ with wearable sensors (we consider a smart shirt with biosensors) and a single PDA device and environmental sensors. The next layer comprises m Data On-Looker nodes $(Ol_1, Ol_2, .; Ol_m)$ and k fog nodes $(F_1, F_2, .; F_k)$. The first layer is responsible for collecting health data from the patients. The second layer involves two different entities, such as data on-lookers and fog nodes. The data on-looker nodes are responsible for redundant data elimination and health status prediction. The health status prediction is the process of the forecasting health status of the user in the next time frame based on the collected time-series data. The result will be added with the current data to increase the accuracy of classification. The fog nodes are responsible for classifying the user's current health status based on the wearable data and predicted report. The final cloud layer consists of a cloud server. The detail of the three layers is provided in the Table 2.

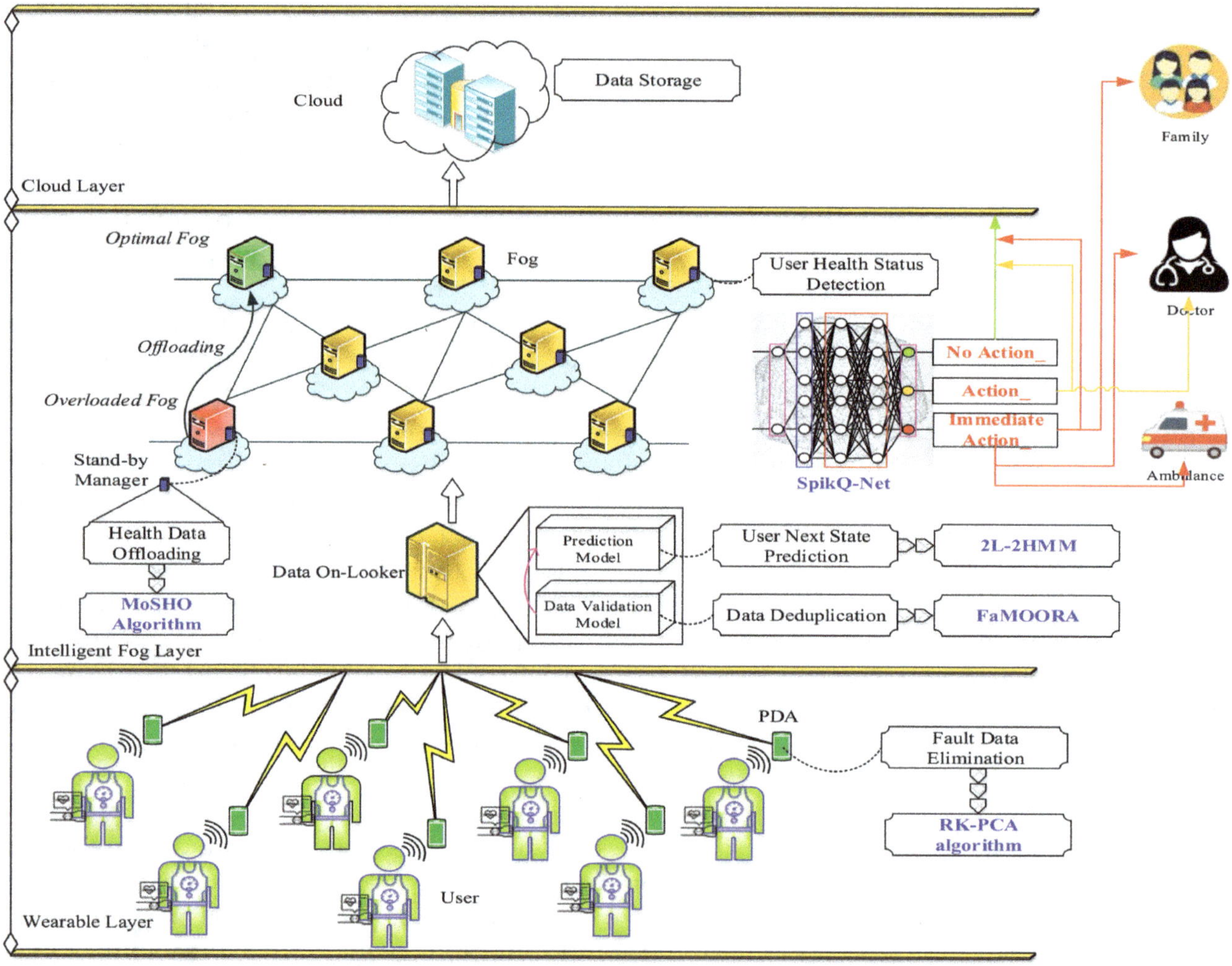

Figure 1. Tri-FogHealth System Architecture.

Table 2. Description of Three Layers in Tri-FogHealth.

Layer	Entities Involved	Functions Incorporated
Wearable Layer	• Users with smart shirts • Wearable Devices with biosensors • PDA	• Data Generation and Aggregation • Fault Data Detection and Elimination by RK-PCA
Intelligent Fog Layer	• Data On-Looker Nodes • Intelligent Fog Nodes	• Redundant Data Elimination by FaMOORA • Health Status Prediction by Temporal Analysis (2L-2HMM) • Health Status Detection by SpikQ-Net • Alert Generation on Emergency Cases
• Cloud Layer	• Cloud Servers	• Data Storage and Retrieval

As shown in the table, each layer works upon different algorithms. Each algorithm is intended for a different process. Each process contributes to improving the quality and accuracy of the healthcare system. On the proposed healthcare system, we make the following assumptions,

- All users have the same number of wearable devices to sense and generate health data;
- The number of fog nodes always equal or higher than the number of data on-looker nodes (i.e.,) $k \geq m$;

By considering the above two assumptions, we designed the tri-foghealth system. Functions carried in each layer of the proposed system are explained in the consecutive subsections.

4.2. Fault Data Elimination in the Wearable Layer

In the device layer, the health data and environmental data are aggregated. The wearable smart shirt is the primary source of health data for each user. Further, the environmental data is collected in every region to detect the user's health status accurately. As the main issue in wearable sensors is fault data generation, the first layer designed in a way such that the fault data problem will be overwhelmed. The fault data is detected and eliminated at the device layer for each user. For that, we present the RK-PCA algorithm in PDA. A fault data in the healthcare system can be detected based on the deviation with the normal data model and the variation with the other sensor data. For instance, the heart rate is generally proportional to the respiratory rate. When there is conflict occurs, then any one of those sensors reported fault data. Thus, the consideration of multiple sensor data models should much support the fault data detection and elimination.

To improve accuracy and processing speed, we present the RK-PCA algorithm. Let u_i wears a smart shirt with w biosensors as $S_1, S_2, \ldots, S_w$. Each biosensor senses the data and reports the data to PDA in a regular time interval. RK-PCA has to find fault data by comparing the current data with the normal data model. To this end, the normal data model is built for the sensor data received from the wearable sensors. The sensor data can be denoted as $\{X = X_1, X_2, .; X_t\}$. The data is captured in d dimensions in t time instances. The data model is represented as the Eigenvector. The Eigenvalue equation is defined as $\sum_{\varphi} e_i = \alpha_i e_i$. In this, e_i is estimated as;

$$e_i = \sum_{j=1}^{t} \alpha_i(j)\varphi(X_i(z)) \quad (1)$$

Here, X_i is the chosen data from the normal data model. Similarly, the eigenvalue is computed for all normal data values. From the normal data model, the fault data is detected, as shown in Figure 2.

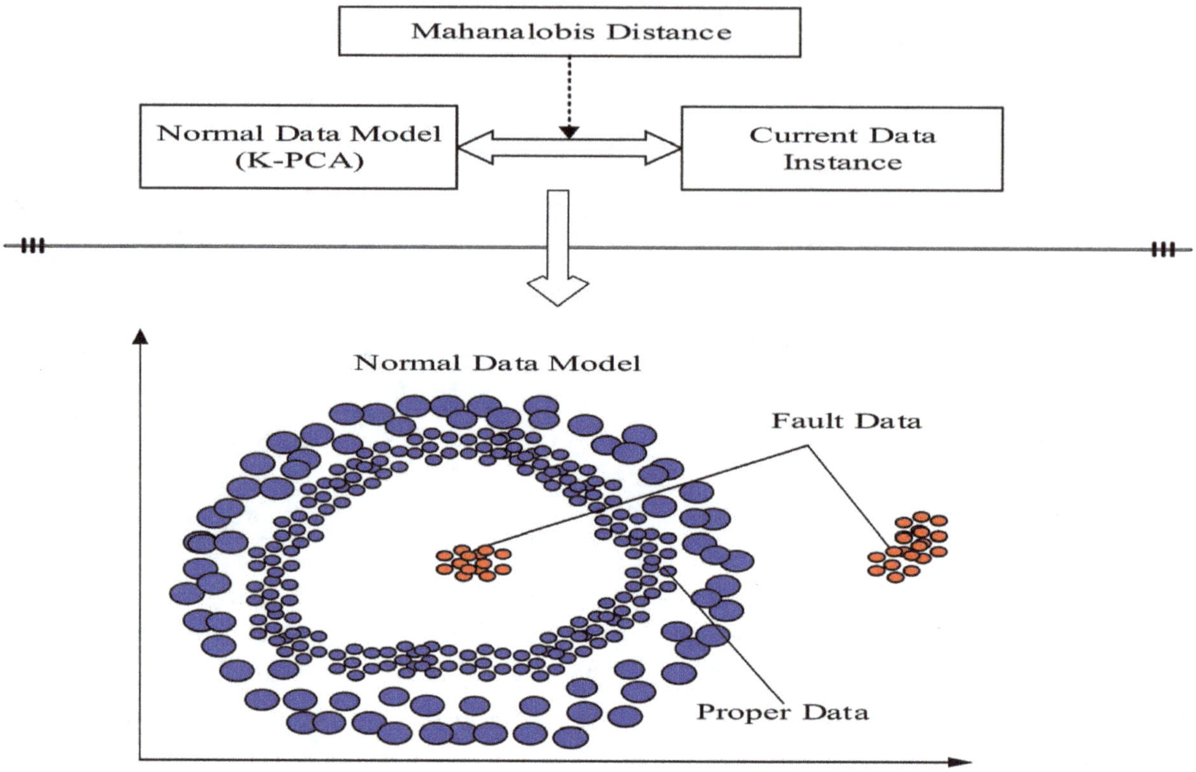

Figure 2. Fault Data Detection by Rapid Kernel Principal Component Analysis (RK-PCA).

As in the figure, the first step is to model the normal data by the RK-PCA algorithm. Here, kernel selection is carried as follows,

$$Ker(X_i, X_j) = \exp\left(\frac{1}{2\sigma^2}(X_i - X_j)^T Q^{-1}(X_i - X_j)\right) \quad (2)$$

The considered kernel is Mahalanobis Kernel (MK) since it supports the non-linear transformations of the data points.

The next step is to compute the similarity between current data instance (S_C) and normal data model (S_{nor}). The similarity is computed as Mahalanobis distance as follows,

$$dis(S_c, S_{nor}) = \sqrt{(S_C - S_{nor})^T CM^{-1}(S_C - S_{nor})} \quad (3)$$

Here, CM defines the covariance matrix defined by the eigenvalues of the normal data model. If the distance is low, then the data is normal. Otherwise, the data is a fault. The PDA carries this process, and the fault data is suppressed in the PDA. In Algorithm 1, we provided a detailed algorithm for RK-PCA algorithm-based fault data detection. The information with no fault is then transmitted to the next layer (i.e.,) intelligent fog layer.

Algorithm 1: RK-PCA for Fault Data Detection.

```
Initialize X_i
For all u ∈ Layer 1
    Get {X_i} from u_i
    Set RK-PCA Dimension
    Select Ker function        //Equation (2)
    Build e_i                  //Normal Data Model
    Construct CM               //From e_i
    Compute (dis)              //Mahanalobis Function
    If X_i to Fault
        Drop X_i
    Else
        Send X_i to Layer 2
    End If
End For
End
```

4.3. Redundant Data Elimination by Data Validation

In the fog layer, two primary functions are performed by the data on-looker nodes. The first process is redundant data elimination, and the next process is the user's health status prediction. The faultless data from PDA is received by the data on-looker nodes in the region. The data on-looker nodes are the special nodes that maintain the previous data records from the wearable devices and environmental sensors. The data on-looker nodes are designed with data validation model and prediction model. The data validation model is responsible for redundant data elimination by comparing the current data with previous data instances. Then, the redundant free data is fed into the prediction model to perform first-level health status prediction. The conceptual structure of the data on-looker node is illustrated in Figure 3.

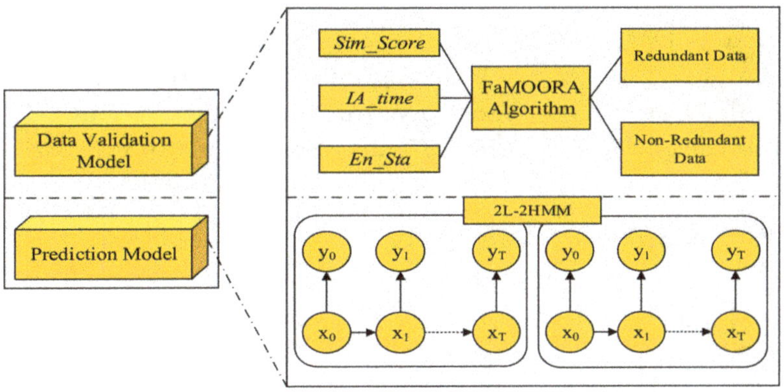

Figure 3. Structure of Data On-Looker Node.

4.3.1. Redundant Data Elimination

In this work, we intend to eliminate redundant data without affecting emergency data. In general, the redundant data elimination is performed if any one of the instances in prior records is matched with the current data. However, in the healthcare system, a redundant may also be emergency data. In this case, the data analysis will be affected. Thus, the problem of redundant data elimination is formulated as a decision-making problem and resolved by a hybrid multi-criteria decision-making algorithm.

We present the FaMOORA algorithm that works upon three major criteria, such as similarity score (Sim_Score), inter arrival time (IA_Time) and environmental status (En_Sta). Each criterion can be defined as follows,

Sim_Score—The current data instance D1 is verified with prior data records from the same user. D1 is the current data instance from the ith user. A data instance is made up of sensor readings sensed by the biosensors incorporated on the user. Thus, D1={Sd1, Sd2, ; Sdw}. Then D1 is compared with succeeding data D2, D3, ... , Dq of the same sensor of the same user:

$$Sim\_Score(D_1, D_j) = \sqrt{(x_1 - x_2)^2 + (y_1 - y_j)^2} \tag{4}$$

The score is computed between all prior data instances.

IA_Time—The inter-arrival time is considered to find whether D_1 is needed to be eliminated or not. If the time between two similar data is relatively less, then the data is duplicate. If the time difference is high, then the data is new, and it is essential for data analysis.

En_Sta—The difference in environmental status also plays a vital role in redundant data elimination. It is because the biosensor data may be the same, but the environmental data may be different. In the worst environmental scenario, the biosensor data will be necessary. In this scenario, data must be preserved.

All three criteria are considered in the FaMOORA algorithm for making decisions on the current data instance. The procedure of the FaMOORA algorithm is detailed below.

Firstly, the decision matrix (DM) is constructed with data upon three criteria as follows,

$$DM = \begin{bmatrix} SS(1,2) & SS(1,3) & SS(1,q) \\ IA(1,2) & IA(1,3) & IA(1,q) \\ EN(1,2) & EN(1,3) & EN(1,q) \end{bmatrix} \tag{5}$$

Then DM is normalized, taking the square root of the sum of all the squares of each alternative per attribute. This ratio can be given as,

$$SS(1,q)^* = \frac{SS(1,q)}{\sqrt{\left[\sum_{q=2}^{q} SS(1,q)^*\right]}} \tag{6}$$

From the normalized DM, the attributes are weighted by using the fuzzy approach. In conventional MOORA [46], the weight value is given for the characteristics based on the analytic hierarchy process (AHP). However, it consumes a significant amount of time. Thus, we present a fuzzy weighting scheme for the FaMOORA algorithm. The weight value of the attribute *SS* is given as,

$$nSS_q = \sum_{q=1}^{g} w_q SS(1,q)^* - \sum_{q=g+1}^{h} w_q SS(1,q)^* \tag{7}$$

Here, g denotes the number of attributes that need to be maximized (beneficial attributes), and h indicates the number of attributes to be minimized (non-beneficial attributes). Further, nSS_q is the normalized attribute value. Then the fuzzy weight value is computed within the range of [0, 1]. The weight value calculated above will be in $[r_1, r_2]$. Then it can be mapped into fuzzy values as,

$$FW(nSS_q) = \frac{|nSS_q - r_1|}{|r_1 - r_2|} \tag{8}$$

For each attribute value, the weight value is computed as above. Thus, the normalized DM becomes the fuzzy weighted DM (FWDM) with the values of [0, 1]. From the FWDM, the decision on the current data instance is made based on the following if-then rule,

$$\text{If } (\text{SS}(1,\text{q}) \text{ to } (>0.5)\ \&\text{IA}(1,\text{q})\&\&\text{EN}(1,\text{q}) \text{ to } (<0.5)$$
$$\text{Then, } \text{D}_1 = \text{Duplicate}$$

By following the above rule, the data duplication decision is made, and the data on-looker nodes suppress the duplicate data. Then, the redundant free data is fed into the nearby fog node for health status prediction.

4.3.2. User Health Status Prediction by Temporal Analysis

The prediction model receives the user's health data from the data on-looker node then analysis the data based on temporal information. The prediction module carries the process of health status prediction. In this section, we introduce the 2L-2HMM model that predicts the users' health status. In this stage, the data instance from biosensors is analyzed with time series. The proposed 2L-2HMM works upon two levels. In the first level, the biosensor data is interpreted as in the HMM model. Let D_i be the data instance of u_i. The fog node first extracts the time series data u_i of the u_i. The next status of u_i upon biosensor data is characterized by $\delta_i(t+1)\ of\ \{\pi, \mathbb{A}, \mathbb{B}\}$. Here, A denotes the transition probability matrix, and B is the observation probability matrix. The observation matrix is composed of the data instances gathered by the biosensors. The initial state distribution is denoted as,

$$\pi_i = P(H_1 = 1), \qquad 1 \le i \ge p \tag{9}$$

where, P is the number of probability distributions, and H denotes the hidden state. The state transition probability of transition from state x to state y is computed as,

$$\mathbb{a}_{x,y} = P(H_t = y|H_{t-1}), \quad 1 \le y \ge p,\ 1 \le k \ge w \tag{10}$$

The observation probability distribution defines the probability of state transition for the observation lk as,

$$\mathbb{b}_k = P(l_k|H_t = y), \quad 1 \le y \ge p,\ 1 \le k \ge w \tag{11}$$

In general, the observation variable lk depends on the hidden state H_k while the hidden state depends on the previous hidden state H_{t-1}. The prediction of the next state of u_i is performed based on the Bayes assumption on observation distribution as follows,

$$P(l_k|H_t = y) = \prod_{w=1}^{|L_k|} P(l_k|H_t = y) \tag{12}$$

The user's health status is determined as normal or emergency based on the time-series data.

In the second level, the location variations of the users are considered. For instance, the set of locations of the user denotes $= \{L_1, L_2, \ldots, L_t\}$. As the tri-foghealth works upon remote monitoring, the user location may cover home, home surroundings, home long-distance. In this level, the user's current location is verified, whether it is frequent or non-frequent. Upon this information and the status predicted from the first level, 2L-2HMM uses the following rules,

- When the user's next status is emergency, and the location is not-frequent of the user, then the user is in a critical situation (C_1).
- When the user's next status is emergency, and the location is a frequent location of the user, then the user is in a near-critical situation (C_2).
- When the user's next status is normal, then the user is in the non-critical situation (C_3).

The user's next health status is appended with the data to increase the accuracy in the fog nodes. In addition, the health status prediction process assists in timely data analysis. In Algorithm 2, we detailed the process carried by data on-looker nodes, including redundant data elimination and user's health status prediction. At the end of this algorithm, the data instance is appended with the user's next state to make health status detection accurate.

Algorithm 2: Process in Data On-Looker.

```
Initialize  D1, D2, ..; Dj, ...
//Start Validation Model→ FaMOORA
For  Di do
    Compute Sim_Score
    Compute IA_Time
    Compute EN_Sta
    Construct DM
    Normalize DM
    Update weights by FW
    Apply IF-THEN Rules
    If Di to Duplicate
        Drop Di
    Else
        Fed  Di to 2L – 2HMM
    End if
End for
//Start Prediction Model →2L-2HMM
For Di do
    Extract μi
    Compute a_{x,y}, b_k                    //Equations (10) and (11)
    Predict Next State
    Extract θ = {L1, L2, ..., Lt}
    Fuse Two Levels
    Append User's Next Status
End for
End
```

4.3.3. User's Health Status Detection by Fog Nodes

After predicting the user's health status by data on-looker, the health data is delivered to the fog nodes. In fog nodes, health status detection is performed based on three categories of attributes by using SpikQ-Net. The proposed SpikQ-Net combines a spiking neural network that mimics the natural neural network [47] and a quantum neural network that works upon quantum mechanics [48]. The fusion of both neural networks results in better accuracy of the user's health status detection process. First, we clearly described the attributes detail in the Table 3.

Table 3. Attributes Description.

Category	Attributes	Description
Behavior	• Cholesterol • Smoke • Cig/Day • Height • Weight • Activity • Chronic_Disease • Location	Attributes are related to the user's normal behavior. We consider the static information like smoke or not and dynamic information like location to monitor the user's health status
Biomedical	• Blood_Pressure • Glucose_Level • Heart_Rate • Respiratory_Rate • Temperature	We consider the data from wearable devices. All data related to the biomedical data that shows the user's current health status
Environmental	• Room_Temperature • Noise_Level • Air_Quality	These data are collected from the regional environmental sensors.

The SpikQ-Net gets the input of these three categories of attributes, such as behavioral, biomedical, and environmental. Generally, the user's health status is detected based on the biomedical data. The reason for considering behavioral and environmental attributes is that both attributes have a high impact on the biomedical sensor data. For example, the heart rate is increased when the user is doing exercise and also in a noisy environment. In this case, the abnormal heart rate is reported by the biomedical sensors due to the tenancy of environmental and behavioral attributes. Thus, we considered all three categories of attributes in the user's health status detection. All three types of attributes are fed into the SpikQ-Net from the current data instance, as shown in Figure 4.

Let the current data instance be $D_i(t)=\{(BD_i)(BMD_i)(EN_i)\}$. The data instance at time t is composed of behavior (BD_i) biomedical (BM_i), and environmental (EN_i) attributes at time instance t. For each user, SpikQ-Net first extracts these attributes by learning the data received. Then, the weight value is adjusted based on the fusion of these attributes to detect health status. Similarly, the instances from various users are fed as input to the SpikQ-Net. The proposed SpikQ-Networks as follows,

1. The set of input functions $(D_1(t),\ D_2(t), .; D_i(t), \ldots, D_n(t))$ is fed into the input layer;
2. Each neuron learns the input to produce output vectors in the hidden layers;
3. The initial weight values (W_i) are initialized as the random numbers;
4. Then the weight values are updated according to the update rule of quantum mechanics;

$$W_i(t+1) = W_i(t) + \eta(|\,o\rangle - |y(t)\rangle)\langle D_j\,| \tag{13}$$

5. Here o is the desired output provided for the training stage, η is step size, and it is set as $0 < \eta < 1$;
6. At last, the out layer learns the output based on the weights learned from hidden layers. The output of the quantum perceptron at the time t is,

$$|y(t)\rangle = \sum_{j=1}^{n} W_i(t)|D_i\rangle \tag{14}$$

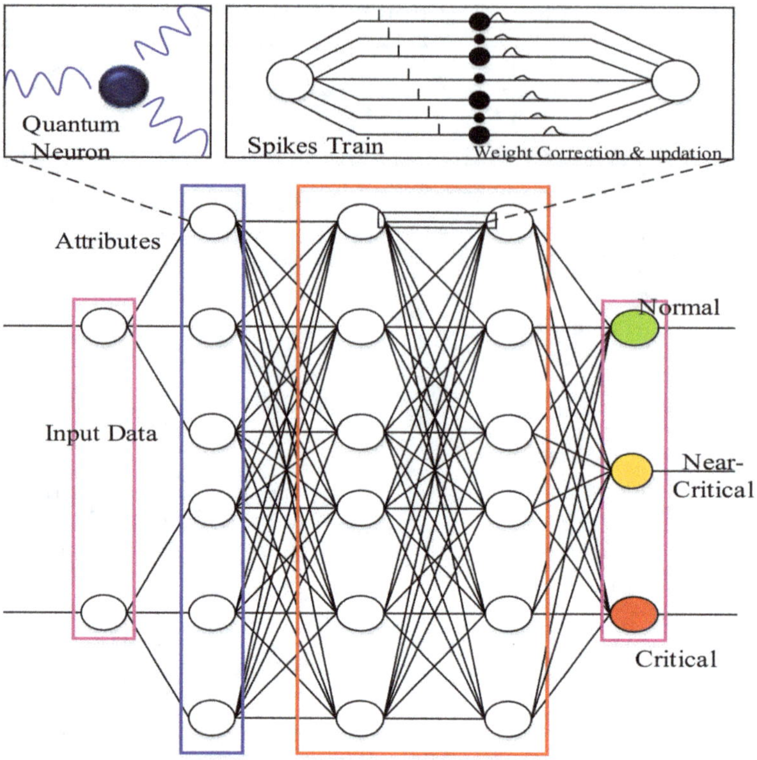

Figure 4. SpikQ-Network for Health Status Detection.

In this procedure, we introduce spikes between quantum neurons. The current activation function value is considered the neuron's state, and the spikes increase its value to achieve better accuracy. The introduction of spikes alters the weight update expression as follows,

$$W_i(t+1) = W_i(t) + \eta\delta_i(t) + v\Delta W_i(t-1) \tag{15}$$

Here, v is the momentum parameter and $\Delta W_i(t-1)$ is the weight correction in the previous iteration. In this manner, the weight values of each neuron are updated for each parameter, and the output layer detects the user's health status.

The main aim of this process is to detect the user's health status as normal, critical, and non-critical classes. As per the class, the necessary action is taken. The fog nodes take all the steps. That is, the latency is relatively low for the users. In addition, emergency actions assist in the timely detection of abnormalities as the process is performed in the fog layer.

4.3.4. Health Data Offloading

The data on-looker node assigns the data for analysis to random fog nodes. Thus, the fog nodes become overloading. To overcome this issue, we present the health off procedure. Although data processing in the fog layer minimizes latency, there has been a huge issue that is fog overloading. Users within the same region often access the same fog node. In such a case, when user density is high in a particular area, the fog node will become overloaded. Besides, if the environmental condition of a specific region becomes worst, then many users in that region will require immediate action. Thus, we present a fog offloading scheme in healthcare services. Each fog node has the stand-by manager who monitors the load of the fog node regularly and makes a decision on fog overloading. The health off decision is made in the following two cases,

Case 1: When the fog node becomes overloaded
Case 2: When the environmental condition becomes worst

If the health off decision is made, the stand-by manager selects an optimal fog node for health data offloading. For optimal fog node selection, we propose the MoSHO algorithm. Consider, f_{ol} becomes overloaded, then it selects the optimal fog node (fopt) from the set of fog nodes. The spotted hyena optimization algorithm is a bio-inspired optimization algorithm that works upon the social behavior of spotted hyenas [49]. As single objective-based offloading is inefficient to maintain the load among fog nodes, we formulate multiple objective functions in the MoSHO algorithm. The proposed MoSHO algorithm works in three steps: searching prey, encircling, and attacking the target. The overall process of the MoSHO algorithm is summarized below.

Fitness Evaluation—Initialize the spotted hyenas' population. The initial population list consists of a set of candidate fog nodes as $IP \in \{F_1, F_2, .; F_k\}$. Then, the fitness value is computed for each node in the IP set. In the MoSHO algorithm, multiple criteria are considered for the computation of the fitness function of jth candidate search agent $Fn(F_j)$. The considered multiple criteria are load value β, distance τ, and energy required ρ. The first objective function computes the current load value of the candidate fog nodes in terms of the number of processing tasks and available resources. The second objective function computes the distance between the current and candidate fog nodes. Thus, the offloading is performed between two nearby fog nodes, which minimizes the offloading time. The third objective function is formulated based on the energy required for offloading the current load from the current fog node to the optimal fog node. Thus, the fitness value is expressed as follows,

$$Fn(F_j) = \frac{1}{\sum(\beta_j, \tau_j, \rho_j)} \tag{16}$$

The fitness function is computed for all fog nodes in the candidate set.

Hunting—From the candidate solutions, the search agent who has the highest fitness value is selected to explore solutions in the given search space. The best search agent has the location of the prey. Thus, the other search agents form a cluster to move towards the best search agent. The cluster and the movement are expressed mathematically as follows,

$$D_h = \left|B.\omega_{h_1} - \omega_{h_2}\right| \tag{17}$$

$$\omega_{h_2} = \omega_{h_1} - E.D_h \tag{18}$$

$$C_{h1} = \omega_{h_2} + \omega_{h_2+1} + \ldots + \omega_{h_2+V} \tag{19}$$

Here, ω_{h_2} defines the position of the first best-spotted hyena, ω_{h_1} represents the position of other spotted hyenas. In addition, V denotes the number of spotted hyenas, and it is computed as follows,

$$V = Count_{nos}(\omega_{h_2} + \omega_{h_2+1} + \ldots + (\omega_{h2} + Ran)) \tag{20}$$

where Ran defines the random vector [0.5, 1], nos represents several solutions and count all candidate solutions.

Attacking Prey (Exploitation)—In this phase, the solutions are updated towards the best search agent. This phase is known as attacking the prey. It can be mathematically formulated as,

$$\omega(b+1) = \frac{C_h}{V} \tag{21}$$

The $\omega(b+1)$ saves the best solution and updates the positions of other search agents. The position updation is performed according to the best search agent. Next, the search agent fitness value is updated towards the ideal solution. This process is iterated until the optimal fog node is selected.

In Algorithm 3, the procedure of MoSHO based health off is proposed. Then, the data is offloaded to the optimal fog node selected by the MoSHO algorithm. The process of emptying prevents the fog nodes from overloading the problem. As offloading is performed between closest fog nodes, the latency is minimized. All three functions are performed in the fog layer to achieve better performance.

Algorithm 3: Procedure of Health Off by MoSHO.

```
Initialize population F_1, F_2, .. F_k ∈ IP
For all F_j ∈ IP
   Compute  Fn(Fj)  using Equation (16)
   Find best search agent
   Moves clusters              //Equations (17)–(19)
   Find number of hyenas    //Equation (20)
   Update solutions            //Equation (21)
   Find F_opt
   Offload data
End for
End
```

5. Experimental Evaluation

In this section, we present the experimental setup and comparative analysis of the proposed smart healthcare system.

5.1. Experimental Setup

In this section, we illustrate the experimental model of the tri-foghealth system. The proposed tri-foghealth is modelled in the iFogSim simulation tool. The iFogSim tool is best to model fog based environments with the functionalities of CoreCloudSim on the top of the cloud layer. For the proposed system, the code is written in Java language. All necessary packages and tools are installed on the PC to make experiments on the proposed tri-foghealth system. The proper software and hardware parameters are provided in the Table 4.

Table 4. Software and Hardware Description.

Software/Hardware	Description
Simulation Tool	iFogSim
Simulator Version	3.0.3
Operating System	Windows 7 Ultimate
Programming Language	Java
Development Kit	JDK 1.8
IDE	NetBeans 8.2
Database	MySQL-5.1.36 (Wamp Server 2.0)

The MySQL database is used to store the healthcare data of users. The other simulation parameters set in the experimentation is provided in the Table 5.

The proposed tri-foghealth system is built up based on the above simulation settings. At first, the users are needed to register with the proposed method by reporting their behaviors in the initial form. Then, the user data is stored in the cloud layer. Data from the same user is stored in a separate database after analysis by the fog nodes. The proposed experimental setup and flow are illustrated in Figure 5. As in Figure 5, we construct our fog topology for the smart healthcare system. The users and the fog nodes are deployed in different regions. The proposed tri-foghealth system analyzes the data from another region.

Table 5. Experimental Settings.

Parameter		Value
Number of users		≅ 50
Number of biosensors in each user		5
Number of data on-lookers		10
Number of fog nodes		10
Fog Node Configuration	Storage	1 GB
	Bandwidth	1000 KBs
	Resource Cost	3.0
	Memory Cost	0.5
Cloud Configuration	MIPS	1000
	Memory	10 MB
	Bandwidth	1000 KBs
SpikQ-Net	Number of neurons	10
	Number of hidden layers	3
	Activation Function	Sigmoid
	Step Size	0.2
MoSHO	Initial Population	100
	Ran	0.3
	Iteration	100

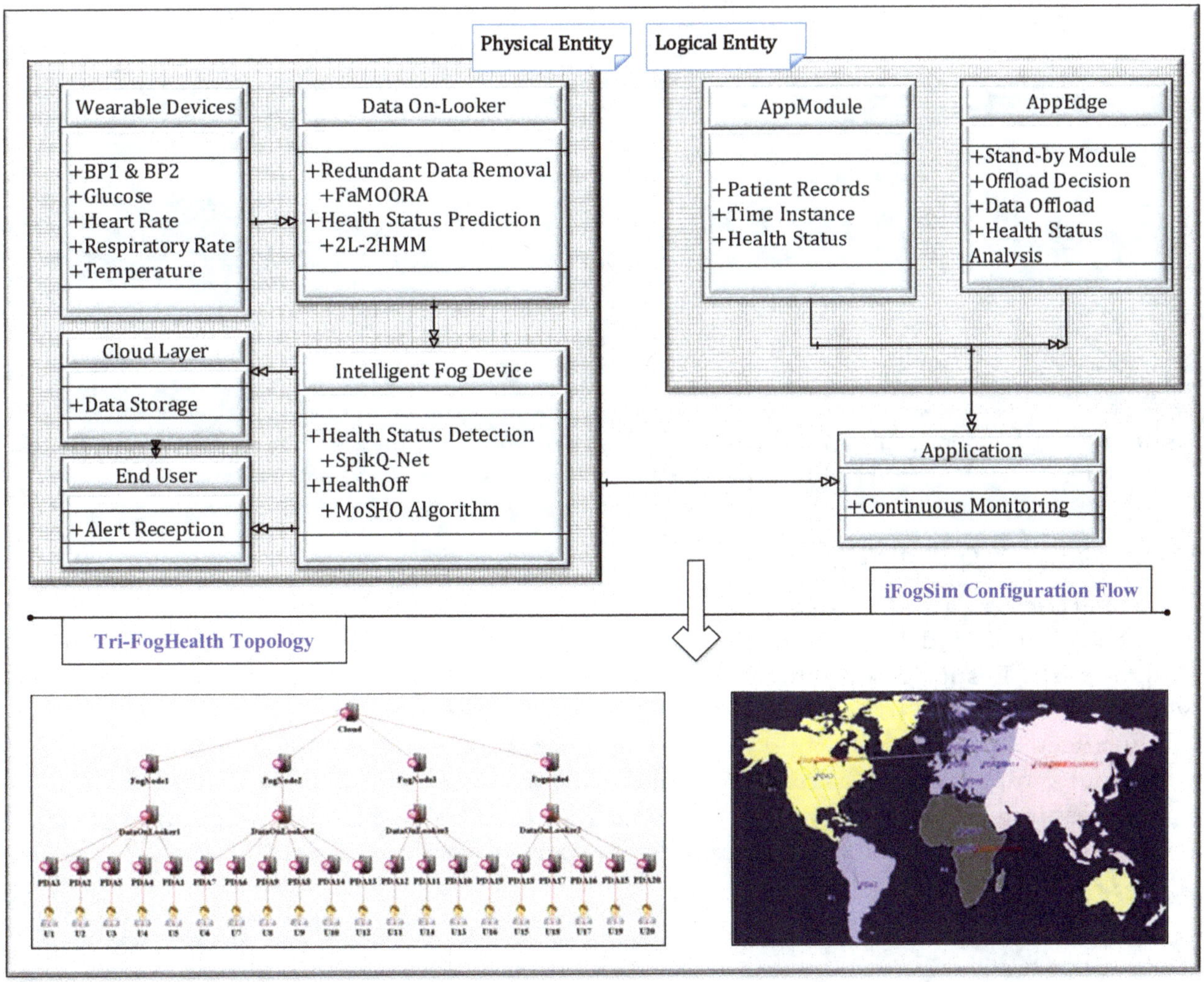

Figure 5. Experimental Setup of Tri-FogHealth System.

Data generation and analysis: in this work, we present a framework for monitoring the user's regular health status. Thus, we generate health data from the sensors. For each user, we create health data as per the considered attributes. The sample data generated for the users in a given time instance in a synchronized manner, as shown in the Figure 6b. In this way, we create nearly 1000 sample data with biomedical, behavior, and environmental attributes (i.e.,) each sample represents the biomedical, behavior and ecological data. The data is generated from 50 users registered in the system. The generated samples are sufficient to train the SpikeQ-Net neural network. Then, we use this data to train our healthcare system. Figure 6c shows the data points classified by the 2L-2HMM algorithm. Then, these data points are fed into SpikQ-Net, which is shown in the Figure 6d. Here, we set the binary values for specific attributes. For instance, we set Activities as Sit_(0), Sleep_(1), and Work_(2). Thus, the data contains either 0 or 1 or 2 at a given time instance. The proposed system also supports a particular disease diagnosis if the proper dataset is used.

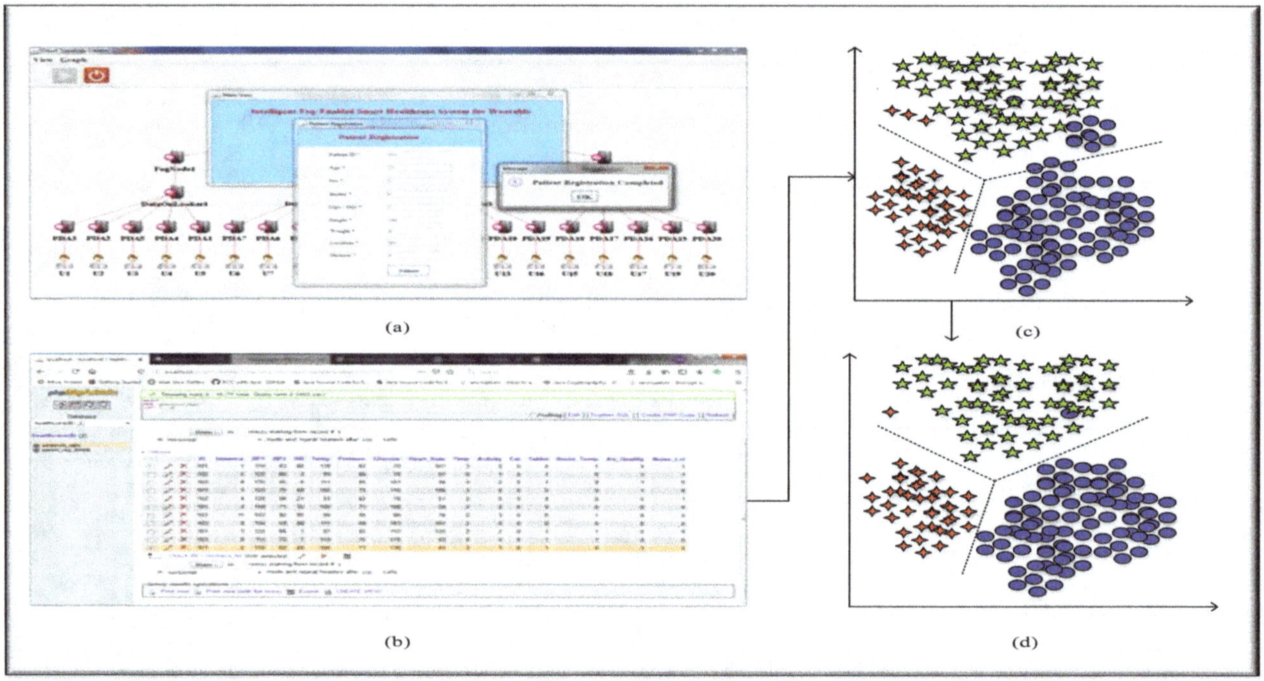

Figure 6. (**a**) User Registration in Tri-FogHealth, (**b**) Sample Data Generated, (**c**) Health Status Prediction (2L-2HMM), (**d**) Health Status Detection (SpikQ-Net).

5.2. Application Scenario: Remote Quarantine Monitoring for Covid-19 Outbreak

The novel corona virus (Covid-19) outbreaks are the significant and severe outbreak that healthcare systems handle. In Covid-19, it is impossible to treat all patients in the hospitals since the count is increasing rapidly. In such cases, remote patient monitoring will be a practical solution [46]. It can be achieved by our proposed tri-fog heath system, which focuses on remote monitoring. In Covid-19, most of the affected peoples have mild external symptoms like fever, cough and throat pain but have severe internal symptoms such as oxygen level reduction. As a result of these symptoms, the patient suffers from respiratory problems. We can apply the proposed tri-fog health for monitoring the patients who are in self-quarantine. The application setup is demonstrated in Figure 7.

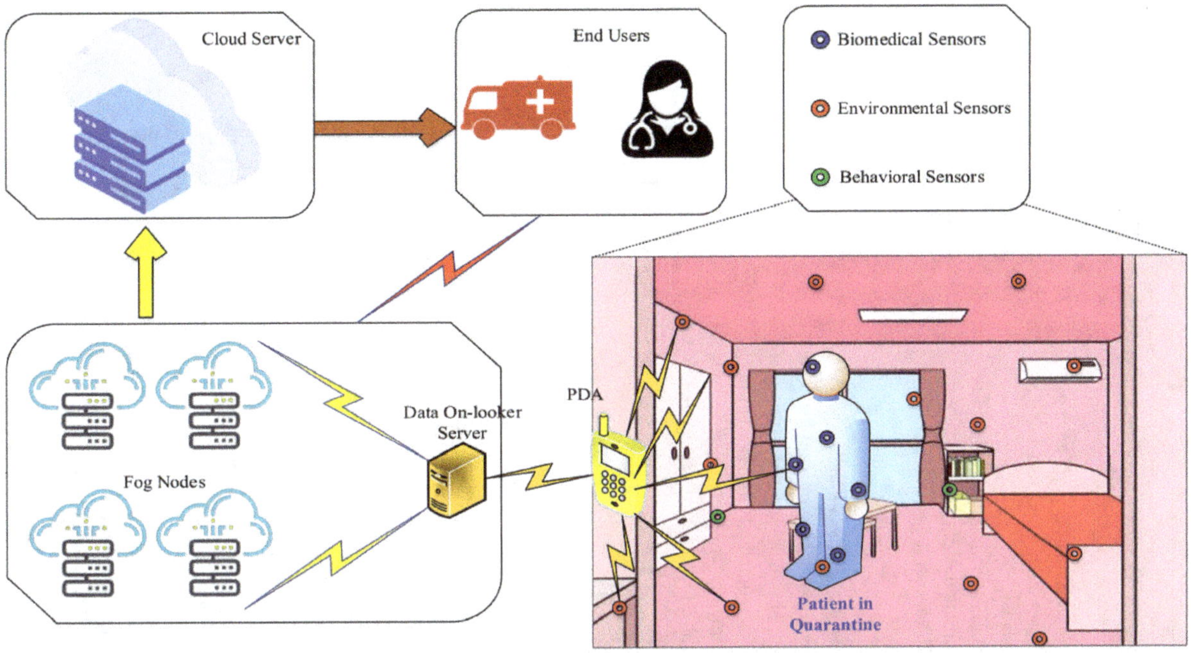

Figure 7. Covid-19 Remote Monitoring by Tri-FogHealth.

As shown in the setup, the patient who is quarantined in a room is equipped with biomedical sensors such as BP, glucose, respiratory rate, and temperature. Additionally, the place is equipped with environmental sensors to measure environmental changes. Before quarantine, the patient must be registered in the system by providing health history, which is further helpful in analyzing health status. The data collected from the quarantine room is sent to the data on-looker node through wireless communication. There, the data is cleaned, and the health status is predicted. Then, the information is fed into the fog nodes, which detect the health status by SpikQ-Net upon all three sets of attributes. It is worth to mention that tri-fog health generates an immediate alert to hospitals and doctors if any abnormality is detected in data. Corresponding government authorities can handle the fog and cloud servers. Thus, patient monitoring will be easy and accurate. Above all, the patients will get timely health services, which prevent early deaths due to Covid-19. In addition, the involvement of the health off procedure assists in offloading data among regions if any one of the regions become more congested. This prototype can be implemented by deploying wearable devices for quarantined patients. Nowadays, the usage of wearable (smart watches) becomes interesting among many users same as smartphones (can be used as PDA). Thus, data collection and analysis is easy in the proposed prototype.

5.3. Comparative Analysis

After setting up all necessary parameters, we generate data in the system to compare the efficiency of the proposed method. The proposed tri-foghealth system is compared with prior healthcare systems. For comparison, we consider fog based healthcare systems such as Fog-BBN [43], Fog-CPE [44], Fog-Smart Office [45] and also cloud-based healthcare systems such as Cloud-CDS [40], Cloud-Gaussian [41], and Cloud-MoPS [42]. We have summarized comparison between all these works in the Table 6. In the considered results, attributes are also varying. Fog-BBN and Fog-Smart Office works have considered all three sets of attributes, including biomedical, behavior, and environmental attributes. The rest of the current research works consider a single set of attributes (i.e.,) biomedical attributes. Besides, none of the existing healthcare works has concentrated on the offloading procedure in fog computing. Thus, the health load among fog nodes is imbalanced, which affects the overall performance.

Table 6. Comparison of Prior Works.

Work	Architecture	Concept	Attributes Considered	Cons	Common Issues
Cloud-CDS [40]	Cloud-based Smart Healthcare System	CDS based Healthcare System Decision Tree-based classification	Biomedical	1 The involvement of decision tree increases latency and also it is not stable 2 The CDS system is unable to handle streaming data for healthcare services	1 Latency is high since the data processing is performed in the cloud layer
Cloud-Gaussian [41]	Cloud-based Physiological Sign Monitoring	Gaussian Model detects health level Patient's Health Trajectory is extracted	Biomedical	1 The high Gaussian parametric approach increases the complexity 2 Single physiological sign consideration limits the accuracy of abnormality detection 3 Not able to support mobile users	2 Processing redundant data in the cloud layer improves execution too 3 Not suitable for emergency services
Cloud-MoPS [42]	Cloud-based Mobile Healthcare System	A smart shirt and Wearable Technology is used for health monitoring	Biomedical	1 Massive data analysis by threshold technique is inefficient 2 Classification accuracy is low, but the latency is high	
Fog-BBN [43]	Cloud-Fog based Patient Health Monitoring	BBN Classifier is used in Fog Layer THI is computed in Cloud Layer	Biomedical Behavior Environmental	1 Processing the same attributes in fog & cloud layer increases latency 2 BBN classifier is hard to complex and analyze 3 Only supports static users	1 Imbalanced load among fog nodes affects the system stability 2 Execution time is high due to the presence of a fault and redundant data from wearable devices
Fog-CPE [44]	Hierarchical Data Fusion Model with Sensor, Fog and Cloud Model	Biosensor Readings are Classified in each Level	Biomedical	Biosensor data alone is insufficient to analyze the health data accurately CPE works upon pre-defined rules which are not efficient for dynamic health data	
Fog-Smart Office [45]	Fog-Cloud Healthcare System for Smart Office	Severity Index is constructed to monitor the health status	Biomedical Behavior Environmental	Bayesian classifier which is used here is complex and has less accuracy Final health status is detected and a decision made in the cloud layer which increases latency	

The proposed tri-foghealth system resolves the major issues encountered in the prior research works. Thus, the proposed work achieves better results. The comparisons are made based on latency, execution time, detection accuracy, and system stability.

5.3.1. Analysis of Latency

Latency is defined as the overall time taken by the system to respond to the user's received data. The latency includes propagation and processing time. Latency (α) is computed as follows,

$$\alpha = \alpha_p + \beta \tag{22}$$

Here, α_P denotes the propagation time taken by the data to reach the fog layer and β indicates execution time (i.e.,) processing time. In Figure 8, we compare the latency achieved by proposed and prior works concerning the number of users.

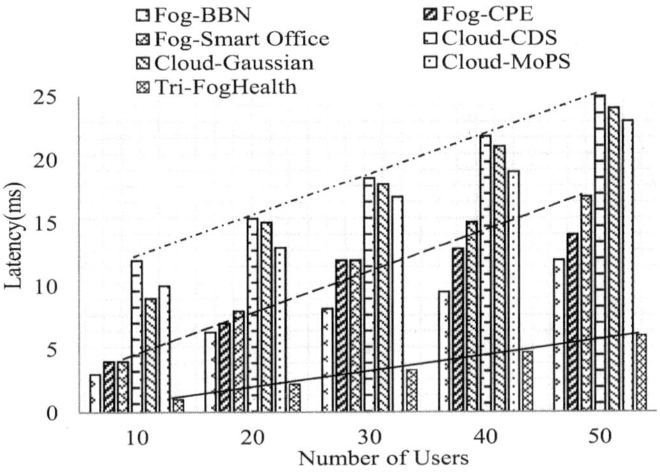

Figure 8. 7 Comparison on Latency upon Number of Users.

The analysis shows that the proposed tri-foghealth system has minimum latency than other cloud-based and fog-based systems. The cloud-based approaches like CDS, Gaussian, and MoPS methods have latency up to 20 ms, which is twice the time higher than the fog-based systems. Among the fog based systems, the proposed Tri-FogHealth system attains latency 6 ms even for 50 users. In the CDS system, a decision tree is used for classification. In general, the decision tree has higher time consumption, which increases the latency for users.

Similarly, the Gaussian approach has high complexity, and the MoPS algorithm works upon a static threshold, which can't handle the massive amount of data. Besides, the cloud-based systems relatively introduce high latency for users. Although BBN, Smart Office, and CPE methods decrease latency better than the cloud systems, still latency is high due to inefficient algorithms.

In Figure 9, we compare the latency achieved by fog-based approaches based on the number of fog nodes. Latency in fog-BBN is high since the second level THI computation is performed in the cloud layer. Thus, the latency is high in fog-BBN. In fog-CPE, rule-based health status detection increases the latency in the presence of a small number of fog nodes. In the fog-smart office, the Bayesian classifier has higher time consumption. Each fog-based approach has some limitations, such as increasing the latency and decreasing the efficiency of fog nodes. In proposed tri-foghealth, the system minimizes the latency with the efficient algorithm. The tri-foghealth system has only 5 ms of latency, even with two fog nodes. The main reason behind this high efficiency is that the tri-foghealth system follows the health off procedure in cases of fog overloading. Therefore, the issue of fog overloading has been overwhelmed. Thus, the proposed tri-foghealth system achieves much better efficiency.

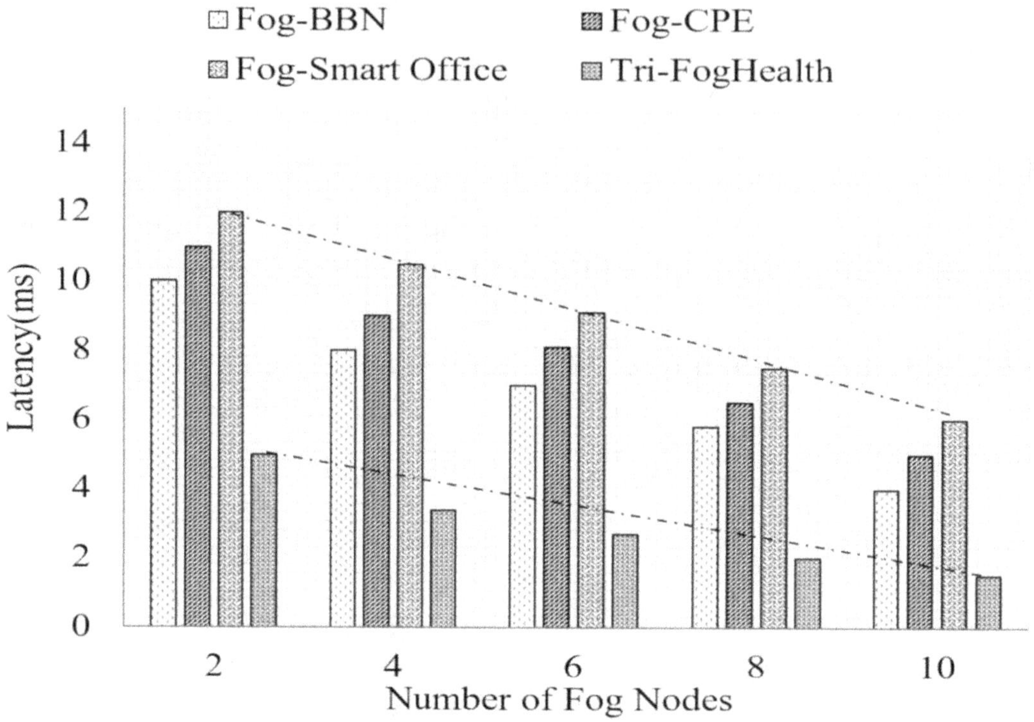

Figure 9. Comparison of Latency upon Number of Fog Nodes.

5.3.2. Analysis of Execution Time

Execution time is defined as the time taken by the healthcare system to predict the users' health status. The execution time measures the health status prediction and detection time.

In Figure 10, we compare the execution time achieved by the proposed tri-foghealth system. And the analysis shows that the execution time performed by the proposed tri-health system is lower. In comparison, the main reason for high execution time is the inefficiency of the algorithm. In fog-BBN, the Bayesian classification and THI computation are performed based on the same attributes (i.e.,) processing the same attributes increases the execution time. In the fog-CPE and smart office, the conventional rule-based algorithms are incorporated. Thus, the execution time is high in all these works. To mention that the Cloud-MoPS method takes 19 ms to process data from 50 users. As MoPS incorporates no algorithm for data analysis, it takes much time, which is nearly thrice time higher than the tri-foghealth system. In Figure 11, we analyzed execution time based on the number of fog nodes.

The comparative analysis shows that all of the fog based approaches suffer from higher execution time. Another leading cause for excessive execution time is that all works analyze fault and duplicate data from wearable devices. This analysis increases the execution time for the user's health data up to 15 ms. In addition, the curve shows that fog-smart office work has 8 ms of execution time, even in 10 fog nodes. The increase in the number of fog nodes alone is ineffective in achieving better efficiency.

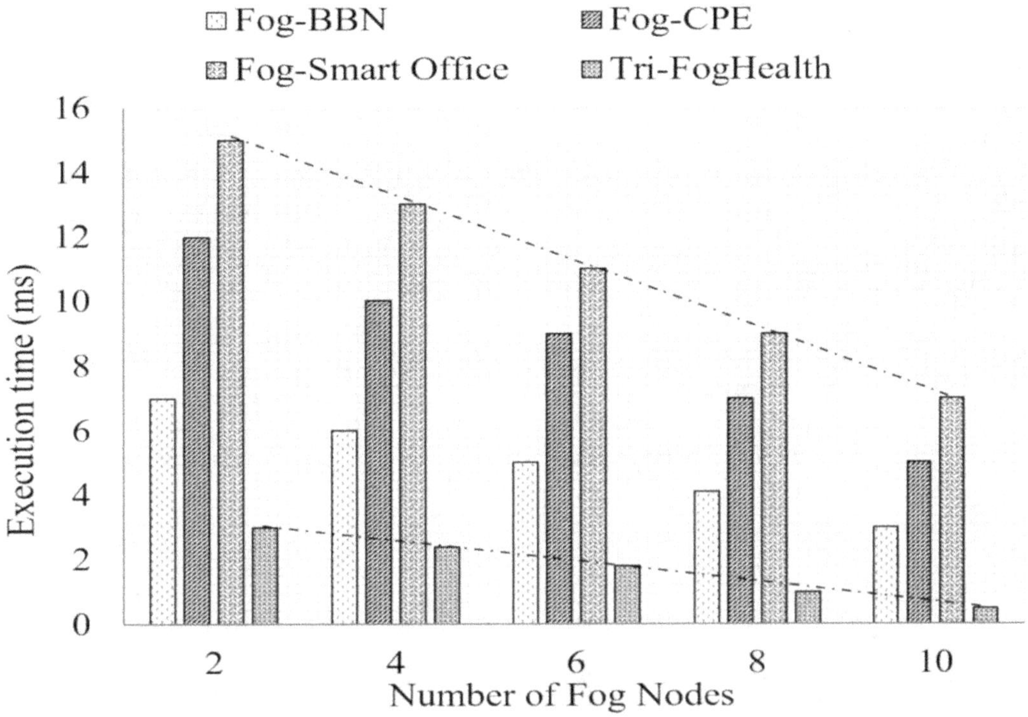

Figure 10. Comparison on Execution Time upon Number of Fog Nodes.

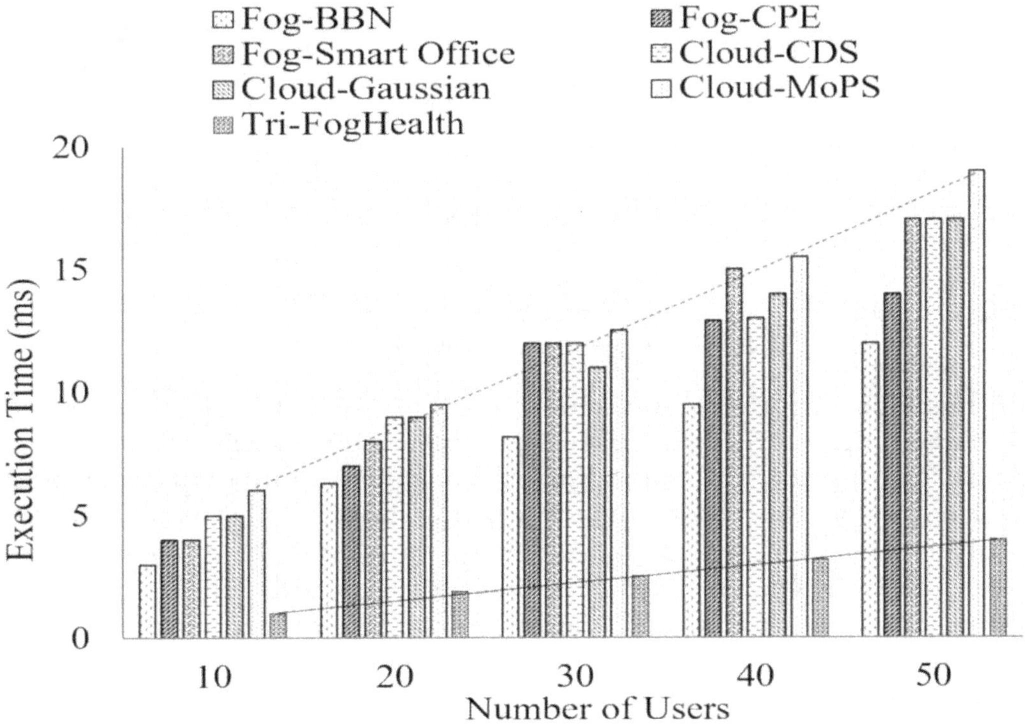

Figure 11. Comparison of Execution Time.

On the other hand, the proposed tri-foghealth system has only 3 ms of execution, even with two fog nodes. And the execution time is 0.5 ms in the presence of 10 fog nodes. This analysis shows that the fault data and redundant data elimination phases play a pivotal role in analyzing health data. With both approaches, we achieve timely detection on the user's health status.

5.3.3. Analysis of Detection Accuracy

Detection accuracy is defined as the number of corrective actions taken by the fog layer after analyzing the user's health status. Accurate detection is the ultimate goal of any smart healthcare system.

In Figure 12, the detection accuracy achieved by tri-foghealth work is compared with all prior research works concerning the number of users. In Figure 13, the detection accuracy is compared with fog based approach based on the number of fog nodes. In both analyzes, we can see that the tri-foghealth system has only slight variations. It maintains the accuracy curve more significantly than 95%.

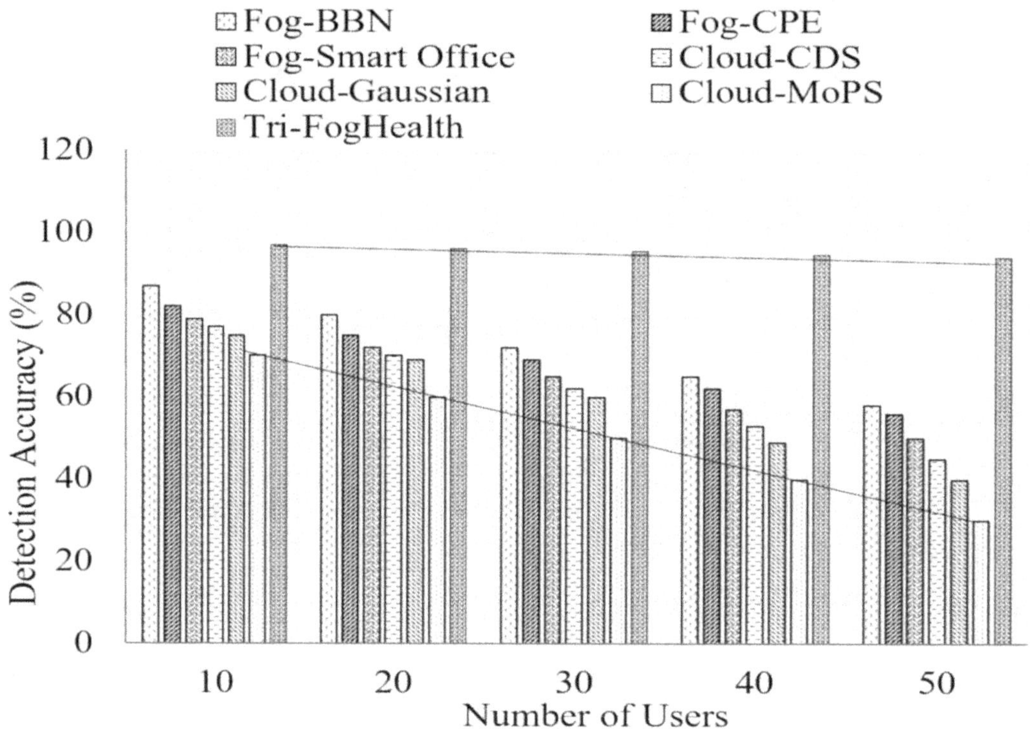

Figure 12. Comparison of Detection Accuracy.

The other methods have lower detection accuracy when the number of users increases. The existing accuracy curve shows that accuracy is decreased linearly. The main reason behind this much accuracy degradation is the algorithms used by the existing works are inefficient. In most cases, the Bayesian classifier is proposed, which has limitations in constructing the classifier model. Besides, most of the current works use the biosensor data for the user's health status detection. For accurate detection, behavior and environmental data are required. Thus, the lack of these data in existing works traps the detection accuracy to 30%. Even for 50 users, the tri-foghealth system achieves 94% in detection accuracy.

On the other hand, accuracy concerning the number of fog nodes shows that the proposed work achieves better accuracy even with two fog nodes. As we suppressed fault data and redundant data in the wearable layer, we make better accuracy greater than 90%, while other fog-based methods acquire lower accuracy, lower than 60%. In addition, the data overloading of fog nodes is a major problem in fog-based ways. Analyzing a massive amount of data in a single fog node makes the fog node inefficient. The presence of the health off procedure in proposed work supports at a high accuracy level.

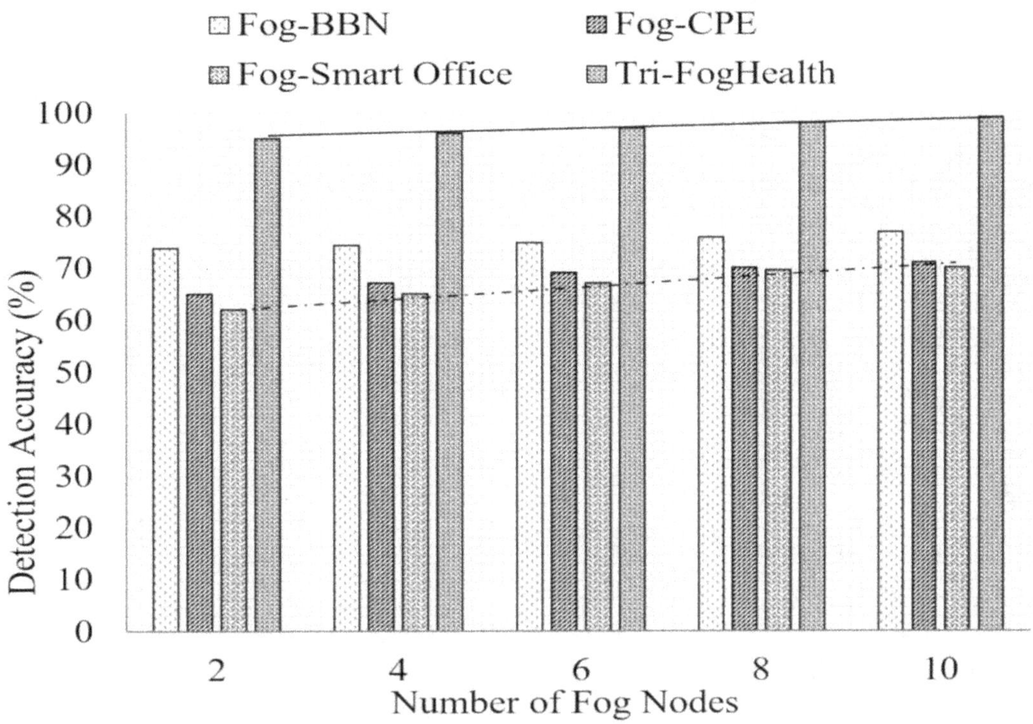

Figure 13. Comparison of Detection Accuracy.

5.3.4. System Stability

System stability is defined as the ability of the healthcare system to support a large number of users without a reduction in its efficiency and accuracy. In precise terms, it validates the scalability of the proposed healthcare system.

The comparative analysis of system stability is shown in Figure 14. Comparison is made for fog-based systems since the cloud-based systems can support a more significant number of users due to resource availability. The main drawback of cloud-based systems is high latency. Although fog-based systems resolve these problems, the stability of the system is still a concern. Since the fog nodes generally have resources lower than the cloud server and most of the users in the same region access the same fog nodes. In this analysis, we consider 50 users in the system.

In the presence of two fog nodes, most of the works have nearly 75% of stability. The stability is then increased linearly concerning the number of fog nodes. However, the highest stability achieved by the existing works is lower than 80% because all these works have an imbalanced load among fog nodes. As a result, the overloading fog nodes become unable to process data requests. On the other hand, the proposed tri-foghealth system achieves 96% for users, even with two fog nodes. The main reason behind these results is (i) fault data elimination by PDA, (ii) redundant data elimination by data on-looker, and (iii) health off by using the MoSHO algorithm. Altogether, tri-foghealth achieves system stability up to 98%. Form the comparison; we can conclude that the proposed tri-foghealth system has much better efficiency.

In Figure 15, system stability is compared between fog based and cloud-based approaches concerning the number of users. For a smart healthcare system, it is necessary to process many users without compromising accuracy. The analysis shows that the proposed foghealth approach achieves better stability regardless of the number of users (i.e.,) it reaches 96% and above strength for a varying number of users. An increase in the number of users and amount of data does not affect the stability of the proposed system. In this case, different fog based and cloud-based approaches achieve the same level of stability, which lies between 65% to 80%.

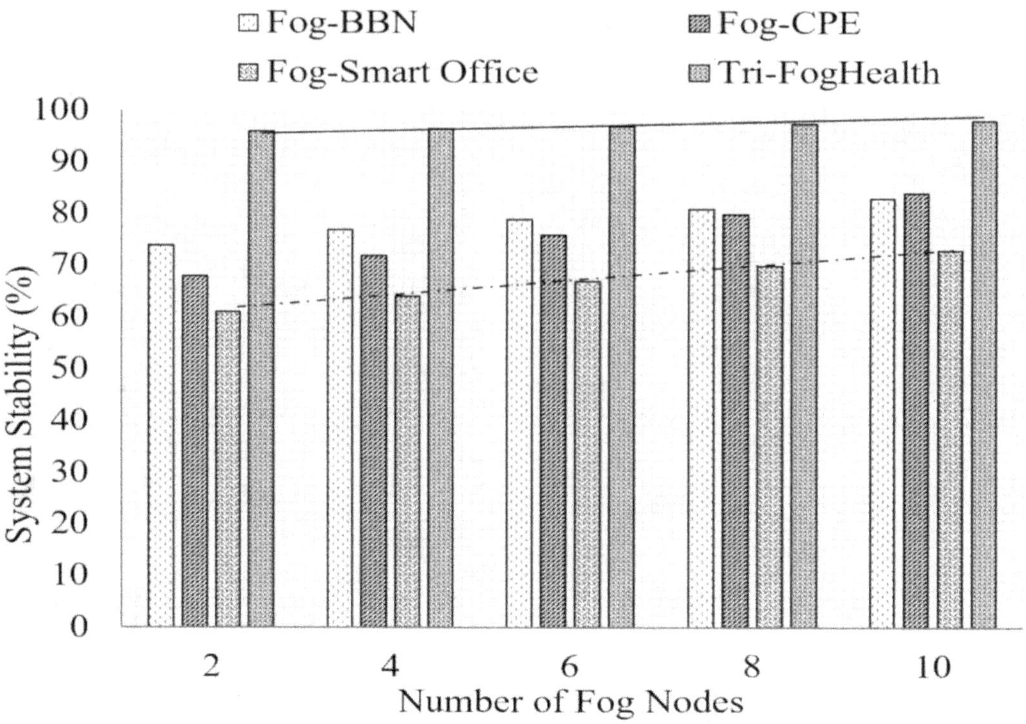

Figure 14. Comparison of System Stability.

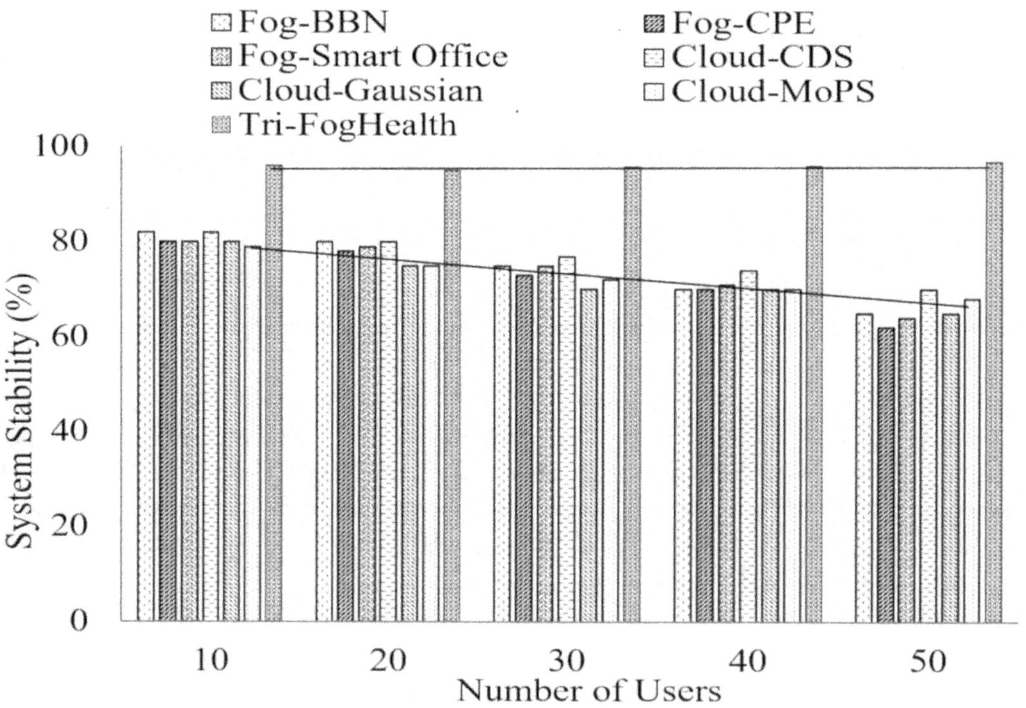

Figure 15. Comparison of System Stability based on Number of Users.

Further, there is a gradual decrease in stability with an increase in the number of users. An increase in the number of users increases the amount of data to be processed in fog and cloud layers. Although the cloud is more scalable than fog nodes, algorithm design also matters in achieving system stability. This analysis shows that the proposed tri-foghealth approach and the algorithms involved are effectual in analyzing the user's health status.

5.3.5. Discussion on Results

In this subsection, we discuss our proposed system. First, we summarize the average results of the proposed tri-foghealth system in Table 7. In this table, we have compared the proposed and existing works based on the average values obtained for each metric. The comparison shows that the proposed work achieves much better performance compared to existing research works. Mainly, the latency and execution time is relatively low in the proposed system without loss in detection accuracy. It shows that the proposed tri-foghealth system is suitable for real-time healthcare analysis.

Table 7. Numerical Comparison on Obtained Results.

Parameter	Cloud-CDS [36]	Cloud-Gaussian [37]	Cloud-MoPS [38]	Fog-BBN [39]		Fog-CPE [40]		Fog-Smart Office [41]		Tri-FogHealth	
				WRT n	WRT m	WRT n	WRT m	WRT n	WRT m	WRT n	WRT m
Latency (ms)	18.52	17.4	16.4	7.8	6.96	9.98	7.92	11.2	9.02	3.44	2.9
Execution Time (ms)	11.2	11.2	12.5	7.8	5.02	9.98	8.6	11.2	11	2.52	1.74
Detection Accuracy (%)	61.6	58.6	50	72.4	75.3	68.8	68.4	64.6	66.7	95.44	97
System Stability (%)	76.6	72	72.8	78.8	74.4	76	72.6	67	73	97	96

In this subsection, we discuss our proposed system. First, we summarize the average results of the proposed tri-foghealth system in Table 7. The comparison shows that the proposed work achieves much better performance compared to existing research works. Mainly, the latency and execution time is relatively low in the proposed system without loss in detection accuracy. It shows that the proposed tri-foghealth system is suitable for real-time healthcare analysis.

In Table 8, we summarize the overall contribution made in this work and its impact on results. We can see that the proposed algorithm supports the system to achieve better results in terms of latency, execution time, detection accuracy, and system stability. Although the proposed approach performs better efficiency, it also achieves tolerable complexity.

Table 8. Summarization of Proposed System.

The Methodology Used in Tri-FogHealth	Contribution in Results
RK-PCA Fault Detection	Eliminates fault data generated by wearable devices Increases detection accuracy since it allows only proper data for analysis Minimizes execution time since a large amount of fault data is suppressed
FaMOORA Redundant Data Elimination	Eliminates redundant data generated by wearable devices Minimizes execution time since the repeated data has been removed
2L-2HMM Health Status Prediction	Predicts user's health status based on temporal variations Increases detection accuracy since it predicts the user's next state Minimizes latency
SpikQ-Net Health Status Detection	Detect user's current health status Minimizes latency since the response is generated in the fog layer Detection accuracy is high since it considers there categories of attributes Execution time is low as the SpikQ-Net which is a machine learning technique that works faster than statistical approaches
MoSHO Health Off	Enable offloading procedure when the fog becomes overloaded Minimizes latency by offloading data to optimal fog nodes Increases system stability by maintaining a balanced load among the fog

The complexity analysis of the proposed system is summarized as follows,

$$Complexity = nT + (n - FD)T + 2T + T$$

As in the above, the complexity is also low in the proposed system. Here, n represents the number of data instances, and FD defines fault data. When compared to Gaussian and BBN classifiers, the complexity is low in the tri-foghealth system.

6. Conclusions

In this paper, we propose a novel tri-foghealth system for the smart healthcare system. The tri-foghealth system has worked upon three main layers by using wearable technology. The biomedical data generated from the wearable layer is processed in PDA to eliminate fault data using the RK-PCA algorithm. Then, the faultless data is fed into the data on-looker node in the intelligent fog layer; the data on-looker node is responsible for predicting the user's health status. For this, it uses temporal data in the 2L-2HMM algorithm. Before prediction, the current data instance is subjected to redundant data elimination process by the FaMOORA algorithm. After health status prediction, the data is processed by the fog nodes using SpikQ-Net, which works upon behavior, biomedical, and environmental attributes. Based on the emergency level of data, the immediate action is taken in the fog layer. Simultaneously, the health off procedure followed with the MOSHO algorithm to prevent the intelligent fog layer from overloading. The experimental results show that the proposed tri-foghealth system outperforms the current research works. In the future, we have planned to test the tri-foghealth system for specific disease diagnosis as the present system is designed to find general abnormalities. In addition, we intend to extend this healthcare system with trusted services as the health data is relatively sensitive. Thus, security provisioning is also a better research direction to extend the tri-foghealth system.

Author Contributions: Conceptualization, M.I. and L.L.; methodology, M.I.; software, M.I.; validation, M.I.; L.L. and A.N.; formal analysis, M.I.; L.L. and A.K.; investigation, L.L.; resources, G.L. and L.L.; data curation, G.L. and H.W.; writing—original draft preparation, M.I.; writing—review and editing, M.I.; A.N. and A.K.; visualization, M.I and Y.M.A.; supervision, L.L.; project administration, L.L.; funding acquisition, A.M.E.-S. All authors have read and agreed to the published version of the manuscript.

Acknowledgments: The authors extend their appreciation to King Saud University for funding this work through Researchers Supporting Project number (RSP-2020/133), King Saud University, Riyadh, Saudi Arabia.

References

1. Mohapatra, S.; Mohanty, S.; Mohanty, S. Smart healthcare: An approach for ubiquitous healthcare management using IoT. In *Advances in Ubiquitous Sensing Applications for Healthcare*; Academic Press: Cambridge, MA, USA, 2019.
2. Ahad, A.; Tahir, M.A.; Yau, K.A. 5G-based smart healthcare network: Architecture, taxonomy, challenges, and future research directions. *IEEE Access* **2019**, *7*, 100747–100762. [CrossRef]
3. Tian, S.; Yang, W.; Grange, J.M.; Wang, P.; Huang, W.; Ye, Z. Smart healthcare: Making medical care more intelligent. *Glob. Health J.* **2019**, *3*, 62–65. [CrossRef]
4. Muzny, M.; Henriksen, A.; Giordanengo, A.; Mužík, J.; Grøttland, A.; Blixgård, H.; Hartvigsen, G.; Årsand, E. Wearable sensors with possibilities for data exchange: Analyzing status and needs of different actors in mobile health monitoring systems. *Int. J. Med. Inform.* **2019**, *133*, 104017. [CrossRef] [PubMed]
5. Papa, A.; Mital, M.; Pisano, P.; Giudice, M.D. E-health and wellbeing monitoring using smart healthcare devices: An empirical investigation. *Technol. Forecast. Soc. Chang.* **2020**, *153*, 119226. [CrossRef]
6. Mutlag, A.A.; Ghani, M.K.; Arunkumar, N.; Mohammed, M.A.; Mohd, O. Enabling technologies for fog computing in healthcare IoT systems. *Future Gener. Comput. Syst.* **2019**, *90*, 62–78. [CrossRef]
7. Mahmud, R.; Ramamohanarao, K.; Buyya, R. Application management in fog computing environments: A taxonomy, review, and future directions. *ACM Comput. Surv.* **2020**. [CrossRef]
8. Zhao, R.; Yan, R.; Chen, Z.; Mao, K.; Wang, P.; Gao, R.X. Deep Learning and Its Applications to Machine Health Monitoring: A Survey. *arXiv* **2016**, arXiv:abs/1612.07640. [CrossRef]

9. Soualhi, M.; Nguyen, K.T.; Soualhi, A.; Medjaher, K.; Hemsas, K.E. Health monitoring of bearing and gear faults by using a new health indicator extracted from current signals. *Measurement* **2019**, *141*, 37–51. [CrossRef]
10. Fu, Y.; Peng, C.; Gomez, F.; Narazaki, Y.; Spencer, B.F. Sensor fault management techniques for wireless smart sensor networks in structural health monitoring. *Struct. Control Health Monit.* **2019**. [CrossRef]
11. Petrovska, B.; Zdravevski, E.; Lameski, P.; Corizzo, R.; Štajduhar, I.; Lerga, J. Deep learning for feature extraction in remote sensing: A case-study of aerial scene classification. *Sensors* **2020**, *20*, 3906. [CrossRef]
12. Munir, M.; Siddiqui, S.A.; Chattha, M.A.; Dengel, A.; Ahmed, S. FuseAD: Unsupervised anomaly detection in streaming sensors data by fusing statistical and deep learning models. *Sensors* **2019**, *19*, 2451. [CrossRef]
13. Merrill, N.; Eskandarian, A. Modified autoencoder training and scoring for robust unsupervised anomaly detection in deep learning. *IEEE Access* **2020**, *8*, 101824–101833. [CrossRef]
14. Ceci, M.; Corizzo, R.; Japkowicz, N.; Mignone, P.; Pio, G. ECHAD: Embedding-based change detection from multivariate time series in smart grids. *IEEE Access* **2020**, *8*, 156053–156066. [CrossRef]
15. Hu, J.; Wu, K.; Liang, W. An IPv6-based framework for fog-assisted healthcare monitoring. *Adv. Mech. Eng.* **2019**, *11*. [CrossRef]
16. Jeyaraj, P.R.; Rajan, S.E.; Martis, R.J.; Panigrahi, B.K. Fog computing employed computer aided cancer classification system using deep neural network in internet of things based healthcare system. *J. Med. Syst.* **2019**, *44*, 34.
17. Nweke, H.F.; Wah, T.Y.; Mujtaba, G.; Al-garadi, M.A. Data fusion and multiple classifier systems for human activity detection and health monitoring: Review and open research directions. *Inf. Fusion* **2019**, *46*, 147–170. [CrossRef]
18. Goschenhofer, J.; Pfister, F.M.; Yuksel, K.A.; Bischl, B.; Fietzek, U.; Thomas, J. Wearable-based Parkinson's Disease Severity Monitoring using Deep Learning. *arXiv* **2019**, arXiv:1904.10829.
19. Mani, N.; Singh, A.; Nimmagadda, S.L. An IoT guided healthcare monitoring system for managing real-time notifications by fog computing services. *Procedia Comput. Sci.* **2020**, *167*, 850–859. [CrossRef]
20. Zheng, H.; Xiong, K.; Fan, P.; Zhong, Z.; Letaief, K.B. Fog-assisted multiuser swipt networks: Local computing or offloading. *IEEE Internet Things J.* **2019**, *6*, 5246–5264. [CrossRef]
21. Runkle, J.; Sugg, M.; Boase, D.; Galvin, S.L.; Coulson, C.C. Use of wearable sensors for pregnancy health and environmental monitoring: Descriptive findings from the perspective of patients and providers. *Digit. Health* **2019**, *5*. [CrossRef]
22. Sangeetha, A.; Thangavel, A. Pervasive healthcare system based on environmental monitoring. *Intell. Pervasive Comput. Syst. Smarter Healthc.* **2019**. [CrossRef]
23. Aboudi, N.E.; Benhlima, L. Big data management for healthcare systems: Architecture, requirements, and implementation. *Adv. Bioinform.* **2018**. [CrossRef]
24. Sun, F.; Zang, W.; Gravina, R.; Fortino, G.; Li, Y. Gait-based identification for elderly users in wearable healthcare systems. *Inf. Fusion* **2020**, *53*, 134–144. [CrossRef]
25. Albahri, A.S.; Albahri, O.S.; Zaidan, A.A.; Zaidan, B.B.; Hashim, M.; Alsalem, M.A.; Mohsin, A.H.; Mohammed, K.I.; Alamoodi, A.H.; Enaizan, O.; et al. Based on multiple heterogeneous wearable sensors: A smart real-time health monitoring structured for hospitals distributor. *IEEE Access* **2019**, *7*, 37269–37323. [CrossRef]
26. Zhang, H.; Liu, J.; Kato, N. Threshold tuning-based wearable sensor fault detection for reliable medical monitoring using bayesian network model. *IEEE Syst. J.* **2018**, *12*, 1886–1896. [CrossRef]
27. Colopy, G.W.; Roberts, S.J.; Clifton, D.A. Bayesian optimization of personalized models for patient vital-sign monitoring. *IEEE J. Biomed. Health Inform.* **2018**, *22*, 301–310. [CrossRef]
28. Liu, Y.; Zhang, L.; Yang, Y.; Zhou, L.; Ren, L.; Wang, F.; Liu, R.; Pang, Z.; Deen, M.J. A novel cloud-based framework for the elderly healthcare services using digital twin. *IEEE Access* **2019**, *7*, 49088–49101. [CrossRef]
29. Anagaw, A.; Chang, Y. A new complement naïve Bayesian approach for biomedical data classification. *J. Ambient Intell. Humaniz. Comput.* **2019**, *10*, 3889–3897. [CrossRef]
30. Pathinarupothi, R.K.; Durga, P.; Rangan, E. IoT-based smart edge for global health: Remote monitoring with severity detection and alerts transmission. *IEEE Internet Things J.* **2018**, *6*, 2449–2462. [CrossRef]
31. Rahmani, A.M.; Gia, T.N.; Negash, B.; Anzanpour, A.; Azimi, I.; Jiang, M.; Liljeberg, P. Exploiting smart e-Health gateways at the edge of healthcare Internet-of-Things: A fog computing approach. *Future Gener. Comput. Syst.* **2018**, *78*, 641–658. [CrossRef]

32. Gai, K.; Lu, Z.; Qiu, M.; Zhu, L. Toward smart treatment management for personalized healthcare. *IEEE Netw.* **2019**, *33*, 30–36. [CrossRef]
33. Hassan, M.K.; El-Desouky, A.I.; Badawy, M.M.; Sarhan, A.M.; Elhoseny, M.; Manogaran, G. EoT-driven hybrid ambient assisted living framework with naïve Bayes–firefly algorithm. *Neural Comput. Appl.* **2018**, *31*, 1275–1300. [CrossRef]
34. Tuli, S.; Basumatary, N.; Gill, S.S.; Kahani, M.; Arya, R.C.; Wander, G.S.; Buyya, R. HealthFog: An ensemble deep learning based smart healthcare system for automatic diagnosis of heart diseases in integrated IoT and fog computing environments. *Future Gener. Comput. Syst.* **2020**, *104*, 187–200. [CrossRef]
35. Muhammed, T.; Mehmood, R.; Albeshri, A.A.; Katib, I.A. UbeHealth: A personalized ubiquitous cloud and edge-enabled networked healthcare system for smart cities. *IEEE Access* **2018**, *6*, 32258–32285. [CrossRef]
36. Khattak, H.A.; Arshad, H.; Islam, S.U.; Ahmed, G.; Jabbar, S.; Sharif, A.M.; Khalid, S. Utilization and load balancing in fog servers for health applications. *Eurasip J. Wirel. Commun. Netw.* **2019**, *2019*, 1–12. [CrossRef]
37. Mutlag, A.A.; Ghani, M.K.; Mohammed, M.A.; Maashi, M.S.; Mohd, O.; Mostafa, S.A.; Abdulkareem, K.H.; Marques, G.; Díez, I.D. MAFC: Multi-Agent fog computing model for healthcare critical tasks management. *Sensors* **2020**, *20*, 1853. [CrossRef]
38. Sharma, S.; Saini, H. A novel four-tier architecture for delay aware scheduling and load balancing in fog environment. *Sustain. Comput. Inform. Syst.* **2019**, *24*, 100355. [CrossRef]
39. Adhikari, M.; Gianey, H.K. Energy efficient offloading strategy in fog-cloud environment for IoT applications. *Internet Things* **2019**, *6*, 100053. [CrossRef]
40. Naghshvarianjahromi, M.; Kumar, S.; Deen, M.J. Brain-inspired intelligence for real-time health situation understanding in smart e-health home applications. *IEEE Access* **2019**, *7*, 180106–180126. [CrossRef]
41. Zhu, T.; Colopy, G.W.; MacEwen, C.; Niehaus, K.E.; Yang, Y.; Pugh, C.W.; Clifton, D.A. Patient-specific physiological monitoring and prediction using structured gaussian processes. *IEEE Access* **2019**, *7*, 58094–58103. [CrossRef]
42. Leu, F.; Ko, C.; You, I.; Choo, K.R.; Ho, C. A smartphone-based wearable sensors for monitoring real-time physiological data. *Comput. Electr. Eng.* **2018**, *65*, 376–392.
43. Verma, P.; Sood, S.K. Fog assisted-IoT enabled patient health monitoring in smart homes. *IEEE Internet Things J.* **2018**, *5*, 1789–1796. [CrossRef]
44. Dautov, R.; Distefano, S.; Buyya, R. Hierarchical data fusion for smart healthcare. *J. Big Data* **2019**, *6*, 1–23. [CrossRef]
45. Bhatia, M.; Sood, S.K. Exploring temporal analytics in fog-cloud architecture for smart office healthcare. *Mob. Netw. Appl.* **2019**, *24*, 1392–1410. [CrossRef]
46. Brauers, W.K.; Zavadskas, E.K. The MOORA method and its application to privatization in a transition economy. *Control Cybern.* **2006**, *35*, 445–469.
47. Xiang, S.; Zhang, Y.; Gong, J.; Guo, X.; Lin, L.; Hao, Y. STDP-based unsupervised spike pattern learning in a photonic spiking neural network With VCSELs and VCSOAs. *IEEE J. Sel. Top. Quantum Electron.* **2019**, *25*, 1–9. [CrossRef]
48. Salahshour, E.; Malekzadeh, M.; Gholipour, R.; Khorashadizadeh, S. Designing multi-layer quantum neural network controller for chaos control of rod-type plasma torch system using improved particle swarm optimization. *Evol. Syst.* **2019**, 1–15. [CrossRef]
49. Dhiman, G.; Kumar, V. Spotted hyena optimizer: A novel bio-inspired based metaheuristic technique for engineering applications. *Adv. Eng. Softw.* **2017**, *114*, 48–70. [CrossRef]

10

Investigation of Vocal Fatigue Using a Dose-Based Vocal Loading Task

Zhengdong Lei [1], Laura Fasanella [1], Lisa Martignetti [2] and Nicole Yee-Key Li-Jessen [2] and Luc Mongeau [1,*,†]

1 Department of Mechanical Engineering, McGill University, Montreal, QC H3A 0C3, Canada; zhengdong.lei@mail.mcgill.ca (Z.L.); laura.fasanella@mail.mcgill.ca (L.F.)
2 School of Communication Sciences and Disorders, McGill University, Montreal, QC H3A 1G1, Canada; lisa.martignetti@mail.mcgill.ca (L.M.); nicole.li@mcgill.ca (N.Y.-K.L.-J.)
* Correspondence: luc.mongeau@mcgill.ca
† Current address: 845 Sherbrooke Street West, Montreal, QC H3A 0G4, Canada.

Abstract: Vocal loading tasks are often used to investigate the relationship between voice use and vocal fatigue in laboratory settings. The present study investigated the concept of a novel quantitative dose-based vocal loading task for vocal fatigue evaluation. Ten female subjects participated in the study. Voice use was monitored and quantified using an online vocal distance dose calculator during six consecutive 30-min long sessions. Voice quality was evaluated subjectively using the CAPE-V and SAVRa before, between, and after each vocal loading task session. Fatigue-indicative symptoms, such as cough, swallowing, and voice clearance, were recorded. Statistical analysis of the results showed that the overall severity, the roughness, and the strain ratings obtained from CAPE-V obeyed similar trends as the three ratings from the SAVRa. These metrics increased over the first two thirds of the sessions to reach a maximum, and then decreased slightly near the session end. Quantitative metrics obtained from surface neck accelerometer signals were found to obey similar trends. The results consistently showed that an initial adjustment of voice quality was followed by vocal saturation, supporting the effectiveness of the proposed loading task.

Keywords: vocal fatigue; vocal distance dose; neck surface accelerometer

---

1. Introduction

Vocal fatigue may be diagnosed through a series of voice symptoms, which include, for example, hoarse and breathy vocal qualities, pitch breaks, reduced pitch and loudness ranges, throat discomfort, and unsteady voice [1]. Vocal fatigue may be experienced by any individuals during their life time, but it is more frequently encountered by professional voice users in occupational settings. Vocal fatigue increases vocal effort and decreases speaking stamina. Ultimately, vocal fatigue can lead to voice disorders, such as vocal hyperfunction or vocal nodules. Vocal fatigue is difficult to define because many factors, such as self-reported feelings, doctor-rated symptoms, and instrumental measures, could be criteria for its determination. For example, a self-reported feeling of vocal fatigue might be due to psychological stress, thereby not causing much detectable change in physiological measures [2]. Standards for assessing vocal fatigue are therefore difficult to establish. Nevertheless, most current research adopted the definition of vocal fatigue as a sense of increased vocal effort [3].

Considerable progress has been made in the evaluation of voice quality. Perceptual, acoustic, and aerodynamic measurements, along with self-administered tests, have been used to characterize changes in voice quality and performance in laboratorial settings [4,5]. The most commonly used method of voice quality evaluation in clinics is auditory perception, which relies on listeners' personal experience and expertise. Commonly used subjective evaluation tools included the GRBAS (Grade,

Roughness, Breathiness, Asthenia and Strain) proposed by the Japan Society of Logopedics and Phoniatrics, the CAPE-V (Consensus Auditory-Perceptual Evaluation of Voice) proposed by the American Speech-Language and Hearing Association, and the SAVRa (Self-Administrated Voice Rating) proposed by the National Center for Voice and Speech in the United States. These tools require specific vocal stimuli. For example, the CAPE-V requires the completion of three defined phonation tasks assessed through perceptual rating. This therefore limits the applicability of these tools in situations where the vocal stimuli are varied or unspecified. Many studies have investigated uncertainties in subjective judgment methodologies for voice quality evaluation. Kreiman and Gerratt investigated the source of listener disagreement in voice quality assessment using unidimensional rating scales, and found that no single metric from natural voice recordings allowed the evaluation of voice quality [6]. Kreiman also found that individual standards of voice quality, scale resolution, and voice attribute magnitude also significantly influenced intra-rater agreement [7]. Objective metrics obtained using various acoustic instruments have been investigated, and attempts have been made to correlate these with perceptual voice quality assessments [8–12].

A plethora of temporal, spectral, and cepstral metrics have been proposed to evaluate voice quality [13,14]. Commonly used features or vocal metrics include fundamental frequency ($f0$), loudness, jitter, shimmer, vocal formants, harmonic-to-noise ratio (HNR), spectral tilt (H1-H2, harmonic richness factor), maximum flow declination rate (MFDR), duty ratio, cepstral peak prominence (CPP), Mel-frequency cepstral coefficients (MFCCs), power spectrum ratio, and others [15–19]. Self-reported feelings of decreased vocal functionality have been used as a criterion for vocal fatigue in many previous studies [1,4,20–22]. Standard self-administered questionnaires, such as the SAVRa and the Vocal Fatigue Index (VFI), have been used to identify individuals with vocal fatigue, and to characterize their symptoms [23–25]. Hunter and Titze used the SAVRa to quantify vocal fatigue recovery based on 86 participants' tracking reports. The results showed a self-reported 50% recovery within 4–6 h, and 90% recovery within 12–18 h [24]. Halpern et al. used one of the three dimensions in SAVRa, i.e., the inability to produce soft voice (IPSV), to track vocal changes in school teachers. The SAVRa scores were then compared with two clinicians' ratings of the participants' $f0$, and loudness [26]. The overall correlation between self-ratings and clinician ratings was not significant. The average absolute difference score was 1.7. This showed that the clinicians and the teachers had different rating standards.

Prolonged or inappropriate voice use is commonly regarded as one of the causes of vocal fatigue. Vocal loading tasks (VLTs) are often used to investigate the relationship between voice use and vocal fatigue in laboratorial settings [1]. Previous VLT studies have typically instructed participants to complete standardized reading tasks of prescribed durations at specific loudness levels [1,4,24]. Perceptual, acoustic, and aerodynamic measurements have been used to evaluate changes in voice quality and performance before and after VLTs [4]. Unfortunately, the findings from these studies were often reported as inconsistent. Comparisons across different studies have been at times contradictory. This may have been caused by multiple factors: (1) the prescribed VLT might not have induced a detectable level of vocal fatigue across individuals, (2) the amount of vocal loading across participants may not have been consistent due to the lack of a universal method to quantify vocal loading, and (3) there may have been variability in experimental settings. A more robust vocal loading protocol for VLT is therefore needed to improve consistency, and to allow comparisons across different studies.

Amongst methods of quantifying voice use for vocal fatigue assessment, the vocal distance dose, D_d, first proposed by Titze et al., was adopted in the present study [27]. The vocal distance dose attempts to approximately quantify the distance traveled by vocal folds during vocal oscillation [27,28]. It is usually calculated in terms of the fundamental frequency, the sound pressure level, the voicing duration, and the vocal duty ratio. Whether D_d correspondes to the true cumulative vocal fold displacement has not yet been verified. But, as a four-parameter estimates, vocal distance dose is more comprehensive than other metrics that are based on one single parameter. Svec et al. described the procedures to calculate the distance dose using synchronized microphone and EGG data [29]. The EGG signal was used to locate the peak position for each vocal cycle in the time domain. The microphone signal was used to quantify loudness. Carroll et al. used cumulative vocal dose data correlations with subjective measurements in vocal fatigue experiments. An abrupt increase in vocal loading was closely related to a harsher subjective self-reported rating [30]. Echternach et al. found that a 10-min intensive VLT with a >80 dB loudness level was comparable to a 45-min teaching task in terms of vocal dose [31]. Remacle et al. showed that kindergarden teachers had significantly greater distance doses than elementary school teachers based on an investigation of 12 kinderdarten and 20 elementary school female teachers [5]. Bottalico and Astolfi calculated the vocal distance dose and the sound pressure level (SPL) for school teachers during their daily teaching assignments. They found that female teachers had on average a higher (>3.4 dB) loudness level than male teachers, but vocal distance doses did not differ very much between female and males teachers [32]. Morrow and Connor used an ambulatory phonation monitor to record and calculate the SPL and the distance dose for elementary music teachers with and without voice amplification [33]. The results showed that voice amplification significantly decreased the average SPL and the distance dose. These studies used the vocal distance dose as a quantitative measure of voice use in the VLTs or routine phonation tasks. Despite progress, no definitive correlations have been yet made between subjective assessments and objective measures in vocal fatigue studies. The distance dose prospectively offers a quantitative metric for vocal loading. Such framework is essential for cross-participants or cross-sessions comparisons to be meaningful and reasonable.

In the present study, a uniquely designed VLT was investigated. Ten human subjects were recruited and participated in the study. The vocal distance dose was used to quantify the participants' vocal loading online during the experiment. Subjective and objective measures were used to assess participants' voice qualities. A cross-session comparison was made to investigate the relationship between total distance dose and voice quality.

2. Research Hypothesis and Objective

We hypothesized that vocal fatigue during dose-based VLT varies with the vocal distance dose, D_d. The objective of this study was to investigate possible correlations between auditory-perceptual ratings, self-reported ratings, and acoustic measures during a dose-monitored VLT.

3. Participant Recruitment

The human research ethics protocol (A09-M46-11A) was approved by the Institutional Review Board at McGill University. No occupational voice users such as singers, teachers, and voice actors were recruited, because previous studies showed that their voice had greater endurance for vocal loadings than normal voice users [1,34]. The purpose of the study was not communicated to the participants before the experiment was concluded. The participants were only informed that they had to perform reading sessions. This was to help reduce the participants' biases towards the SAVRa ratings. For example, if the participants were aware that the study was measuring vocal fatigue, they would expect their voice quality to degrade throughout the sessions. This may increase the risk of biased ratings through the introduction of a psychological variable into the cross-session analysis of the participants' voice quality.

Participants were recruited in Montreal, Canada. The inclusion criteria were that the participants should be female, native English speakers with no history of voice disorders. Sex and gender differences in voice performance were found to be significant by Hunter et al. [35,36]. The present study only used female participants to exclude sex as a variable in the pilot study. Male participants will be used in future experiments. The participants' demographic information is shown in Table 1. The experiments were conducted in a sound-proof voice recording studio located in the Centre for Interdisciplinary Research in Music Media and Technology (CIRMMT). All experiments took place in the morning, around 9:00 a.m. The participants were instructed not to use their voice often over a period of 8 h before the experiments. The participants were required to withdraw from the study if they were found to have a voice problem, such as cough and cold, in the early morning. During the experiment, participants who reported any severe physical discomforts, such as unceasing cough and voice loss, were asked to withdraw from the recording session.

Table 1. Personal information about the participants.

ID	Age	Occupation
1	32	SLP
2	22	psychology student
3	38	psychology student
4	25	engineering student
5	23	SLP student
6	22	nutrition student
7	24	SLP student
8	26	engineering student
9	31	arts student
10	26	psychology student

4. Experimental Protocol Design and Data Acquisition

4.1. Vocal Loading Protocol

The VLT protocol is illustrated in Figure 1. Before the formal recording, the participants were required to attend a preparation session, during which they learned how to use a voice biofeedback monitor for the experiment. The VLT was structured as a series of six successive sessions ($S_i(i = 1, 2, .., 6)$). The participants were asked to read loudly the novel "Harry Potter and the Sorcerer's Stone" [37]. For each session, the participants were required to reach a D_d of 500 m within 25 min. After this reading task, the participants were required to finish a voice quality evaluation test with in 5 min. In preliminary study, a D_d of 500 m in 25 min was found to be intensive enough to induce vocal fatigue on participants, as self-reported. All the participants' voice was fully recovered after one day. This indicated that the selected D_d level did not induce any long-term vocal damage to the participants. The preliminary study also showed that the distance dose was sensitive to $f0$, loudness and phonatory style. A reading task using a habitual $f0$ and SPL yielded a distance dose of approximately 5 m per 20 s. But a note sung with similar $f0$ and SPL yielded a distance dose over 20 m per 20 s. Therefore, singing was prohibited in this experiment. The participants were asked to use a daily speech communication style.

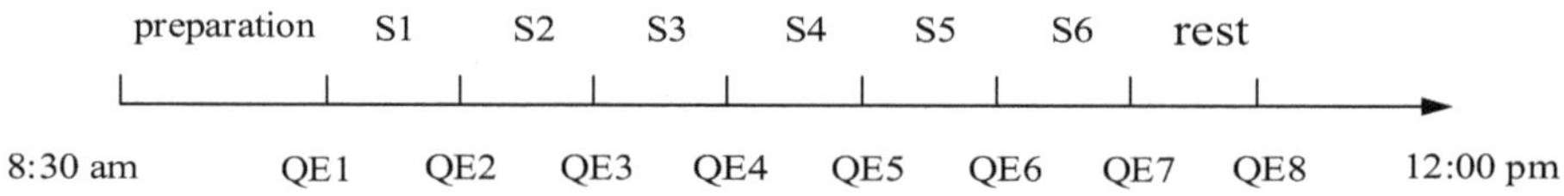

Figure 1. Measurement protocol of the vocal loading task in the vocal fatigue study. $QE_i(i = 1, 2, .., 8)$: Quality Evaluation; $S_i(i = 1, 2, .., 6)$ represents each vocal loading task session.

4.2. Voice Biofeedback Monitoring

The participants were seated in front of a microphone, and wore a neck surface accelerometer (NSA) mounted using adhesive (*Tensive*) [38]. The NSA recorded the neck surface vibration and streamed it on a hard disk [39–41]. During recording, the participants were asked to remain stationary, with the microphone at a distance of 50 cm from their mouth. The VLT sessions were monitored using a short-time (20 s long) distance dose calculator and a accumulative distance dose calculator in *LabView* (2018, NI, TX, US). A screenshot of the tool is shown in Figure 2. When the cumulative distance dose reached 500 m, the circular progress LED indicator turned from green to red, indicating the completion of one VLT session. The square-shaped LED indicator turned from green to red if the participant's previous 20 s distance dose did not reach a threshold value of 11 m. The threshold value was adjusted by trial-and-error to be high enough to induce vocal fatigue while ensuring that all participants could complete the VLT sessions. The participants were asked to keep an eye on the two indicators during the VLT sessions, so that they could adjust their vocal effort online, in real time. The virtual vocal distance dose monitoring tool prompted participants to read intensively throughout the VLT sessions. The 20 s distance dose calculation algorithm is illustrated in Figure 3. The total distance dose was calculated as the sum of all previous 20 s distance doses. The recording devices were a condenser acoustic microphone (Type 4178, *Brüel & Kjær*, Denmark) and the NSA. The microphone sensitivity was verified using a calibrated precision sound pressure level meter (Type 2250-L, *Brüel & Kjær*, Denmark).

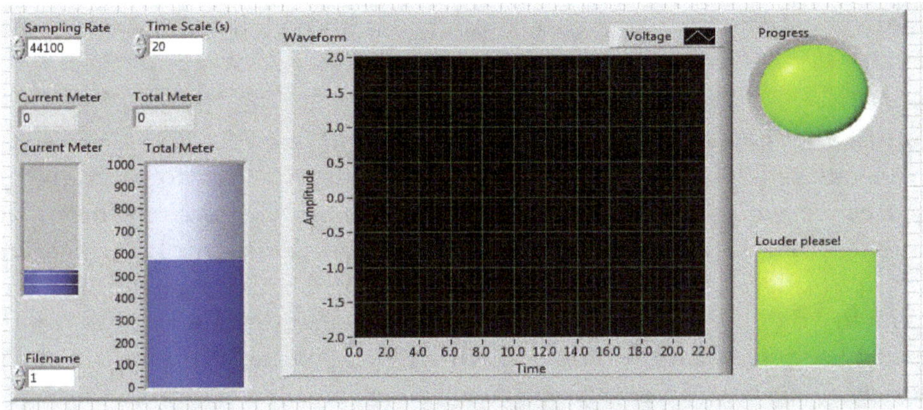

Figure 2. Virtual vocal distance dose monitor.

1: segment the entire recording into uniform-length (100 ms) frames;
2: remove unvoiced utterances from each frame using a zero-cross-rate based vocal activity detection method;
3: locate the position (x_i,y_i) of the vocal cycle peak for each frame, $i = [1, 2, ..., n]$ where n is the number of cycles for each frame;
4: calculate the SPL (dB ref. 20μ Pa) for each peak value using the formula: $\mathrm{SPL} = 1.108 \times 20 \times \log10(|\mathrm{y_i}|) + 89.25$;
5: calculate $f0$ in Hz using $44100/(x_{i+1} - x_i)$;
6: calculate the phonation threshold pressure in kPa using $P_{th} = 0.14 + 0.06(f0/f_{0N})^2$, where f_{0N} was 190 Hz for females [48];
7: calculate the lung pressure in kPa using $P_L = P_{th} + 10^{(\mathrm{SPL}-78.5)/27.3}$ [40];
8: calculate the amplitude of vocal fold vibration in m using $A_i = 0.05 \times 0.01 \times [(P_L - P_{th})/P_{th}]^{1/2}$ [33];
9: calculate the distance dose in m for each frame using $D_d = \sum_{i=1}^{n-1} 4A_i$ [35].

Figure 3. Procedure for the 20 s distance dose calculation.

4.3. Subjective and Objective Measures of Vocal Fatigue

Three subjective methods of voice quality assessment were used in the experiment. They were the fatigue-indicative symptom documentation, the CAPE-V rating, and the SAVRa. Fatigue-indicative symptoms, such as cough, swallowing, and voice break, were recorded manually. Before, between, and after each VLT session, the participants performed a voice quality evaluation (QE) task, rated using the CAPE-V rating [42] and the SAVRa rating [23]. The CAPE-V ratings included six dimensions: overall severity, roughness, breathiness, strain, pitch, and loudness. The SAVRa ratings included three dimensions: speaking effort level (EFFT), laryngeal discomfort level (DISC), and inability to produce soft voice (IPSV). The QE took less than 5 min to complete. After completion, the participants remained silent until the start of the next session. A fixed volume (100 mL) of water was given to the participants immediately before each QE. No drinking was allowed during the VLT sessions. After the experiment, the microphone recordings of the CAPE-V task were sent to four certified speech language pathologists (SLPs) for auditory-perceptual rating. The four SLPs had more than 3 years of experience on voice research and clinical diagnosis, and they used the CAPE-V on voice patients and experimental participants quite often during the past three years. Three of them were voice doctors in the McGill University Health Centre, and the other one was a voice research associate in

McGill University. The CAPE-V recordings were blindly rated by the SLPs. There were eight audio recordings for each participant. The order of within-participant files was randomized to reduce the SLPs' rating bias. The audio files were rated participant by participant, so that the SLPs could identify the participant-specific baseline of voice quality for each rating task.

Voice features, such as $f0$, SPL, duty ratio, CPP, spectral tilt, HRF, jitter, and shimmer extracted from the recorded NSA and microphone signals, were labeled with the corresponding session numbers. These voice features were compared across sessions to track the variations between the participants' voice qualities. These vocal metrics were also compared with the CAPE-V and SAVRa ratings.

4.4. Data Analysis

The mean values and standard deviations of the normalized SAVRa and the original CAPE-V rating scores were calculated. The SAVRa scores were first normalized for each participant, and then the normalized scores were clustered for statistical analysis. The scores in the SAVRa and CAPE-V ratings are inversely related to the voice quality, i.e., a higher score implies lower voice quality and vice-versa. This rule applies to all dimension ratings of the SAVRa and CAPE-V. For correlation analysis, all voice quality data were assumed to obey a Gaussian distribution. A rigorous validation of this assumption would require a larger data set, which was beyond the scope of the present study. A Pearson correlation analysis was done between each pairs of dimensions of the SAVRa rating scores and the CAPE-V rating scores.

Fifteen acoustic features were calculated from the microphone and the NSA data using Matlab (2018a). The symbols and a description of the features are shown in Table 2. Features commonly used in previous vocal fatigue studies were selected. The original microphone and NSA signals were segmented into uniform frames of duration 100 ms (20–40 vocal cycles). Frames that were too short (20–30 ms) were insufficient for extracting effective jitter and shimmer, and frames that were too long (>500 ms) could not satisfactorily resolve $f0$ variations. The unvoiced frames were detected and removed using the zero-cross rate method [43].

Table 2. List of features extracted from the microphone and NSA signals.

Symbols	Explanation	Source
$f0$	fundamental frequency	microphone
SPL	sound pressure level	microphone
duty ratio	voicing percentage in recording time	microphone
CPP_MIC	cepstral peak prominence	microphone
jitter_MIC	pitch perturbation	microphone
shimmer_MIC	loudness perturbation	microphone
CPP_NSA	cepstral peak prominence	NSA
jitter_NSA	pitch perturbation	NSA
shimmer_NSA	loudness perturbation	NSA
TILT_MIC	spectral tilt	microphone
HRF_MIC	harmonic richness factor	microphone
H1H2_MIC	different between H1 and H2 magnitudes	microphone
TILT_NSA	spectral tilt	NSA
HRF_NSA	harmonic richness factor	NSA
H1H2_NSA	different between H1 and H2 magnitudes	NSA

The procedure of multivariate analysis in the present study was that a trend was searched in SAVRa scores at first to build a baseline of identifying vocal fatigue. A similar trend in the CAPE-V scores was then searched to verify the consistency between self-administered and SLP-rated methods. Finally, this trend was searched in the fifteen acoustic features to demonstrate some specific features have the potential of indicating vocal fatigue.

5. Data Analysis Results and Discussions

5.1. SAVRa and CAPE-V Rating Results

The mean values and standard deviations of the normalized SAVRa and the original CAPE-V rating scores are shown in Figures 4 and 5, respectively. The Pearson correlation coefficients for SAVRa rating results (mean values) were 0.957 (EFFT vs. DISC), 0.834 (EFFT vs. IPSV), and 0.852 (DISC vs. IPSV), respectively. The average variation trajectories of these three dimensions are well correlated with each other. The EFFT and the DISC scores increased rapidly from QE1 to QE2, as shown in Figure 4. The IPSV score increased mildly at the beginning of the VLT sessions, which indicated that the soft phonation quality decreased slightly for S1. The average score increased for the EFFT, DISC, and IPSV from QE1 to QE2 were 0.52, 0.38, and 0.07, respectively. The effect of rest on self-reported voice quality ratings was notable for all dimensions. The mean and the standard deviation values of the three dimensions of the SAVRa ratings are shown in Table 3. The EFFT, the DISC, and the IPSV decreased by 50.0%, 59.3%, and 50.9%, respectively, from QE7 to QE8. In general, the high score ratings for all three dimensions occurred late in the sessions. The maximum (0.88) EFFT scores occurred at QE6, the maximum (0.88) DISC scores occurred at QE7, and the maximum (0.82) IPSV scores occurred at QE5. This indicated a cumulative effect, i.e., vocal fatigue increased over time during VLT sessions. In general, all three dimensions of the SAVRa ratings followed a similar trend across sessions.

Table 3. SAVRa mean and deviation values in terms of VLT session. The display format was $x(y)$, where x was the mean and y was the standard deviation. QE_i (i = 1...8): quality evaluation. EFFT: speaking effort level. DISC: laryngeal discomfort level. IPSV: inability to produce soft voice.

	EFFT	DISC	IPSV
QE1	0.08 (0.25)	0.02 (0.07)	0.23 (0.39)
QE2	0.61 (0.38)	0.40 (0.27)	0.30 (0.28)
QE3	0.54 (0.20)	0.52 (0.27)	0.46 (0.28)
QE4	0.66 (0.27)	0.48 (0.22)	0.71 (0.31)
QE5	0.80 (0.14)	0.76 (0.13)	0.82 (0.19)
QE6	0.88 (0.25)	0.83 (0.14)	0.67 (0.30)
QE7	0.84 (0.26)	0.88 (0.26)	0.72 (0.36)
QE8	0.42 (0.38)	0.36 (0.32)	0.35 (0.45)

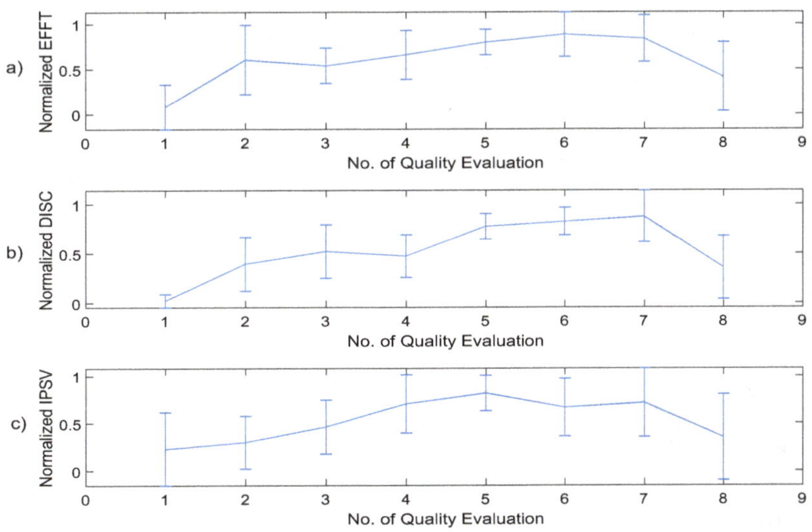

Figure 4. Cross-session variations mean and standard deviation values of SAVRa ratings for all participants (n = 10). (**a**) speaking effort level (EFFT); (**b**) laryngeal discomfort level (DISC); (**c**) inability to produce soft voice (IPSV).

The Pearson correlation coefficients between the overall severity trace and other dimensions in the CAPE-V ratings are shown in Table 4. This indicated that the overall severity, roughness, and strain variations were well correlated. The mean values of the overall severity, the roughness, and the strain scores followed a trend similar to that of the SAVRa results, as shown in Figure 5. They increased rapidly after S1 (QE1–QE3), remained constant for several sessions, and decreased over the remainder of the session. This trend was generally consistent with those of all three dimensions in SAVRa ratings, which showed a vocal 'transition' or 'adjustment' period in the first session and a vocal 'recovery' period during the final session. The maximum values of these three dimensions, shown in Figure 5, occurred at QE6. The mean and deviation values of the three dimensions of the SAVRa ratings are shown in Table 5. Other dimensions in the CAPE-V ratings followed different trends. The standard deviations of the CAPEV ratings across SLPs were larger than those of SAVRa ratings.

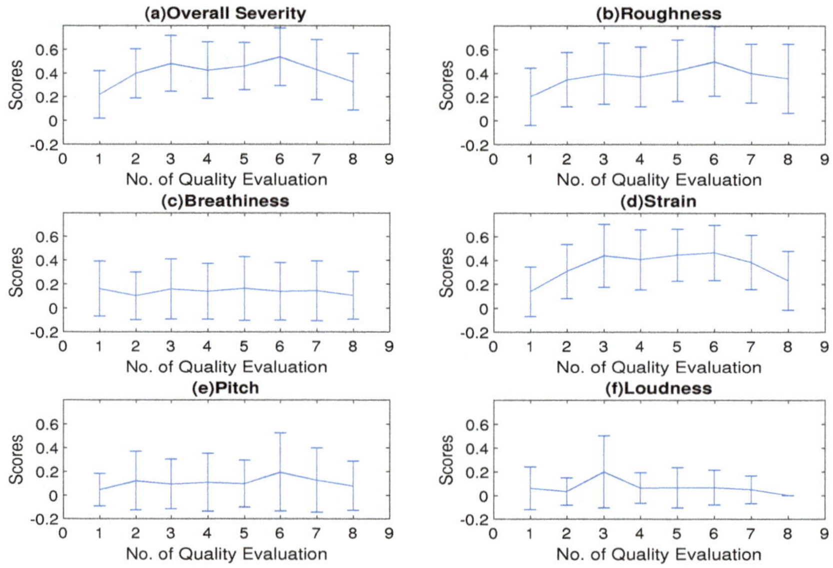

Figure 5. Cross-session variations mean and standard deviation values of CAPE-V ratings for all participants (n = 10).

Table 4. Pearson correlation coefficients between the overall severity and other dimensions.

With Overall Severity	r	p
Roughness	0.948	0.00
Breathiness	0.103	0.81
Strain	0.969	0.00
Pitch	0.810	0.01
Loudness	0.402	0.32

Table 5. CAPEV mean and deviation values in terms of VLT session. The display format was $x(y)$, where x was the mean and y was the standard deviation. OS: overall severity, RG: Roughness, BT: Breathiness, ST: Strain, PT: Pitch, LD: Loudness.

	OS	RG	BT	ST	PT	LD
QE1	0.22 (0.20)	0.20 (0.24)	0.16 (0.23)	0.14 (0.21)	0.04 (0.14)	0.06 (0.18)
QE2	0.39 (0.21)	0.34 (0.23)	0.10 (0.20)	0.31 (0.23)	0.12 (0.25)	0.03 (0.12)
QE3	0.48 (0.23)	0.39 (0.26)	0.15 (0.25)	0.44 (0.27)	0.09 (0.21)	0.20 (0.30)
QE4	0.42 (0.24)	0.37 (0.25)	0.14 (0.23)	0.41 (0.25)	0.11 (0.24)	0.06 (0.13)
QE5	0.46 (0.20)	0.42 (0.26)	0.16 (0.27)	0.44 (0.22)	0.10 (0.20)	0.07 (0.17)
QE6	0.53 (0.24)	0.50 (0.29)	0.14 (0.24)	0.46 (0.23)	0.19 (0.33)	0.07 (0.15)

5.2. Vocal Fatigue Symptoms Recordings

The participants' vocal fatigue-indicative symptoms during the six VLT session are shown in Figure 6. The cross-participant discrepancy in the vocal symptoms is notable. For example, participant No. 4 was found to display much more (+47) symptoms than participant No. 8. One cough by participant No. 5 occurred for 4 VLT sessions, but no cough was observed for participants No. 3, No. 7, and No. 8 during any VLT sessions. The mean counts of vocal fatigue symptom appearances for all participants are shown in Figure 6. The average counts of swallowing increased by a factor of 1.8 from S1 to S2, then decreased to a relatively stable level (4–4.5 times). This trend is consistent with that of the overall severity, the roughness, and the strain in the CAPE-V ratings, and the EFFT in the SAVRa ratings. This finding validated the previous study results, which showed that re-hydration could relieve vocal fatigue, and allow voice to be sustained over longer time periods [44,45]. No similar trends were observed for any other symptoms, nor any dimensions in the CAPE-V and the SAVRa.

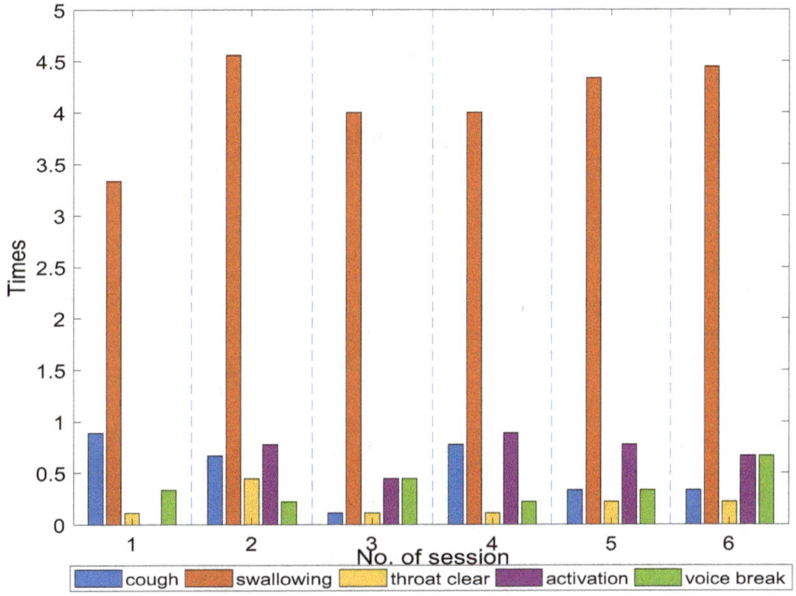

Figure 6. Mean counts of vocal fatigue symptom appearances for all participants during the VLTs in terms of session. The vertical blue dash lines separate different VLT sessions.

5.3. Acoustic Feature Analysis

The cross-session variations of the mean and confidence level (95%) of the features for all participants are shown in Figure 7. The NSA data of participant No.1 was unavailable due to sensor failure. The $f0$, SPL, and duty ratio in Figure 7 follow a similar trend. They increase rapidly at the beginning, reach a certain saturation level over the remaining sessions. $f0$, SPL, and duty ratio indicated a vocal adjustment over session S1. The mean value variations of these three features from S1 to S2 were at least 100% larger than those of any other following VLT session. The $f0$ had the minimal mean value variation (<2 Hz) in the last three sessions. The SPL mean value decreased by 2 dB after S4 and increased by 1 dB after S5. The duty ratio mean value increased by 2% from one plateau (S2–S4) to another (S5–S6). The trends in $f0$, SPL and duty ratio were largely consistent with the trends in CAPE-V and SAVRa ratings.

A considerable decrease in CPP was found to be related to the presence of dysphonia by Heman-Ackah [16]. The CPP_MIC in Figure 7 showed a slight increase (0.15 dB) from S1 to S2, and a decrease (0.3 dB) from S3 to S4. The fluctuation of the CPP_MIC from S1 to S6 was less than 2%, which means that the variation of CPP_MIC was not significant. The CPP_NSA showed a sharp increase (2 dB) in the late session after sustaining a relatively low level for the first three sessions. The jitter_MIC increased rapidly from S1 to S4 by 10% but decreased by 5% afterwards, which was not well correlated with the subjective rating results for the VLT sessions. The jitter_NSA showed a trend similar to jitter_MIC, but with a larger decrease after S3. The mean values of the shimmer_MIC and shimmer_NSA were well correlated ($r = 0.91, p = 0.987$). Their progressions were similar to that of the $f0$. This indicates that the loudness perturbation increased rapidly in the early sessions, and saturated at a high level over the last sessions.

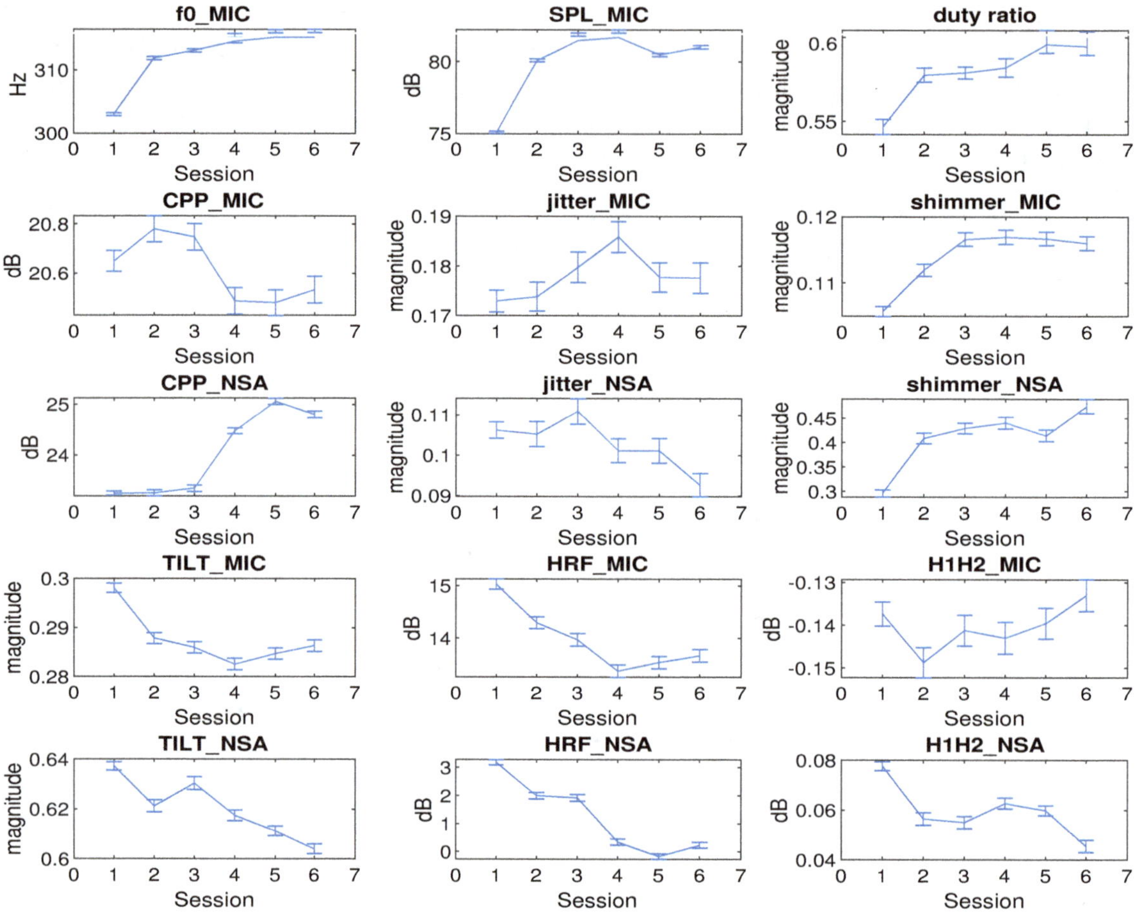

Figure 7. Cross-session variations of means and confidential levels in terms of feature for all participants.

A decrease in spectral tilt slope was found to correlate with stressed phonation by Sluijter and Heuven [46]. A decrease in spectral tilt slope indicates that higher frequencies are increased more than lower frequencies. In Figure 7, the TILT_MIC slopes and the TILT_NSA slopes decreased from S1 to S6 in general. Thus, the high frequencies of both the microphone and NSA spectra increased throughout VLT sessions. Childers and Lee found that vocal fry had a higher HRF value than modal and breathy voice [47]. The HRF_MIC and the HRF_NSA obeyed similar trends than TILT_MIC and TILT_NSA. The HRF_MIC was well correlated ($r = 0.94, p = 0.98$) with HRF_NSA. These two features showed identical trends. The HRF mean values decreased from S1 and converged to S6. The H1H2_NSA decreased by 50% from S1 to S6, and remained constant from S2 to S5. A comprehensive analysis of the Pearson correlation between each pair of features is shown in Table 6. There are two groups of well correlated (>90%) features. The first group includes $f0$, SPL_MIC, duty ratio, shimmer_MIC, and shimmer_NSA. The first group shows a rapid increase in early session followed by saturation. The second group includes TILT_MIC, TILT_NSA, HRF_MIC, and HRF_NSA and shows a general decrease from S1 to S6.

Table 6. Pearson correlation coefficients for each pair of features. The fi (i = 1, ..., 15) represents *f*0, SPL, duty ratio, CPP_MIC, jitter_MIC, shimmer_MIC, CPP_NSA, jitter_NSA, shimmer_NSA, TILT_MIC, HRF_MIC, H1H2_MIC, TILT_NSA, HR_NSA, and H1H2_NSA, respectively.

	f1	f2	f3	f4	f5	f6	f7	f8	f9	f10	f11	f12	f13	f14	f15
f1	1	*	*	*	*	*	*	*	*	*	*	*	*	*	*
f2	0.95	1	*	*	*	*	*	*	*	*	*	*	*	*	*
f3	0.97	0.86	1	*	*	*	*	*	*	*	*	*	*	*	*
f4	−0.39	−0.20	−0.45	1	*	*	*	*	*	*	*	*	*	*	*
f5	0.61	0.69	0.44	−0.51	1	*	*	*	*	*	*	*	*	*	*
f6	0.96	0.96	0.90	−0.40	0.74	1	*	*	*	*	*	*	*	*	*
f7	0.68	0.46	0.76	−0.91	0.46	0.63	1	*	*	*	*	*	*	*	*
f8	−0.44	−0.24	−0.56	0.70	−0.15	−0.30	−0.78	1	*	*	*	*	*	*	*
f9	0.95	0.94	0.90	−0.28	0.59	0.91	0.57	−0.51	1	*	*	*	*	*	*
f10	−0.96	−0.97	−0.87	0.37	−0.75	−0.96	−0.59	0.29	−0.89	1	*	*	*	*	*
f11	−0.95	−0.89	−0.89	0.62	−0.79	−0.95	−0.79	0.49	−0.87	0.95	1	*	*	*	*
f12	−0.06	−0.20	0.08	−0.50	−0.04	−0.01	0.45	−0.54	0.03	0.22	−0.03	1	*	*	*
f13	−0.80	−0.63	−0.89	0.62	−0.30	−0.67	−0.86	0.87	−0.79	0.67	0.77	−0.26	1	*	*
f14	−0.88	−0.72	−0.91	0.77	−0.59	−0.83	−0.94	0.69	−0.77	0.82	0.94	−0.21	0.90	1	*
f15	−0.82	−0.80	−0.83	0.03	−0.23	−0.73	−0.40	0.47	−0.92	0.68	0.63	−0.10	0.73	0.58	1

6. Discussion and Conclusions

The primary finding in the SAVRa results was that the ratings show an arch-shaped variation trajectory from QE1 to QE8. This trend was also observed in the CAPE-V rating results. In the SAVRa ratings, the rapid increase of the vocal effort, the vocal discomfort level, and the severity of the soft phonation quality indicated a voice adjustment period. Over this period, the participants' vocal folds were abruptly exposed to a heavy vocal loading, and thus the subjects' feelings of vocal fatigue were strong over this period. After this period, the degrees of the participants' perceived vocal fatigue remained constant at a high level, or increased moderately from QE2 to QE7. The vocal loading intensity for each VLT session was identical. The participants gradually adapted to the vocal loading intensity, thus the increasing rate slowed down after this period. After the S1, the accumulation effect of the vocal loading led to a slow and persistent increase of the participants' perceived vocal fatigue in the late sessions. This indicates that, given constant vocal stimuli for different sessions, the participants' perceived vocal fatigue increased over time (or vocal distance dose). The notable decrease of the SAVRa scores from QE7 to QE8 reflects the effect of vocal rest on participants' vocal fatigue feelings. This indicates that the participants felt much better about their vocal functionalities after the 15-min rest session, but the rest was not sufficient to completely recover to the original status at QE1. A longer rest session was thus presumed to enhance the vocal recovery process. The findings in the CAPE-V rating results show that the overall severity, roughness, and strain ratings have the same arch-shaped variation trend with the SAVRa results. This indicates that vocal fatigue degraded the participants' voice performance by increasing roughness and strain.

The data for the fatigue-indicative symptoms obeyed different trends than the SAVRa results. Previous studies showed that these symptoms were frequently observed on vocally fatigued participants. However, a quantitative relationship between the number of occurrences of these symptoms and the degree of vocal fatigue could not be established. Individual discrepancies in the counts of these symptoms showed varied sensitivities to vocal fatigue. Some participants coughed frequently during the VLT, while others did not cough at all. Swallowing was much more frequently observed than other symptoms for all participants. This finding further validated the results of previous studies on the effect of hydration on vocal fatigue [44,48], i.e., superficial vocal fold hydration (swallowing or drinking) could help relieve vocal dysfunction and improve vocal efficiency.

Fifteen voice metrics (features) were studied to track voice quality variation across VLT sessions. The statistical analysis results in Figure 7 did not include the rest session. The $f0$, SPL_MIC, duty ratio, shimmer_MIC, and shimmer_NSA rapidly increased in early sessions, and remained constant afterwards. The variation of $f0$ in Figure 7 was consistent with the results of previous studies, which found that participants' $f0$ increased with vocal fatigue [49,50]. The shimmer_MIC and shimmer_NSA showed an increase after the VLT session. This finding contradicts Laukkanen's one-day vocal fatigue study results [51], but it is consistent with Gelfer's 60-min vocal fatigue study results [49]. This might be caused by the different phonation durations.

One limitation of the present study was that the voice type was not considered as a parameter in the voice use quantification. For example, breathy voice obviously had a different vocal loading intensity from pressed voice when the $f0$, SPL, duty ratio, and duration were identical for these two voice types. The impact stress between vocal folds for these two voice types were different. The feelings of vocal fatigue that the breathy and pressed voice brought to participants were therefore different. An improved method of calculating D_d that considers voice quality is therefore needed to make the voice use quantification more accurate. Another limitation was that calculation of the D_d from the NSA may be not very accurate because of the rather large uncertainty in the SPL ($\pm$ 5 dB) estimates from the NSA data [40]. The accuracy of calculating D_d would thus be influenced. This issue limits the use of the dose-based voice use quantification method in long-term voice monitoring. The monitoring of neck surface acceleration is preferable to minimize the influence of extraneous noise and potentially reduce discomfort in occupational settings. A method for directly deriving the magnitude of the vocal fold vibration from the skin acceleration level is therefore needed. The last limitation is that normal swallowing on a daily basis was not measured, and thus the fatigue-indicative symptom analysis lacked a baseline to refer to. This baseline could be established in future work.

Author Contributions: Conceptualization, Z.L., N.Y.-K.L.-J. and L.M. (Luc Mongeau); methodology, Z.L. and L.M. (Luc Mongeau); software, Z.L.; validation, Z.L., N.Y.-K.L.-J. and L.M. (Luc Mongeau); formal analysis, Z.L.; investigation, Z.L.; resources, L.M. (Lisa Martignetti), N.Y.-K.L.-J. and L.M. (Luc Mongeau); data curation, Z.L., L.F. and L.M. (Lisa Martignetti); writing—original draft preparation, Z.L.; writing—review and editing, Z.L., L.F., L.M. (Lisa Martignetti), N.Y.-K.L.-J. and L.M. (Luc Mongeau); visualization, Z.L.; supervision, N.Y.-K.L.-J. and L.M. (Luc Mongeau); project administration, L.M. (Luc Mongeau); funding acquisition, N.Y.-K.L.-J. and L.M. (Luc Mongeau). All authors have read and agreed to the published version of the manuscript.

Acknowledgments: The financial support of of the National Science and Engineering Research Council of Canada is gratefully acknowledged.

Abbreviations

The following abbreviations are used in this manuscript:

CAPE-V	Consensus Auditory-Perceptual Evaluation of Voice
SAVRa	Self-Administrated Voice Rating
GRABAS	Gradem Roughness, Breathiness, Asthenia, Strain
NSA	Neck Surface Accelerometer
SLP	Speech Language Pathologist
MFDR	Maximum Flow Declination Rate
MFCC	Mel-Frequency Spectral Coefficients
VLT	Vocal Loading Task
EGG	Electroglottograph
SPL	Sound Pressure Level
CIRMMT	Centre for Interdisciplinary Research in Music Media and Technology
QE	Quality Evaluation
IPSV	Inability to Produce Soft Voice
CPP	Cepstral Peak Prominence
HRF	Harmonic Richness Factor

References

1. Welham, N.V.; Maclagan, M.A. Vocal Fatigue: Current Knowledge and Future Directions. *J. Voice* **2003**, *17*, 21–30. [CrossRef]
2. Thomas, G.; de Jong, F.; Kooijman, P.G.C.; Donders, A.R.T.; Cremers, C.W. Voice complaints, risk factors for voice problems and history of voice problems in relation to puberty in female student teachers. *Folia Phoniatr. Logop.* **2006**, *58*, 305–322. [CrossRef]
3. Solomon, N.P. Vocal fatigue and its relation to vocal hyperfunction. *Int. J. -Speech-Lang. Pathol.* **2008**, *10*, 254–266. [CrossRef]
4. Remacle, A.; Morsomme, D.; Berrué, E.; Finck, C. Vocal Impact of a Prolonged Reading Task in Dysphonic Versus Normophonic Female Teachers. *J. Voice* **2012**, *26*, 820.e1–820.e13. [CrossRef]
5. Remacle, A.; Morsomme, D.; Finck, C. Comparison of Vocal Loading Parameters in Kindergarten and Elementary School Teachers. *J. Speech Lang. Hear. Res.* **2014**, *57*, 406–415. [CrossRef]
6. Kreiman, J.; Gerratt, B.R. Sources of listener disagreement in voice quality assessment. *J. Acoust. Soc. Am.* **2000**, *108*, 1867–1876. [CrossRef] [PubMed]
7. Kreiman, J.; Gerratt, B.R.; Ito, M. When and why listeners disagree in voice quality assessment tasks. *J. Acoust. Soc. Am.* **2007**, *122*, 2354–2364. [CrossRef] [PubMed]
8. Pabon, J.P.H. Objective acoustic voice-quality parameters in the computer phonetogram. *J. Voice* **1991**, *5*, 203–216. [CrossRef]

9. Roy, N.; Barkmeier-Kraemer, J.; Eadie, T.; Sivasankar, M.P.; Mehta, D.; Paul, D.; Hillman, R. Evidence-Based Clinical Voice Assessment: A Systematic Review. *Am. J. -Speech-Lang. Pathol.* **2013**, *22*, 212–226. [CrossRef]
10. Awan, S.N.; Roy, N. Toward the development of an objective index of dysphonia severity: A four-factor acoustic model. *Clin. Linguist. Phon.* **2006**, *20*, 35–49. [CrossRef] [PubMed]
11. Godino-Llorente, J.I.; Gómez-Vilda, P.; Cruz-Roldán, F.; Blanco-Velasco, M.; Fraile, R. Pathological Likelihood Index as a Measurement of the Degree of Voice Normality and Perceived Hoarseness. *J. Voice* **2010**, *24*, 667–677. [CrossRef] [PubMed]
12. Halberstam, B. Acoustic and Perceptual Parameters Relating to Connected Speech Are More Reliable Measures of Hoarseness than Parameters Relating to Sustained Vowels. *Orl Otorhinolaryngol. Relat. Spec.* **2004**, *66*, 70–73. [CrossRef] [PubMed]
13. Holmberg, E.B.; Hillman, R.E.; Perkell, J.S. Glottal airflow and transglottal air pressure measurements for male and female speakers in soft, normal, and loud voice. *J. Acoust. Soc. Am.* **1988**, *84*, 511–529. [CrossRef] [PubMed]
14. Holmberg, E.B.; Hillman, R.E.; Perkell, J.S.; Guiod, P.C.; Goldman, S.L. Comparisons Among Aerodynamic, Electroglottographic, and Acoustic Spectral Measures of Female Voice. *J. Speech Lang. Hear. Res.* **1995**, *38*, 1212–1223. [CrossRef]
15. Anita Mcallister, Johan Sundberg, S.R.H. Acoustic measurements and perceptual evaluation of hoarseness in children's voices. *Logop. Phoniatr. Vocology* **1998**, *23*, 27–38. [CrossRef]
16. Heman-Ackah, Y.D.; Michael, D.D.; Baroody, M.M.; Ostrowski, R.; Hillenbrand, J.; Heuer, R.J.; Horman, M.; Sataloff, R.T. Cepstral Peak Prominence: A More Reliable Measure of Dysphonia. *Ann. Otol. Rhinol. Laryngol.* **2003**, *112*, 324–333. [CrossRef]
17. Godino-Llorente, J.I.; Gomez-Vilda, P.; Blanco-Velasco, M. Dimensionality Reduction of a Pathological Voice Quality Assessment System Based on Gaussian Mixture Models and Short-Term Cepstral Parameters. *IEEE Trans. Biomed. Eng.* **2006**, *53*, 1943–1953. [CrossRef]
18. Fang, S.H.; Tsao, Y.; Hsiao, M.J.; Chen, J.Y.; Lai, Y.H.; Lin, F.C.; Wang, C.T. Detection of Pathological Voice Using Cepstrum Vectors: A Deep Learning Approach. *J. Voice* **2018**. [CrossRef]
19. Klatt, D.H.; Klatt, L.C. Analysis, synthesis, and perception of voice quality variations among female and male talkers. *J. Acoust. Soc. Am.* **1990**, *87*, 820–857. [CrossRef]
20. Kitch, J.A.; Oates, J. The perceptual features of vocal fatigue as self-reported by a group of actors and singers. *J. Voice* **1994**, *8*, 207–214. [CrossRef]
21. Kitch, J.A.; Oates, J.; Greenwood, K. Performance effects on the voices of 10 choral tenors: Acoustic and perceptual findings. *J. Voice* **1996**, *10*, 217–227. [CrossRef]
22. Welham, N.V.; Maclagan, M.A. Vocal fatigue in young trained singers across a solo performance: A preliminary study. *Logop. Phoniatr. Vocology* **2004**, *29*, 3–12. [CrossRef] [PubMed]
23. Hunter, E.J. General Statistics of the NCVS Self-Administered Vocal Rating (SAVRa). *Natl. Cent. Voice Speech Online Tech. Memo* **2008**, *11*, 1–10.
24. Hunter, E.J.; Titze, I.R. Quantifying Vocal Fatigue Recovery: Dynamic Vocal Recovery Trajectories after a Vocal Loading Exercise. *Ann. Otol. Rhinol. Laryngol.* **2009**, *118*, 449–460. [CrossRef]
25. Nanjundeswaran, C.; Jacobson, B.H.; Gartner-Schmidt, J.; Abbott, K.V. Vocal Fatigue Index (VFI): Development and Validation. *J. Voice* **2015**, *29*, 433–440. [CrossRef]
26. Halpern, A.E.; Spielman, J.L.; Hunter, E.J.; Titze, I.R. The inability to produce soft voice (IPSV): A tool to detect vocal change in school-teachers. *Logop. Phoniatr. Vocology* **2009**, *34*, 117–127. [CrossRef]
27. Titze, I.R.; Svec, J.G.; Popolo, P.S. Vocal Dose Measures: Quantifying Accumulated Vibration Exposure in Vocal Fold Tissues. *J. Speech Lang. Hear. Res.* **2003**, *46*, 919–932.[CrossRef]
28. Titze, I.R.; Hunter, E.J. Comparison of Vocal Vibration-Dose Measures for Potential-Damage Risk Criteria. *J. Speech Lang. Hear. Res.* **2015**, *58*, 1425–1439. [CrossRef]
29. Švec, J.G.; Popolo, P.S.; Titze, I.R. Measurement of vocal doses in speech: experimental procedure and signal processing. *Logop. Phoniatr. Vocol.* **2003**, *28*, 181–192. [CrossRef]
30. Carroll, T.; Nix, J.; Hunter, E.; Emerich, K.; Titze, I.; Abaza, M. Objective Measurement of Vocal Fatigue in Classical Singers: A Vocal Dosimetry Pilot Study. *Otolaryngol. Neck Surg.* **2006**, *135*, 595–602. [CrossRef]
31. Echternach, M.; Nusseck, M.; Dippold, S.; Spahn, C.; Richter, B. Fundamental frequency, sound pressure level and vocal dose of a vocal loading test in comparison to a real teaching situation. *Eur. Arch. -Oto-Rhino-Laryngol.* **2014**, *271*, 3263–3268. [CrossRef] [PubMed]

32. Bottalico, P.; Astolfi, A. Investigations into vocal doses and parameters pertaining to primary school teachers in classrooms. *J. Acoust. Soc. Am.* **2012**, *131*, 2817–2827. [CrossRef] [PubMed]
33. Morrow, S.L.; Connor, N.P. Voice Amplification as a Means of Reducing Vocal Load for Elementary Music Teachers. *J. Voice* **2011**, *25*, 441–446. [CrossRef] [PubMed]
34. Titze, I.R.; Sundberg, J. Vocal intensity in speakers and singers. *J. Acoust. Soc. Am.* **1992**, *91*, 2936–2946. [CrossRef]
35. Hunter, E.J.; Banks, R.E. Gender Differences in the Reporting of Vocal Fatigue in Teachers as Quantified by the Vocal Fatigue Index. *Ann. Otol. Rhinol. Laryngol.* **2017**, *126*, 813–818. [CrossRef]
36. Hunter, E.J.; Tanner, K.; Smith, M.E. Gender differences affecting vocal health of women in vocally demanding careers. *Logop. Phoniatr. Vocology* **2011**, *36*, 128–136. [CrossRef]
37. Rowling, J.K. Harry Potter and the Sorcerer's Stone. 2001. Available online: http://www2.sdfi.edu.cn/netclass/jiaoan/englit/download/Harry%20Potter%20and%20the%20Sorcerer's%20Stone.pdf (accessed on 4 February 2020).
38. Lei, Z.; Kennedy, E.; Fasanella, L.; Li-Jessen, N.Y.K.; Mongeau, L. Discrimination between Modal, Breathy and Pressed Voice for Single Vowels Using Neck-Surface Vibration Signals. *Appl. Sci.* **2019**, *9*, 1505. [CrossRef]
39. Mehta, D.D.; Zañartu, M.; Feng, S.W.; Cheyne, H.A.; Hillman, R.E. Mobile Voice Health Monitoring Using a Wearable Accelerometer Sensor and a Smartphone Platform. *IEEE Trans. Biomed. Eng.* **2012**, *59*, 3090–3096. [CrossRef]
40. Švec, J.G.; Titze, I.R.; Popolo, P.S. Estimation of sound pressure levels of voiced speech from skin vibration of the neck. *J. Acoust. Soc. Am.* **2005**, *117*, 1386–1394. [CrossRef]
41. Zanartu, M. Acoustic Coupling in Phonation and Its Effect On Inverse Filtering of Oral Airflow and Neck Surface Acceleration. Ph.D. Thesis, Purdue University, West Lafayette, IN, USA, 2010.
42. Zraick, R.; Kempster, G.; Connor, N.; Thibeault, S.; Klaben, B.; Bursac, Z.; Thrush, C.; Glaze, L. Establishing validity of the consensus auditory-perceptual evaluation of voice (CAPE-V). *Am. J. -Speech-Lang. Pathol.* **2011**, *20*, 14–22. [CrossRef]
43. Rabiner, L.; Schafer, R. *Digital Processing of Speech Signals*; Prentice-Hall Signal Processing Series; Prentice-Hall: Englewood, NJ, USA, 1978.
44. Yiu, E.M.L.; Chan, R.M. Effect of Hydration and Vocal Rest on the Vocal Fatigue in Amateur Karaoke Singers. *J. Voice* **2003**, *17*, 216–227. [CrossRef]
45. Solomon, N.P.; Glaze, L.E.; Arnold, R.R.; van Mersbergen, M. Effects of a Vocally Fatiguing Task and Systemic Hydration on Men's Voices. *J. Voice* **2003**, *17*, 31–46. [CrossRef]
46. Sluijter, A.M.C.; van Heuven, V.J. Spectral balance as an acoustic correlate of linguistic stress. *J. Acoust. Soc. Am.* **1996**, *100*, 2471–2485. [CrossRef] [PubMed]
47. Childers, D.G.; Lee, C.K. Vocal quality factors: Analysis, synthesis, and perception. *J. Acoust. Soc. Am.* **1991**, *90*, 2394–2410. [CrossRef]
48. Sivasankar, M.; Leydon, C. The role of hydration in vocal fold physiology. *Curr. Opin. Otolaryngol. Head Neck Surg.* **2010**, *18*, 171–175. [CrossRef]
49. Gelfer, M.P.; Andrews, M.L.; Schmidt, C.P. Effects of prolonged loud reading on selected measures of vocal function in trained and untrained singers. *J. Voice* **1991**, *5*, 158–167. [CrossRef]
50. Hunter, E.J.; Titze, I.R. Variations in Intensity, Fundamental Frequency, and Voicing for Teachers in Occupational Versus Non-Occupational Settings. *J. Speech Lang. Hear. Res.* **2010**, *53*, 862–875. [CrossRef]
51. Laukkanen, A.M.; Ilomäki, I.; Leppänen, K.; Vilkman, E. Acoustic Measures and Self-reports of Vocal Fatigue by Female Teachers. *J. Voice* **2008**, *22*, 283–289. [CrossRef]

11

A Synchronized Multi-Unit Wireless Platform for Long-Term Activity Monitoring

Giuseppe Coviello *, Gianfranco Avitabile and Antonello Florio

Department of Electrical and Information Engineering, Polytechnic University of Bari, 70126 Bari, Italy; gianfranco.avitabile@poliba.it (G.A.); antonello.florio@poliba.it (A.F.)
* Correspondence: giuseppe.coviello@poliba.it

Abstract: One of the objectives of the medicine is to modify patients' ways of living. In this context, a key role is played by the diagnosis. When dealing with acquisition systems consisting of multiple wireless devices located in different parts of the body, it becomes fundamental to ensure synchronization between the individual units. This task is truly a challenge, so one aims to limit the complexity of the calculation and ensure long periods of operation. In fact, in the absence of synchronization, it is impossible to relate all the measurements coming from the different subsystems on a single time scale for the extraction of complex characteristics. In this paper, we first analyze in detail all the possible causes that lead to have a system that is not synchronous and therefore not usable. Then, we propose a firmware implementation strategy and a simple but effective protocol that guarantees perfect synchrony between the devices while keeping computational complexity low. The employed network has a star topology with a master/slave architecture. In this paper a new approach to the synchronization problem is introduced to guarantee a precise but not necessarily accurate synchronization between the units. In order to demonstrate the effectiveness of the proposed solution, a platform consisting of two different types of units has been designed and built. In particular, a nine Degrees of Freedom (DoF) Inertial Measurement Unit (IMU) is used in one unit while a nine-DoF IMU and all circuits for the analysis of the superficial Electromyography (sEMG) are present on the other unit. The system is completed by an Android app that acts as a user interface for starting and stopping the logging operations. The paper experimentally demonstrates that the proposed solution overcomes all the limits set out and it guarantees perfect synchronization of the single measurement, even during long-duration acquisitions. In fact, a less than 30 μs time mismatch has been registered for a 24 h test, and the possibility to perform complex post-processing on the acquired data with a simple and effective system has been proven.

Keywords: IMU; gait analysis; sEMG; long-term monitoring; multi-unit; multi-sensor; time synchronization; Internet of Medical Things; body area network; MIMU

1. Introduction

In many areas of research, medicine, and sport it is important to collect data on particular parameters concerning a subject to obtain information on his/her health condition. Normally, detailed measurements are performed for short periods and in a controlled laboratory environment. With the advent of micro-electro-mechanical system (MEMS) technology and thanks to the non-invasiveness of the equipment available today, a great step forward has been made, allowing acquisitions for long time intervals, during individual procedures in normal daily life. An important task to perform in order to make the procedural steps effective is to check whether the patient is correctly following the doctor's treatment instructions. Nowadays, Information and Communication Technologies' (ICT) progress allows the doctors to remotely follow their patients. Furthermore, thanks to the availability of new

ICT tools, it is possible to study the long-term evolution of particular symptoms related to specific diseases, without affecting patients' everyday lives. They are real on-body laboratories that belong to the field of the Internet of Medical Things (IoMT). For example, considering specific units equipped with heartbeat sensors, it is possible to analyze a patient's heart health in different time slots during the day, monitoring for the presence or insurgence of anomalies [1].

Complex systems are usually needed when monitoring the symptoms of a disease requires verification of several parameters and requires flow algorithms capable of taking into account the evolution of data for recognizing changes in them [2,3], or efficiency optimization algorithms [4] or systems that improve wireless communications [5]. A possible field of application of such a complex system, for instance, could be the study of patients with precocious diagnoses of Parkinson's Disease (PD) [6,7]. Its main symptoms induce motor issues, such as tremor, rigidity, and instability. Thus, a gait analysis or posture monitoring could be helpful to identify those symptoms' progression or regression. Gait analysis can be conducted in several ways [8]—for example, with video frame analysis. The case of kinematic gait analysis is brought out using multiple sensor units. Thanks to information coming from accelerometers and gyroscopes, it is possible to identify an object's motion in the space; in our case those pieces of information are related to an arm or a leg movement.

Advanced forms of PD involve the possibility for the patient to alternate phases in which motor muscles are operative (ON) to phases in which they stop to work (OFF) [9]. This can be related to an ineffective or changed drug therapy and only platforms for long-term monitoring of the patient can be helpful for identifying these types of issues. Those platforms usually match the already mentioned set of gyroscopes and accelerometers for gait characterization with sensors for the sEMG.

Many implementations rely on multiple units with a single sensor as an alternative to a single unit equipped with the whole sensors set. Additionally, especially for sEMG, it is important to monitor points that may be distant in space, so two or more units may be needed. We introduce, in this way, the concept of the multi-unit acquisition system.

From the networking point of view, for a multi-board acquisition system, we talk about Body Area Networks (BANs) [10], which are networks usually with a star topology and connected by wireless protocols, whose coverage is of the order of 1–2 m [11] (that is, the necessary area to cover the entire body).

The length of the time interval used to perform the analysis should be carefully considered. In some cases, it is necessary to do real-time (online) monitoring while in other cases *a posteriori* (offline) monitoring is required. In the first case, the central node (BAN coordinator) is in charge of collecting, processing, and matching the data, before exposing them to the external network to the BAN—the Internet. It is important to have a persistent connection between the BAN coordinator and the Internet. According to [12], this may lead to a significant power consumption associated with the RF portion of the sensing device. Since we are considering wearable motes, it is unfeasible for the devices to use expensive batteries or overly heavy batteries. Additionally, it may be useless to expose very frequently data on the Internet during long-term monitoring.

A better solution seems to be represented by offline processing, in which every mote saves the results of its surveys on a persistent memory and after gathering the data from the whole set of units the data collection is processed. This final step calls for the BAN coordinator to be in charge of strict time synchronization between all motes. In this scenario, the timestamp of each measure is crucial, since the possibility of correctly analyzing the measures by referring them to the same instant depends on it. Some off-the-shelf solutions give the opportunity to store the measured data in a memory. They usually require some extra non-portable and complex hardware, and either their specified accuracy is too low [13] or no details are given regarding the accuracy itself [14].

The paper aims to present a time-synchronized multi-unit, multi-sensor, and multi-rate acquisition system for kinematic and static analysis. The data are collected from different sensors, even using different data rates, over a long time interval of observation during normal daily activities of the patient. The system can be employed for many specific applications, depending on the virtually unlimited number of boards used, the sensors they are equipped with, and their positioning on the body. Because of this, the experiments validating the proposed platform will aim to prove the effectiveness of the approach, generalizing and not specifying a precise operating scenario.

The organization of this paper is as follows: Section 2 reviews related works, while Section 3 formulates the operating problems. Section 4 describes the platform developed, and in Section 5 some experimental results, validating the system, are reported. Finally, conclusions are given in Section 6.

2. Related Work

2.1. Gait Analysis through sEMG

The EMG is the measurement of the electrical activity of a muscle. EMG actually gives only minor information about the contraction of individual muscles, but it provides a visible indication of the muscle activity. The information provided can be extremely interesting when considering the time instance in which a muscle activates [8].

Many methods are available for EMG. The least invasive one, but also one of the most subject to interference, is the surface EMG (sEMG). In fact, first of all, it is not always possible to distinguish one muscle's activity from that of the adjacent ones (the so-called "cross-talk" phenomenon [8]). Moreover, since there is a thick layer of skin covering the muscle, the voltage signal arrives at the electrodes with a significant attenuation that must be compensated with specific preamplification techniques.

However, the sEMG is the preferable way of performing gait activity monitoring over a long time period as it only requires the patient to have some surface electrodes on specific parts of its body.

In the literature, it is possible to find some examples of gait characterization through sEMG-based systems. For example, in [15], the authors propose a gait cadence analysis performed through sEMG. The system is in charge of acquiring electrode signals and processes them according to a first-order statistic, in order to characterize the periodicity of gait in healthy patients.

In [16], a more complicated analysis involving deep learning is presented. In fact, still employing sEMG, the author provides a method to identify and classify two sub-phases of gait (proper stance and swing phases) based on an artificial neural network approach.

In [17], another gait sub-phase recognition system is proposed, with an inferential algorithm for studying and characterizing the sub-phases. The great advantage of this latter approach is its reduced cost, since it is based on Arduino Mega 2560 for signal processing, and it is wearable, thereby allowing one to perform non-invasive remote analysis of gait.

2.2. Multi-Board Acquisition Systems

This work presents a wearable multi-board acquisition system for offline activity monitoring. In the literature, other systems with the same purpose are present, with similar characteristics but with some issues that our design aims to mitigate.

In [9], a wearable system for long-term monitoring of gait is presented. The board has the advantage of being an "add-on" to the patient, unlike others described in the literature that require the patient to wear specific shoes or other specifically designed clothes. Salarian et al.'s work, instead, allows one to equip the patient with the system and remove it when the monitoring is over. The board employed for testing is equipped only by gyroscopes. Nevertheless, the authors claim to have reached interesting results. Note that the proposed system works for offline monitoring, thanks to the fact that the motes store their revelations on 8 MB memory cards.

Laerhoven et al. [18] focused their attention on how to reduce the power consumption for wearable devices of this type. Toward that purpose, they first check for the presence of motion using a set of tilt switches, and then activate an accelerometer to track the motion itself. This latter sensor, indeed, drains far more current than a tilt switch. Moreover, since tilt switches furnish a binary output, it is possible to reduce the computational power required to reveal the presence of motion. Actually, due to the nature of the tilt switches, this system does not guarantee a reduced number of false positive or false negative events of motion, thereby preventing the achievement of high levels of accuracy.

In 2011, Cancela et al. [19] presented a distributed wearable system for online gait analysis in PD made with five 3-axial accelerometers put on limbs and a gyroscope with accelerometer put on the belt. Zigbee protocol is used as the telecommunications standard between the motes and to communicate with a personal computer (PC) that receives and stores the data. The main issues of the approach arise from the fact that online monitoring can be power hungry, as already discussed. Nevertheless, it is useless to collect and process data immediately in long-term monitoring. Moreover, the proposed system requires a PC that must be specifically equipped with algorithms and telecommunication standards transceivers in order to work and collect data, and this may be an obstacle for doctors and patients.

Finally, Oniga et al. [20] developed a solution for studying motion activity/inactivity for a subject in the long term. Wearable motes equipped with only gyroscopes and 3-axis accelerometers are considered and coordinated by a smartphone, in charge of receiving and processing data, before storing them in a persistent online database. The proposed solution is an online monitoring system. It is still capable of reducing some sources of power consumption, thanks to intelligent (triggered) activation of the motes by the smartphone. Nevertheless, the patients must have a smartphone equipped with a specific application and a persistent internet connection to store data on the remote database, accessible to the doctor.

The system presented in this paper allows a more complete analysis of systems of the type previously described in terms of completeness of the measurements that can be made thanks to the variety of sensors used, and by the simplicity and versatility of use. The approach ensures a longer battery life as it minimizes the computational complexity of the synchronization process. Moreover, it allows an easy reconfiguration and expansion of the group of units without any change in the settings, as the synchronization protocol is quite simple and does not involve any bidirectional communication.

2.3. Time Synchronization Protocols

The main issue when analyzing multi-unit (i.e., distributed) systems consists of the physical clocks synchronization. The sub-elements themselves of a multi-board system are not synchronized. It is mandatory that each and every subsystem has the same vision of the time domain, as the units are meant to capture events that later must be cross-correlated. Even assuming the theoretical possibility that every device turns on at at the same time, it is well known that the natural clock drift due to environmental changes may lead to time mismatches in the run-time phase. As a consequence, the need for a time synchronization algorithm arises.

Time synchronization protocols belong either to the distributed protocols (DPs) (consensus-based) or to the centralized protocols (CPs) classes. In the DPs, the decision on the global system time is made by specific algorithms aiming to solve the problem of consensus. The latter, in distributed systems, calls to the single nodes to "agree" on a given property, decision, or quantity [21] (in our case, time). A consensus algorithm has the following properties:

- Termination: after ending, every node makes a decision;
- Agreement: every couple of nodes agrees on the same decision;
- Validity: every decided value is a proposed one;
- Integrity: every node makes a decision at least once.

Obviously, a time synchronization algorithm based on consensus guarantees a high level of accuracy, at the cost of long computation time needed to reach the consensus itself. As a consequence, a DP could be unacceptably heavy in time-critical systems and in fast-changing-events observing systems.

In CPs, the decision is made by a single node, called the leader, that we will identify as the BAN coordinator in our context. Note that backup-leaders can be considered to implement fault tolerance. Some algorithmic solutions are directly inheritable from classical distributed systems theory, while other techniques are specially designed for BANs and other kinds of ad-hoc networks.

The simplest example is constituted by the algorithm proposed by Cristian in [22]. This algorithm operates in two stages: first, the peer node N asks the coordinator C to be time-synchronized; then, after, the coordinator sends a message containing its local time (that will become the network global time) T_C. Once the peer has received this message, it sets its local time to be:

$$T_N = T_C + \widetilde{\tau} \tag{1}$$

with $\widetilde{\tau}$ an estimation of the actual communication delay detailed in Section 3.2.2. The algorithm furnishes a good approximation when the random components of τ are negligible when compared to the deterministic ones.

Another solution is presented in [23], the so-called Berkeley algorithm, adopted in Unix 4.3 BSD. Here, the coordinator observes message exchange containing local clock values T_N^i still to estimate τ_i for each node i, as in the previous case. Then, it averages the clock values. Instead of sending the decided time, the coordinator sends to each node how much it should increase or decrease its clock according to the global decided time.

The presented algorithms are more suitable than the consensus-based synchronization algorithms, but still, they face a time latency in which the event cannot be located in a precise global time instant, that is, until the whole network agrees on a specific timestamp. This issue suggests the need for a new class of algorithms, specifically designed for BANs, that is, more time bound. In fact, since BANs for event sensing must cope with physical quantity measurements which can vary very rapidly, or have to deal with strict energy constraints [24], it is necessary to introduce new strategies.

Let us consider the class of broadcast-based time synchronization algorithms. In this case, the BAN coordinator periodically sends the same message to all the BAN nodes (i.e., a broadcast message). Once each node has received the message, they adjust their internal time according to the specific algorithm procedures.

The reference broadcast synchronization (RBS) algorithm proposed in [24] offers a solution in which the leader sends a broadcast message to all the nodes. These latter register the time in which they received the message as a function of their local clock and inform the other nodes about their local time computation. A global time consensus is reached in a way similar to Berkeley algorithm—that is, once the relative time difference computation in each node is known. Unfortunately, a simpler approach with faster convergence would be needed in some applications.

A lightweight solution is represented by the Flooding Time Synchronization Protocol (FTSP) [25,26]. FTSP sends the MAC layer timestamp to all the nodes in the flooding mode. Each node that received the message computes the local drift as a function of the global time and aligns its local time to it. Linear regression is used for compensating clock skewing and drifting. The main con of the approach is the large amount of exchanged information [26].

In this scenario, our algorithm is a simplified version of the fusion of RBS and FTSP protocols. In fact, we eliminated the clock skewing and drifting compensations needed in FTSP. Furthermore, the message sent in the broadcast will contain the value of the real-time clock (RTC) as payload, instead of taking the time value from the MAC layer, as in the RBS protocol.

3. Problem Formulation

In this section the most important error sources for the time synchronization mismatch will be discussed. They can be divided into two main categories: errors related to the hardware implementation and errors related to other sources that we will call non-hardware implementation.

3.1. Hardware Implementation

3.1.1. RTC Mismatch

In most of the low-cost/low-power systems, the RTC accuracy is guaranteed by using a 32.768 kHz crystal oscillator. Several aspects must be considered when choosing this component for the project;

one of them is the frequency tolerance declared by the manufacturer. Low-cost 32.768 kHz crystals usually have a frequency tolerance of about ±20 parts per million (ppm) that introduces an intrinsic delay of ±10 min/year at its maximum.

Another source of frequency drift is the crystal capacitive loading mismatch. The effective load of a PCB mounted crystal depends on the external loading capacitance tolerance, the PCB parasitics, and the oscillator circuit parasitics. The difference from the load capacitance specified by the manufacturer can lead to an error up to ±200 ppm [27], which introduces a further delay of ±100 min/year at its maximum. Probably, this is the most important error source, so the design phase is very crucial; a typical characteristic is shown in Figure 1.

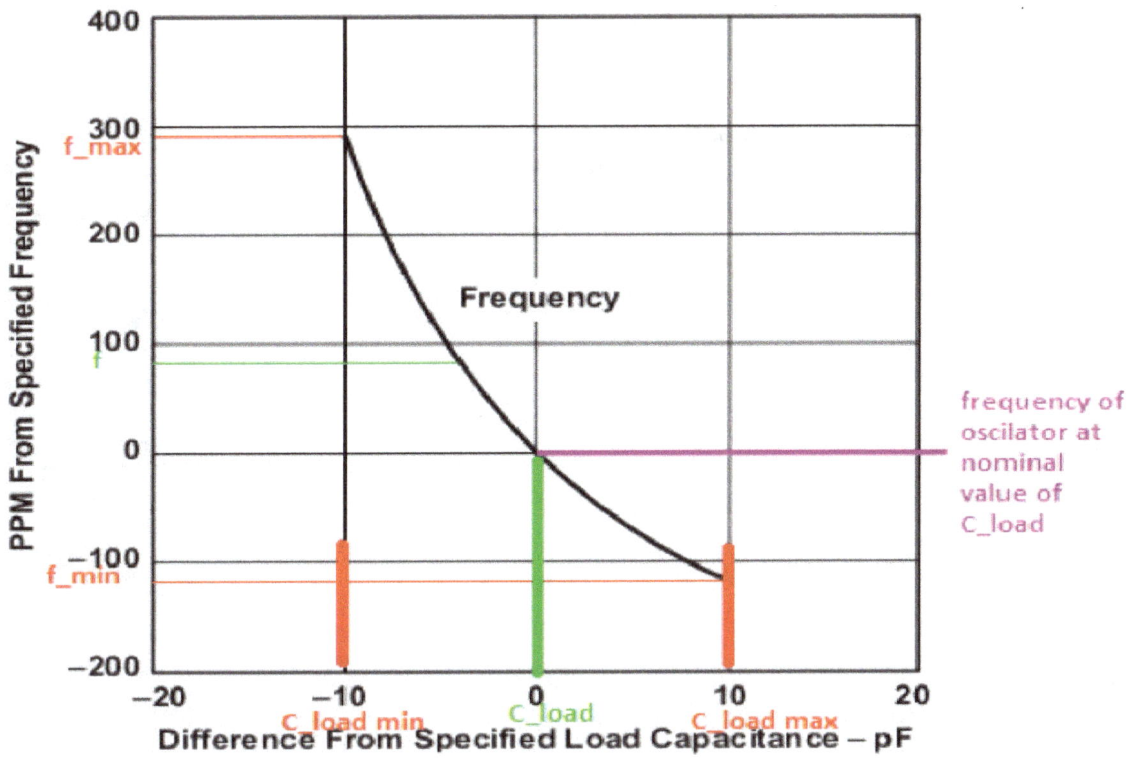

Figure 1. Crystal frequency drift with load capacitance.

It is common for crystal manufacturers to specify the drift due to aging in the first year without specifying the trend for subsequent years because it is unpredictable. This value is around ±3 ppm which means about ±90 s/year at its maximum.

The last source of inaccuracy is represented by the temperature changes that, for quartz, have a trend represented by a parabola whose vertex is the so-called turnover temperature (TOT). Figure 2 shows the graph for crystal ABS07-32.768KHZ-9-T [28] from Abracon (Spicewood, TX, USA) used in the project. In this case, the turnover temperature is around 25 °C. The effect is that the oscillator slows down when the temperature changes around the TOT. It is important to underline that the drift could be significant. Let us consider a 55 °C temperature; the frequency drift is about ±26 ppm which means a delay of about ±13 min/year.

All these aspects lead to the consideration that a calibration or synchronization technique is mandatory. Many calibration techniques are present in literature [29] and producers' data sheets [30,31]. Even though those techniques compensate the clock drift with very little battery power drain, they still require the presence of an external temperature sensor, and most of all, the final accuracy is around ±3.5 ppm which means a delay of about ±0.2 ms/min.

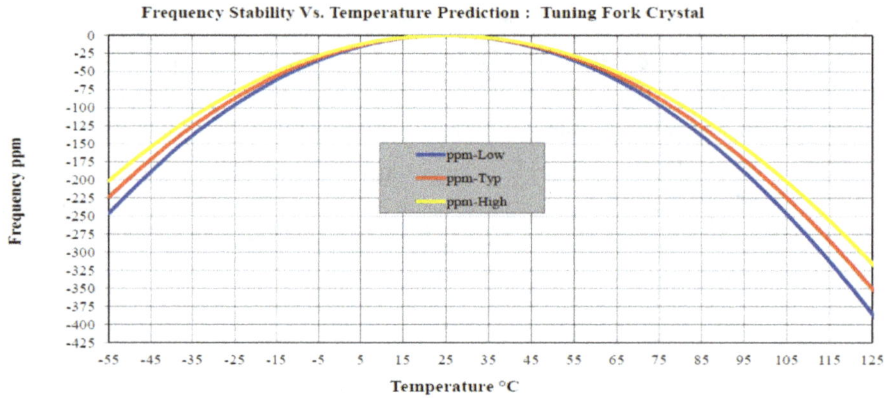

Figure 2. Crystal frequency drift with temperature.

We compared the performances of the RTCs of two identical boards for a 14 h log at a constant temperature of 30 °C. As expected, the mismatch grows linearly and at the end of the observation interval it is around 12 k milliseconds, as shown in Figure 3. That means a total mismatch between the boards of about 238 ppm; that is a delay of about 119 min/year.

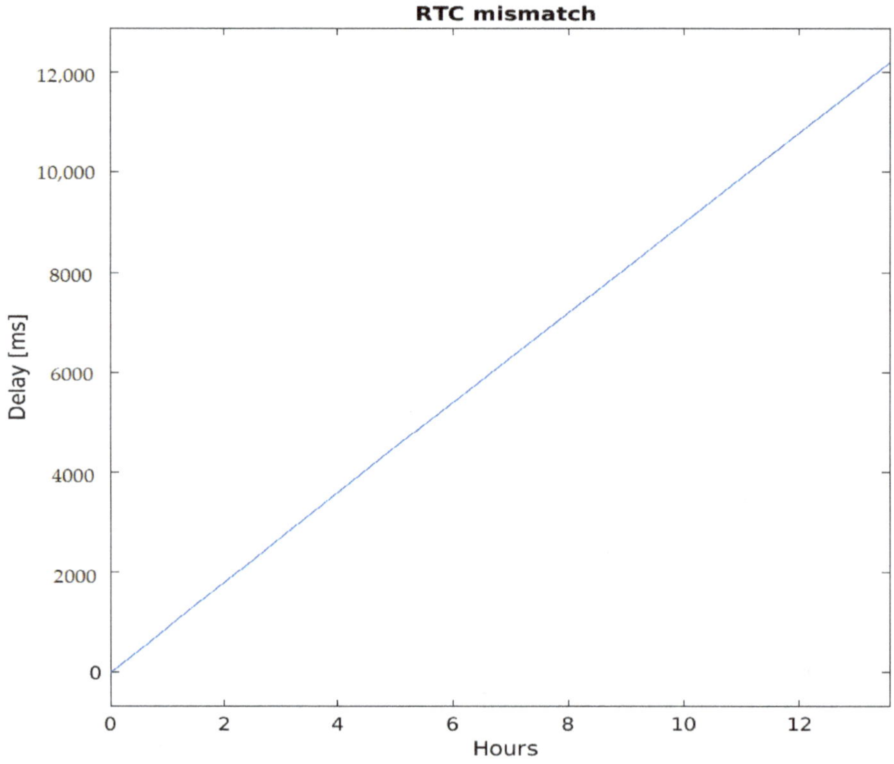

Figure 3. Real-time clock (RTC) difference between two identical boards.

3.1.2. IMUs Sampling Frequency Differences

IMUs with analog-to-digital converters (ADCs) for digitizing the gyroscope, accelerometer, and magnetometer outputs, have several interesting features, such as the selection of the sampling rate, the interrupt feature to alert the processor that a value is exceeding a user-programmable threshold or that a new data are available to read. The sampling frequency of a typical low-cost unit is in the range of a few Hz up to a few kHz. The right sampling frequency could be chosen as a function of the application requirements [32]. Usually, for gait analysis, postural monitoring, or activity monitoring, the frequency of 100 Hz is the right choice [33]. Even in this case, the clock accuracy is important since timing errors directly affect the distance and angle calculations performed by the processor.

In order to show this clock diversity, we use two identical units with a sampling frequency of 100 Hz and the interrupt feature enabled. The output pin is active low and is triggered as soon as the processor reads the data. In Figure 4 it can be noticed that the mismatch is about 57 mHz, while the time needed for the processor to read the data is about 80 μs. This means that the measured frequency differences should be attributed only to the frequency clock tolerance, which is about ±2% for the IMU used [34], and to the internal delays.

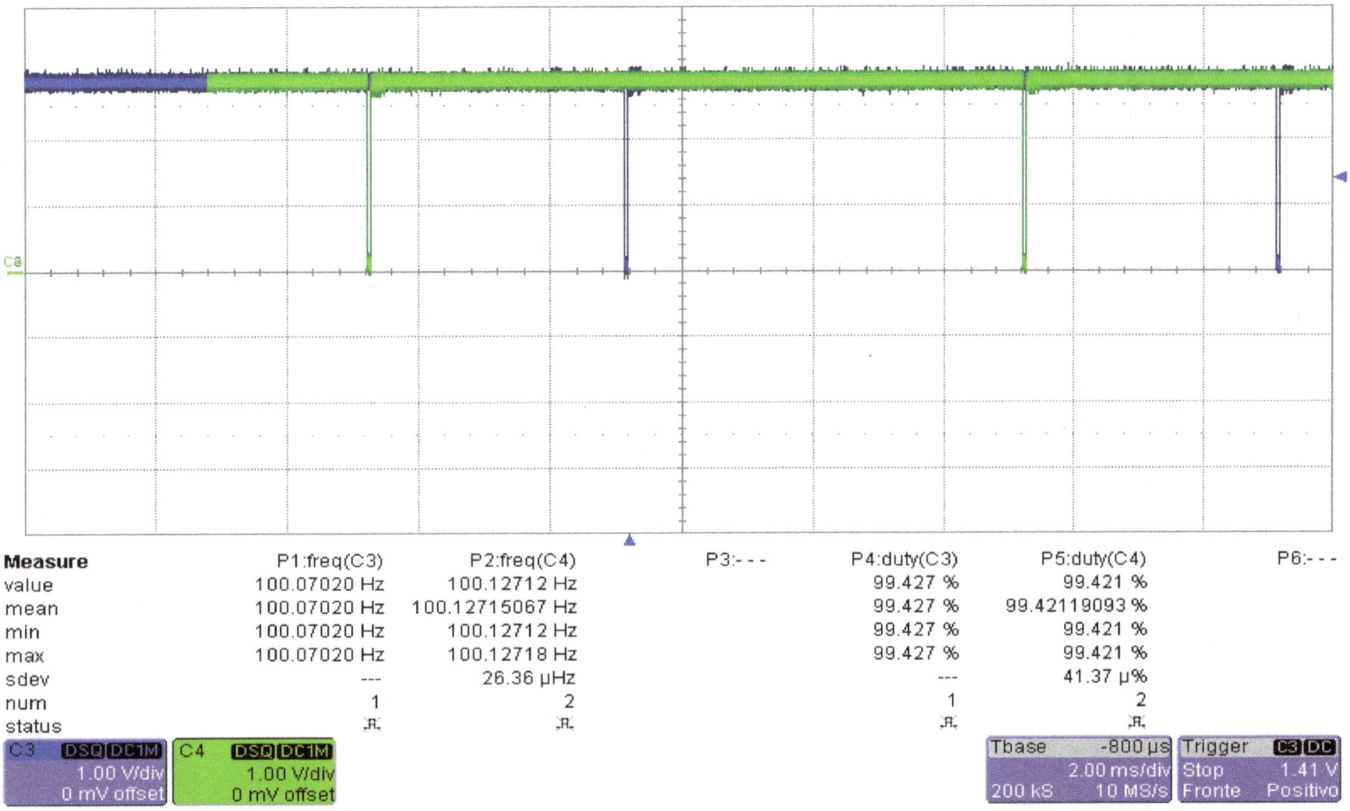

Figure 4. inertial measurement unit (IMU) clock misalignment for two different boards.

As a consequence, it cannot be used as a reference time generator, creating a serious problem. In fact, let us consider the measured IMU clock of 100.12712 Hz as in Figure 4 and an ideal system clock with a resolution of 10ms. In such a situation, every sample from the IMU is associated with a system timestamp. Nevertheless every 7.88 s there is ambiguity and two samples are associated with the same timestamp. The situation is shown in Figure 5. Instead, if the measured clock is smaller than the ideal system clock, we have sampling events without a sample.

This issue can be overcome simply by imposing an oversampling at the IMUs, as discussed in the next section.

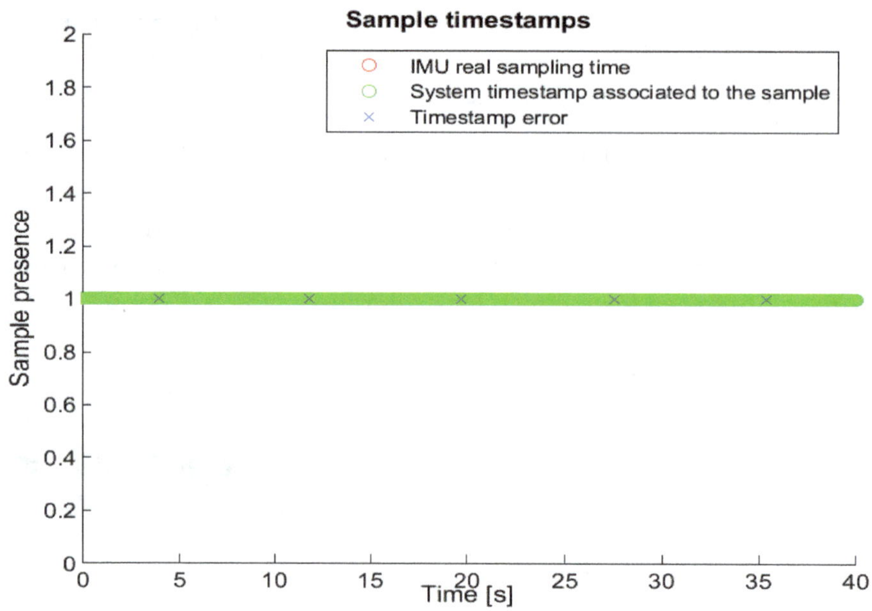

(a)

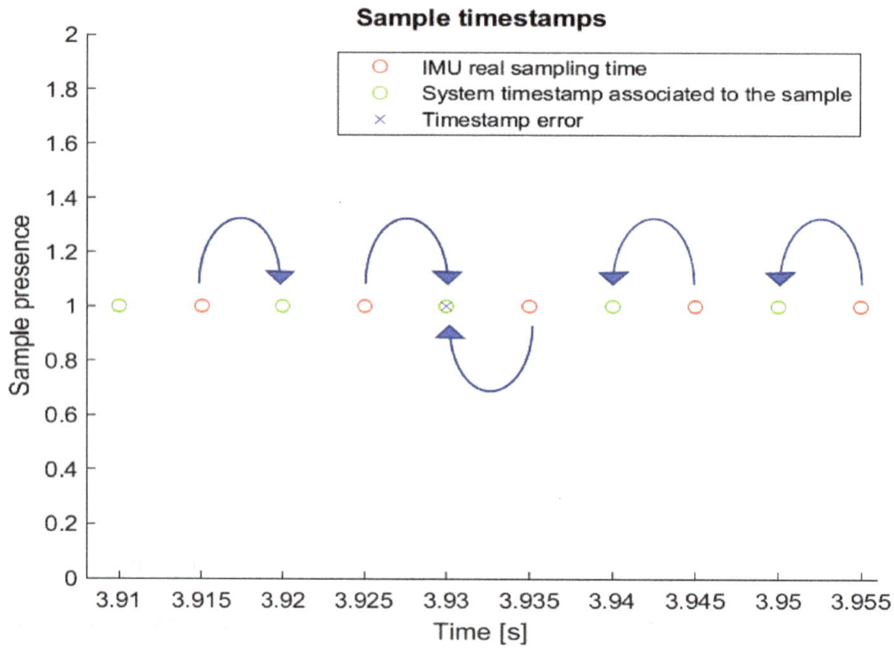

(b)

Figure 5. IMU timestamp error: (**a**) global view and (**b**) zoom.

3.2. Non-Hardware Implementation

This section will describe the problems that are not related to the hardware realization, but, rather, to the firmware implementation or the network topology choice and so on.

3.2.1. Micro SD Card Speed Classes

In applications of the type described in this paper, it is necessary to provide a local data storage system. The use of micro SD card memories represents the simplest and most economical solution, due to their reduced cost and dimensions. In order to simplify the data analysis on a PC, the FAT32 file system has been chosen. The drawback is that the writing process is slower than raw writing without a file system. For example, in our tests, closing a file and opening a new one may require several tens of seconds and it depends on the micro SD card speed class. The goal is not to miss any measurement coming from the IMU but at the same time to guarantee the right timestamp for each measurement. Two simple actions allow one to reach the goal: the first, to put the writing on micro SD card at a low priority, favoring the RTC and the communication with the IMU; the second, to prefer burst writing, correctly sizing the vectors to store in the RAM for the temporary storage of the values coming from the IMU or sensors in general while writing on the micro SD card.

3.2.2. Network Topology

The majority of time synchronization algorithms deal with message exchange. In particular, since we are coping with a wireless connected system, along with the non-determinism coming with clock drift, other sources of synchronization noise must be taken into account, directly depending on the random nature of the radio medium.

In general, the time interval required for the synchronization message to be received from the time instance in which it leaves its source (denoted as τ) can be decomposed into five parts [25]:

- Send time (t_S): the time from the instant the message is composed to that in which it arrives to the network interface;
- Access time (t_A): waiting time for the shared communication channel to be free;
- Transmission time (t_{TX}): time needed for the sender to put the message on the communication channel;
- Propagation time (t_P): traveling time of the electromagnetic signal from the sender to the receiver.
- Reception time (t_R): the dual time of t_S

The overall delay can be expressed as in (2):

$$\tau = t_S + t_A + t_{TX} + t_P + t_R \tag{2}$$

Recalling that in a BAN we are dealing with very short distances (in 1–2 m range), the propagation time difference between two nodes can be neglected. Hence:

$$\tau \approx t_S + t_A + t_{TX} + t_R \tag{3}$$

In this paper, we consider the class of broadcast-based time synchronization algorithms. For these algorithms, the BAN coordinator sends, under some conditions, a message for triggering the correct time setting. In this way, some terms of τ can be neglected. In fact, since we have only one access to the channel, i.e., the one for sending the broadcast message, t_A can be neglected. Additionally, the message is equal for each node, so also t_S can be neglected. Then, the expression (3) further reduces in:

$$\tau \approx t_{TX} + t_R \tag{4}$$

Under these hypotheses, the greatest non-deterministic synchronization artefact is represented by t_R; it should be reduced as much as possible.

4. Platform Presentation

In this section, the synchronized multi-board wireless platform for long-term activity monitoring is discussed. The general idea is to build a flexible and expandable system composed by a wireless network of sensor nodes simultaneously providing multiple measures of different physiological and environmental signals. The organization of the used units will be discussed at a block diagram level as these were designed using standard commercial components configured according to the producers' recommendations. The core system is the synchronization mechanism which makes possible the correlation of the offline post-processed measurements made by different units that are fused for more complex analysis.

It is important to underline that this solution does not necessarily guarantee an absolute timestamp but guarantees an identical timestamp for all slaves. The accuracy of the entire system depends on the accuracy of the RTC implemented on the master. This is because in many cases it is not important to have an accurate absolute RTC system, but it is very important that for each sample of each unit there is a common synchronized timestamp that allows an *a posteriori* perfect alignment of the samples. For example, if we consider a 24 h long posture or step monitoring, an absolute delay of tens of seconds is absolutely not a problem if and only if this delay is present on all the units that compose the system. However, it is possible to change the precision of the system simply by acting on the master hardware implementation, keeping the complexity and cost of the slaves low.

In the next subsections a complete description of the system is presented, starting from the two different units used in this paper, through the architecture used for protocol implementation and the Android app used for managing the execution of the measurements.

4.1. Hardware of IMU Board

The custom designed IMUboard-HW-1-0-0 allocates a nine degrees of freedom (DoF) MPU-9250 nine-axis MEMS MotionTracking™ device from TDK-InveSense (San Jose, CA, USA). The MPU-9250 integrates on the same chip, the TDK-INV 6-axis IMU MPU-6500 and the AKM magnetometer AKM-8963 mutually connected using the AUX-I2C of the MPU-6500 [34]. The angular velocity ranges from ±250 (deg/s) to ±2000 (deg/s), while the measurement range of the acceleration is from ±2 (g) to ±16 (g). The measurement range of the magnetometer is about ±4800 (uT), the sampling rate is up to 8 kHz, and the communication clock frequency is up to 20 MHz for the Serial Peripheral Interface (SPI) reading protocol. The system core is the Nordic Semiconductor (Trondheim, Norway) SoC nRF52832 that integrates a 64 MHz ARM®Cortex™-M4 CPU with 512 kB Flash memory and 64 kB RAM. The SoC manages a multiprotocol Bluetooth 5, ANT/ANT+, and proprietary 2.4 GHz. The processor uses a micro SD card for data logging and it communicates with it in SPI bus mode using the FAT32 file system to allow direct download of the data onto a PC. The user interface uses a couple of LEDs (green and red), two push-button switches for user interaction, and one main power switch. Finally, the power is supplied to the entire system either with a CR2450 coin cell battery, using a proper battery holder on the board, or with an external battery, using the JST connector on the board. The IMUboard-HW-1-0-0 unit is depicted in Figure 6 and the block diagram shown in Figure 7 depicts its structure.

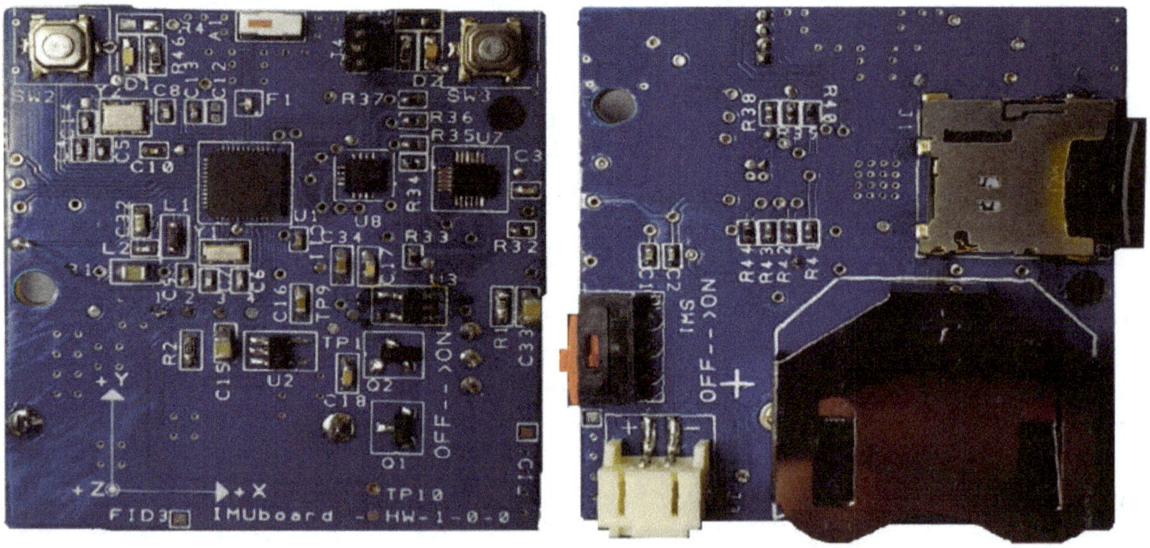

Figure 6. Top and bottom view of IMUboard-HW-1-0-0 unit.

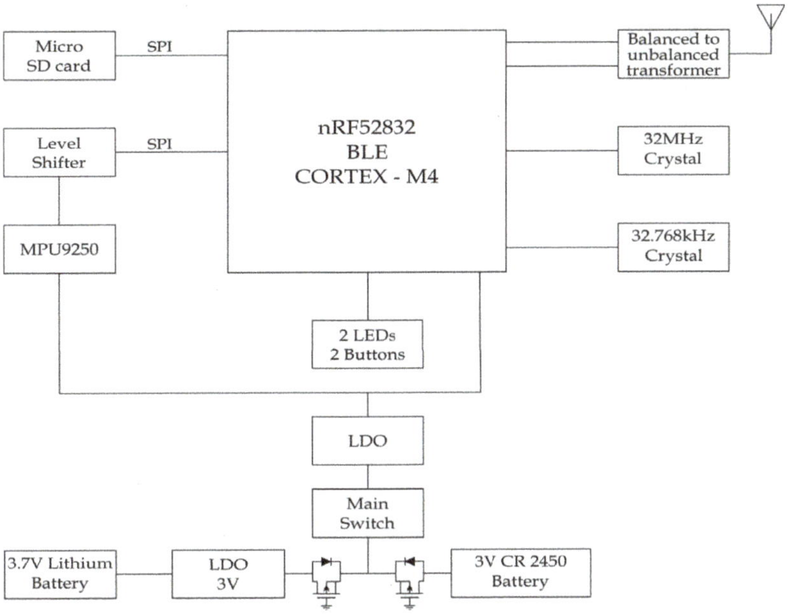

Figure 7. IMUboard-HW-1-0-0 unit block diagram.

4.2. Hardware of sEMG Board

The custom designed sEMG-HW-1-0-0 is an extension of the IMUboard-HW-1-0-0 previously described. It has onboard the circuital part for detecting and conditioning the muscle activity signal. The sEMG-HW-1-0-0 unit is depicted in Figure 8 and the block diagram is shown in Figure 9.

Figure 10 shows the circuit block schematic of the sEMG. The first stage is a differential instrumentation amplifier with a gain of about 300 *V/V*. Its output can be routed to the ADC of a processor to analyze the raw data. The second stage is a rectifier block. The signal, then, is fed to a low-pass filter (LPF) with a cut-off frequency at 3 Hz to suppress the rapid muscle contraction. The fourth stage is an amplifier with a variable gain controlled by the processor to equalize the signal amplitude coming from different quality electrodes or different muscles. The final stage is a comparator whose digital output is sampled at 50 Hz by the microprocessor and indicates that there is muscle activity. The sampling frequency used for the sEMG is independent of the IMU sampling frequency. In fact, two different threads are used for acquisitions and writing takes place on two different files. It is important to underline that each measurement is referenced over time, thereby allowing the correct temporal location of the stored measurements.

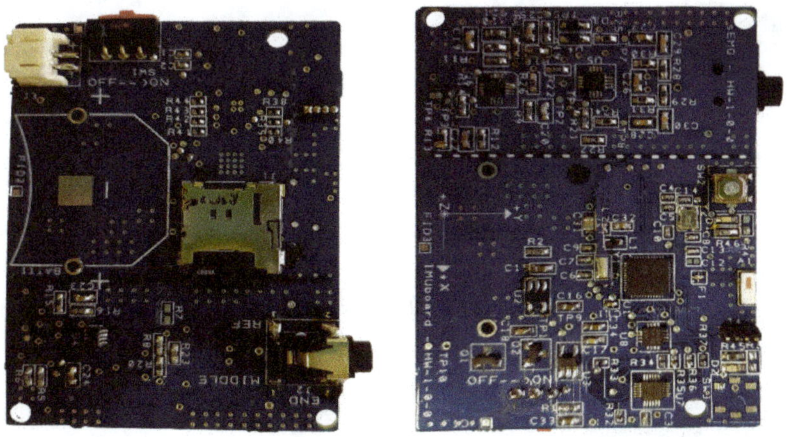

Figure 8. Top and bottom view of sEMG-HW-1-0-0 unit.

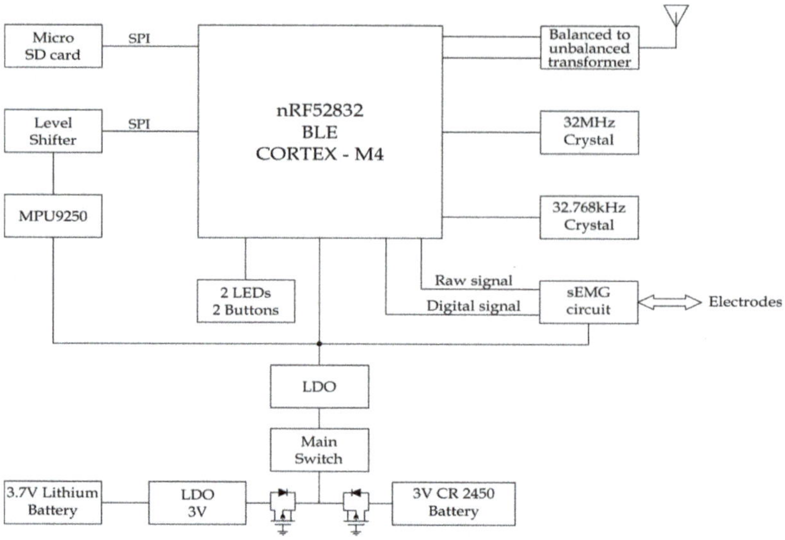

Figure 9. sEMG-HW-1-0-0 unit block diagram.

The circuital simulation performed in Keysight Advanced Design System (ADS) is reported in Figure 11. This circuit allows one to monitor the muscle activity and trigger a specific action without using the microprocessor resources.

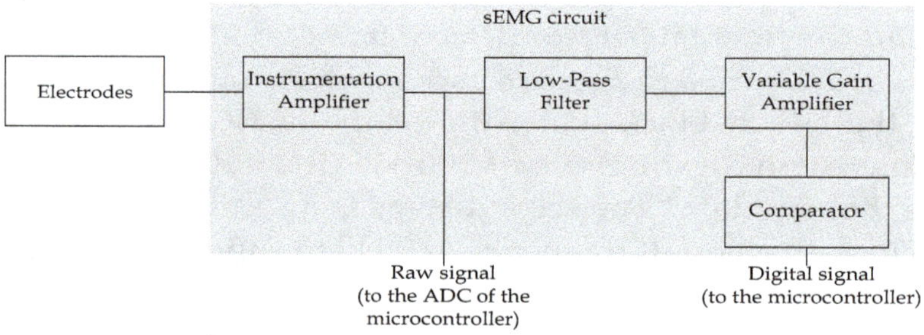

Figure 10. Superficial electromyography (sEMG) circuit block diagram.

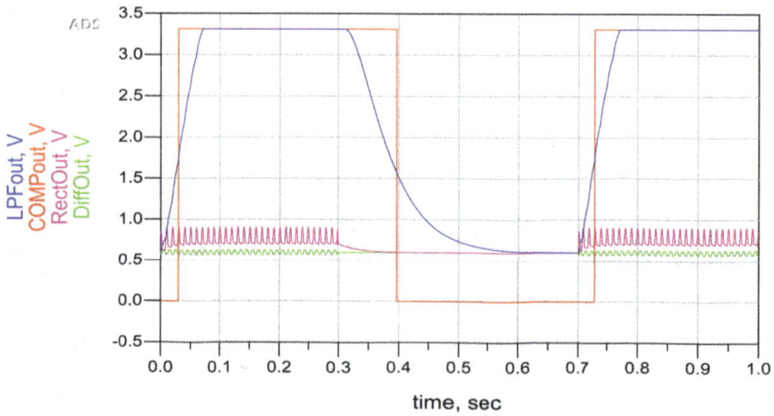

Figure 11. sEMG Advanced Design System (ADS) simulation.

4.3. Master–Slave Architecture

The protocol proposed in this work can be described as a simplified version of the fusion of RBS and FTSP protocols described in Section 2.3. The architecture used is a master–slave architecture, sketched in Figure 12, where the single master node acts as the BAN coordinator. Each BAN has a unique two-byte network ID included in the packets and used for packet filtering. Two types of messages are possible: broadcast messages with no acknowledgment feature which are used when the master needs to communicate with all the slaves in its sub-network and slaveID-oriented messages with an acknowledgment feature for any other communication. The master uses a broadcast message to send its own RTC value at predefined intervals depending on the actual hardware implementation, as it will be discussed in the preceding sections. The slaves refresh their own RTC values according to the values received by the master.

The advantage shared with the RBS protocol is that it eliminates any non-deterministic behavior introduced by the transmitter t_{TX}. The only critical issue is represented by the reception time t_R, defined in [25] as the time interval from the message reception up to the end of its processing. Differently from FTSP protocol, a simple update of the RTC register is the only task to perform during the receiving interval. Therefore, the firmware organization is quite critical because it must guarantee that computational delays are reduced to the minimum possible value.

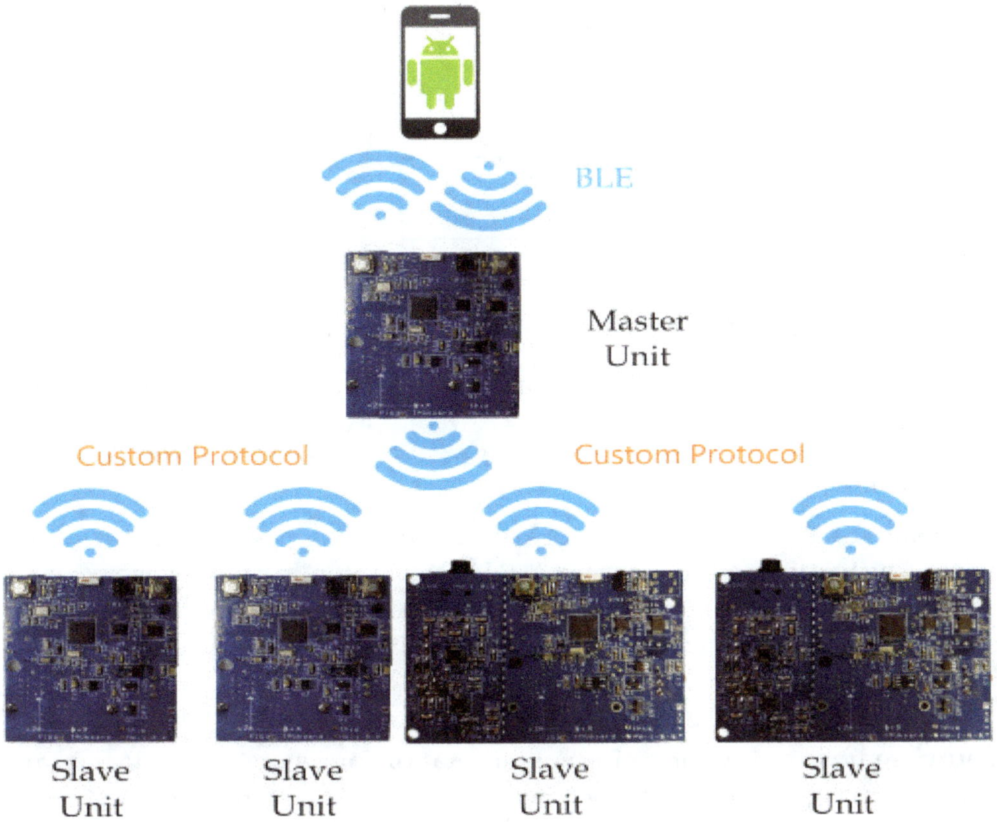

Figure 12. Master–slave architecture.

4.4. Android App

The Android app communicates with the master through Bluetooth Low Energy (BLE) protocol. It represents the user interface for starting, pausing, and stopping the local data logging for the entire system. Finally, it gives the actual RTC value at the start-up, as the units have no backup battery for keeping track of the time when switched off.

4.5. Firmware Considerations

As stated in previous sections, the greatest non-deterministic synchronization artifact is represented by t_R. The firmware should be organized while striving to reduce the elaboration time of the synchronization packet received by the slaves. The flowchart of the packet reception routine is illustrated in Figure 13 where it can be noticed that the synchronization packet is immediately processed.

Further, the micro SD card R/W interrupt level is lower than the one of the RTC module.

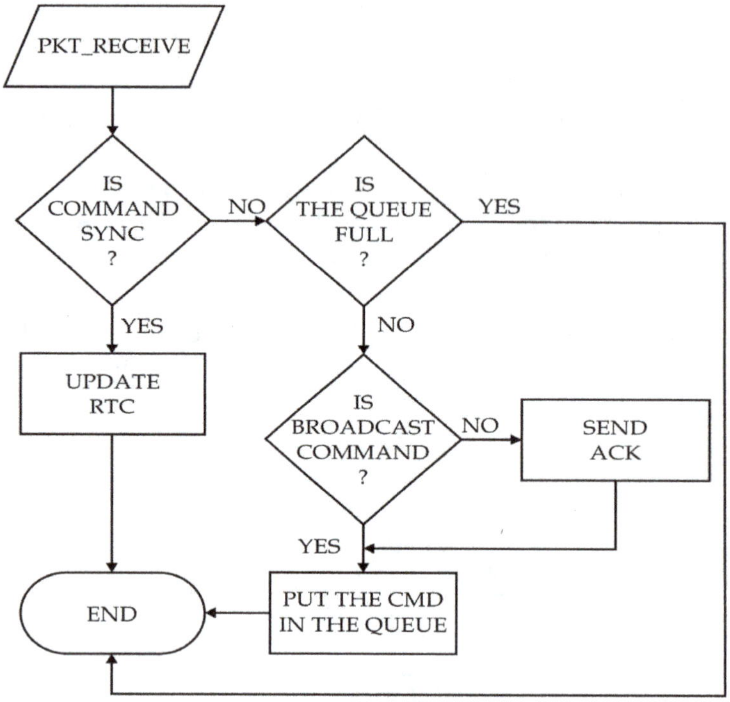

Figure 13. Flowchart of the packet reception routine.

Finally, in order to overcome the issue explained in the Section 3.1.2, the sampling frequency imposed at the IMU is about 200 Hz.

5. Experimental Results

In order to validate the platform performance, different tests were carried out in several application contexts. The hardware settings were: 200 Hz IMU sampling frequency; ≈5 ms RTC resolution; 10 ms IMU sample interval storage in the micro SD card (100 Hz equivalent sampling frequency); 20 s synchronization packet rate; ±250 dps gyroscope sensitivity; ±2 g accelerometer sensitivity.

5.1. Rotating Platform

The first setup is shown in Figure 14 where a total of four slaves, two IMUs, and two sEMGs, were mounted on a rotating platform. A microcontroller drives a stepper motor that rotates the disc according to very specific routines quasi-randomly alternating movements and pauses.

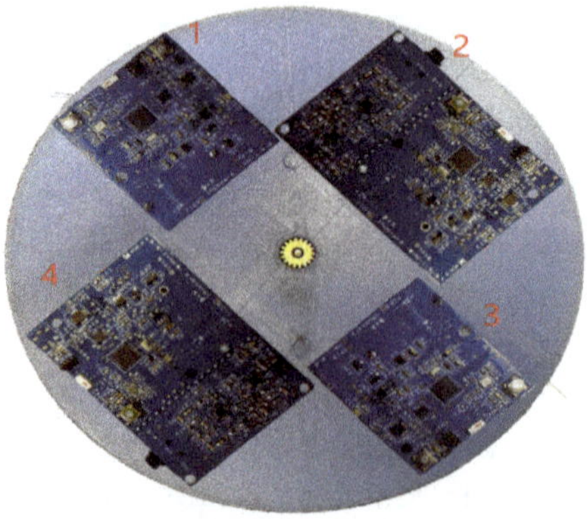

Figure 14. Experimental arrangement on a rotating platform.

Figure 15 reports the analysis of the variance (ANOVA) of the delays for each slave. To that end, the firmware has been modified, lowering the RTC resolution to 10 μs and introducing a routine for memorizing the time difference between the local and the received timestamp. The test lasted 24 h. The figure evidences that the error distribution is comparable for the four slaves used, its mean value being around 25–30 µs, and the 25th and 75th percentiles are about 15 µs and 40 µs, respectively. The reported results demonstrate that the proposed system can be used in applications with much more stringent synchronization requirements.

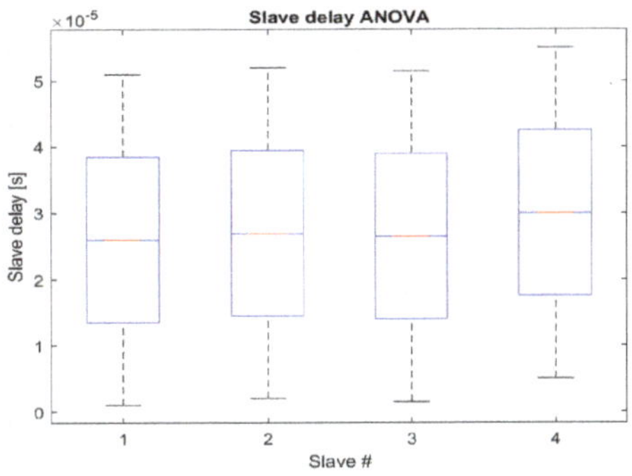

Figure 15. Analysis of the variance (ANOVA) test.

Figure 16 shows the raw values along the z-axis for each unit after about 2.5 h. Each waveform is shifted along the y-axis to improve visibility. Perfect synchronization was noticed along the x-axis, as expected. Even in this case the synchronization was perfect, and duplicate samples were not generated, nor was any missing sample reported, demonstrating the effectiveness of the proposed strategy.

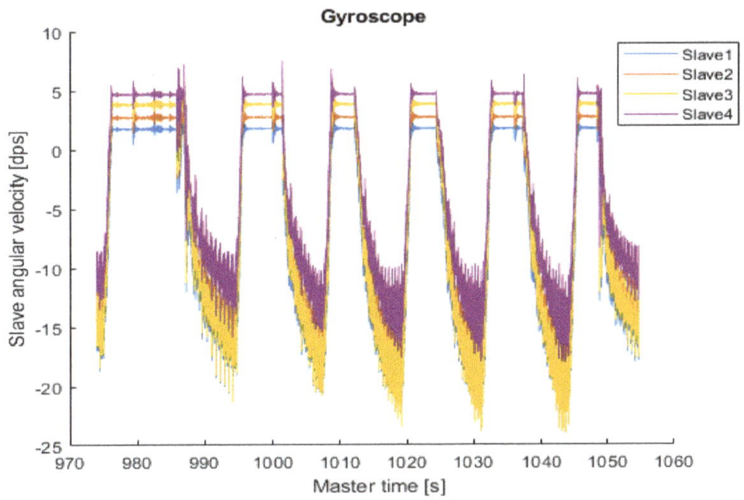

Figure 16. Gyroscope raw data.

5.2. *Walking*

As stated in the introduction, the proposed system gives the main advantage of cross-relating not only the signals coming from different similar units but even signals coming from units equipped with different sensors, allowing one, thus, to correlate heterogeneous signals and perform more complex processing.

In this configuration, one sEMG unit (slave 1) was placed on the tibia of the right leg and one IMU unit (slave 2) on the tibia of the left leg; the IMU orientation for both legs is shown in Figure 17. The electrodes were positioned, as an exercise, as in Figure 17 to analyze the relationship between muscle activity in the area of the Achilles tendon rather than that of a single muscle. Finally, the master is worn by the user in his pocket. For sake of clarity, an extract of the elaborations made on the data of a walk of a healthy individual during a 24 h logging of his daily activities will be reported and discussed below.

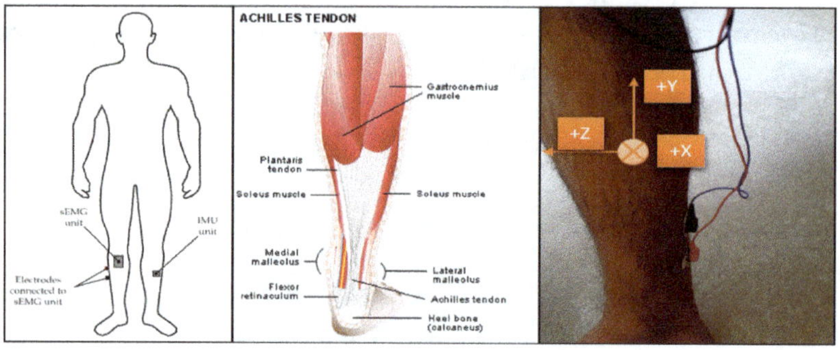

Figure 17. Units placement, achilles tendon area detail, electrode placement, and IMU orientation.

Figure 18 reports the data coming from the gyroscopes, filtered with a bandpass filter with the upper and lower cut-off frequencies of 100 Hz and 2 Hz respectively, along with the electromyography. The figure evidences both the symmetry in the movements of the two lower limbs and the presence of a periodicity in the muscles' activity in the examined region. In particular, the symmetry can be noticed in the regular zero-crossing moment distribution and in the maximum/minimum values of the measured angular speed. The sEMG ON curve has been normalized to the maximum absolute value of the other waveforms reported in the figure to better visualize it.

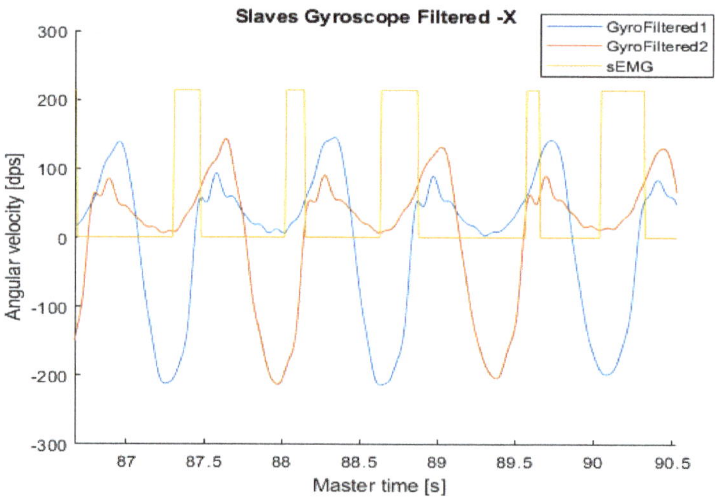

Figure 18. Gyroscope x-axis filtered data for slaves 1 and 2.

The analysis of the angles formed by the tibia in relation to electromyographic data is more relevant. In Figure 19 it is evident that in the analyzed area there is brief muscle activity both in the heel strike and midstance. In this representation the almost-perfect symmetry of the movements of the two limbs is more evident; meanwhile, the measured muscular activity is slightly variable, as it is associated with the walk of a healthy individual during his/her normal day-life, and thus not necessarily following a straight path. This implies that several distinct muscles are involved in the movements. The figure reports the overall activity in the Achille's tendon area.

Finally, as a last example, Figure 20 shows the raw data of the z-axes of the accelerometers with muscle activity. As in the previous case, the figure evidences the symmetry in the two limbs' movements. Much more interesting is the difference in the waveform reporting the accelerations along the z-axis that implies a different intensity of the two foot rests.

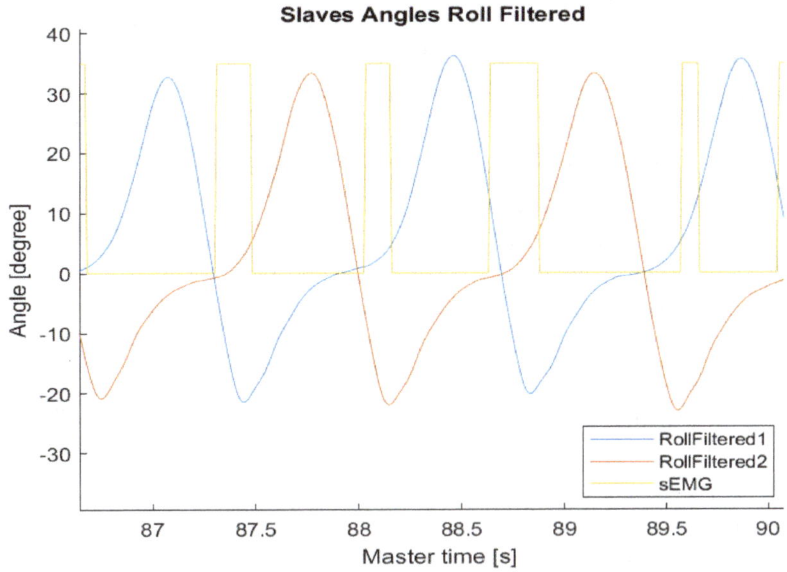

Figure 19. Roll angles for slaves 1 and 2.

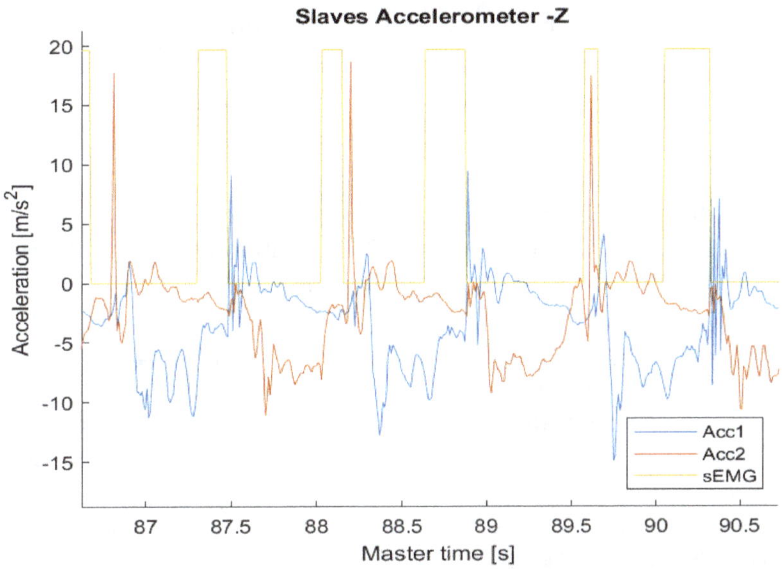

Figure 20. Accelerometer z-axis raw data for slaves 1 and 2.

6. Conclusions

The paper described a platform composed by different units and sensors to be used for long duration monitoring of daily activities. The currently installed and tested sensors are an IMU with nine DoF and a unit for sEMG capable of storing raw data or ON/OFF muscle activation information. The system uses an extremely simple synchronization protocol based on a master–slave architecture, in which the master regularly transmits the reference timestamp. Each slave of the same subnet uses the reference timestamp to avoid time-mismatches.

The reported results aim to demonstrate that all the error sources due to the time synchronization mismatch presented in Section 3 are resolved and overcome. In fact, the synchrony error is below 30 μs, a value that is far beyond the real needs in this type of application related to human activities.

It is important to underline that the measured time mismatch quantifies the slaves' ability to align with the master timestamp. We reiterate once again that it is not necessary that the master timestamp has absolute accuracy, but as demonstrated by the reported experiments, it can itself be affected by all the errors exposed in the Section 3.

The reported results demonstrated the effectiveness of the proposed approach, and most of all, its enormous potential, as it allows one to obtain even more complex processing by correlating apparently unrelated measurements by inserting different sensor types.

As a matter of fact, different in-depth analyses are possible by varying the unit number, the sensor types, the positions, and the post-processing of the measurements, allowing one to correlate apparently uncorrelated parameters. The proposed approach allows the use of non-invasive wearable units for long time periods that could evidence any possible anomaly. Usually, it is quite difficult to observe them in a regular laboratory visit where such anomalies are not detected both due to their their sporadic insurgency and the unconscious attitude to correct them while the patient focuses his/her attention on them.

An important evolution of the platform currently under analysis elects the master unit to decision hub rank, appointing him a real-time analysis of a subset of data arriving from the sensor nodes. In this scenario, the master acts as a time coordinator and decision hub. The evolution does not greatly affect the slave units moving the computational complexity to the master.

Author Contributions: Conceptualization, G.C.; Investigation, G.C.; Resources: A.F.; Validation, G.C.; Writing—original draft: G.C. and A.F.; Writing—review & editing: G.C., G.A. and A.F.; Supervision, G.A. All authors have read and agreed to the published version of the manuscript.

References

1. Giorgio, A.; Guaragnella, C. ECG Signal Denoising using Wavelet for the VLP effective detection on FPGA. In Proceedings of the 2018 AEIT International Annual Conference, Bari, Italy, 3–5 October 2018; pp. 1–5.
2. Casalino, G.; Castellano, G.; Mencar, C. Data Stream Classification by Dynamic Incremental Semi-Supervised Fuzzy Clustering. *Int. J. Artif. Intell. Tools* **2019**, *28*, 1960009. [CrossRef]
3. Ahmed, M.U.; Brickman, S.; Dengg, A.; Fasth, N.; Mihajlovic, M.; Norman, J. A machine learning approach to classify pedestrians' events based on IMU and GPS. *Int. J. Artif. Intell.* **2019**, *17*, 154–167.
4. Carli, R.; Dotoli, M.; Pellegrino, R.; Ranieri, L. Using multi-objective optimization for the integrated energy efficiency improvement of a smart city public buildings' portfolio. In Proceedings of the 2015 IEEE International Conference on Automation Science and Engineering (CASE), Gothenburg, Sweden, 24–28 August 2015; pp. 21–26.
5. Bianchi, A.; Pizzutilo, S.; Vessio, G. CoreASM-based evaluation of the N-AODV protocol for mobile ad-hoc networks. *J. Mob. Multimed.* **2016**, *12*, 31–51.
6. Parkinson, J. An essay on the shaking palsy. *J. Neuropsychiatry Clin. Neurosci.* **2002**, *14*, 223–236. [CrossRef]
7. Margiotta, N.; Avitabile, G.; Coviello, G. A wearable wireless system for gait analysis for early diagnosis of Alzheimer and Parkinson disease. In Proceedings of the 2016 5th International Conference on Electronic Devices, Systems and Applications (ICEDSA), Ras Al Khaimah, UAE, 6–8 December 2016; pp. 1–4.
8. Whittle, M.W. Chapter 4—Methods of gait analysis. In *Gait Analysis*, 4th ed.; Butterworth-Heinemann: Oxford, UK, 2007; pp. 137–175.
9. Salarian, A.; Russmann, H.; Vingerhoets, F.J.; Dehollain, C.; Blanc, Y.; Burkhard, P.R.; Aminian, K. Gait assessment in Parkinson's disease: Toward an ambulatory system for long-term monitoring. *IEEE Trans. Biomed. Eng.* **2004**, *51*, 1434–1443. [CrossRef]
10. Coviello, G.; Avitabile, G. Multiple Synchronized Inertial Measurement Unit Sensor Boards Platform for Activity Monitoring. *IEEE Sens. J.* **2020**, *20*, 8771–8777. [CrossRef]
11. Chen, M.; Gonzalez, S.; Vasilakos, A.; Cao, H.; Leung, V.C. Body area networks: A survey. *Mob. Netw. Appl.* **2011**, *16*, 171–193. [CrossRef]
12. Martinez, B.; Monton, M.; Vilajosana, I.; Prades, J.D. The power of models: Modeling power consumption for IoT devices. *IEEE Sens. J.* **2015**, *15*, 5777–5789. [CrossRef]
13. Wearable IMU Sensor | Motion Sensor | 9DOF-Shimmer3 IMU Unit. Available online: http://www.shimmersensing.com/products/shimmer3-imu-sensor (accessed on 28 May 2020).
14. NGIMU x-io Technologies. Available online: https://x-io.co.uk/ngimu/ (accessed on 28 May 2020).

15. Sun, Q.; Zhou, Z.; Jiang, J.; Hu, D. Gait cadence detection based on surface electromyography (sEMG) of lower limb muscles. In Proceedings of the 2014 International Conference on Multisensor Fusion and Information Integration for Intelligent Systems (MFI), Beijing, China, 28–29 September 2014; pp. 1–4.
16. Morbidoni, C.; Cucchiarelli, A.; Fioretti, S.; Di Nardo, F. A Deep Learning Approach to EMG-Based Classification of Gait Phases during Level Ground Walking. *Electronics* **2019**, *8*, 894. [CrossRef]
17. Luo, R.; Sun, S.; Zhang, X.; Tang, Z.; Wang, W. A Low-Cost End-to-End sEMG-Based Gait Sub-Phase Recognition System. *IEEE Trans. Neural Syst. Rehabil. Eng.* **2020**, *28*, 267–276. [CrossRef] [PubMed]
18. Laerhoven, K.V.; Gellersen, H.W.; Malliaris, Y.G. Long term activity monitoring with a wearable sensor node. In Proceedings of the International Workshop on Wearable and Implantable Body Sensor Networks (BSN'06), Cambridge, MA, USA, 3–5 April 2006; pp. 4–174.
19. Cancela, J.; Pastorino, M.; Arredondo, M.T.; Pansera, M.; Pastor-Sanz, L.; Villagra, F.; Pastor, M.A.; Gonzalez, A.P. Gait assessment in Parkinson's disease patients through a network of wearable accelerometers in unsupervised environments. In Proceedings of the 2011 Annual International Conference of the IEEE Engineering in Medicine and Biology Society, Boston, MA, USA, 30 August–3 September 2011; pp. 2233–2236.
20. Oniga, S.; Tisan, A.; Bólyi, R. Activity and health status monitoring system. In Proceedings of the 2017 IEEE 26th International Symposium on Industrial Electronics (ISIE), Edinburgh, UK, 8 August 2017; pp. 2027–2031.
21. Fischer, M.J. The consensus problem in unreliable distributed systems (a brief survey). In *Foundations of Computation Theory*; Karpinski, M., Ed.; Springer: Berlin/Heidelberg, Germany, 1983; pp. 127–140.
22. Cristian, F. Probabilistic clock synchronization. *Distrib. comput.* **1989**, *3*, 146–158. [CrossRef]
23. Gusella, R.; Zatti, S. The accuracy of the clock synchronization achieved by TEMPO in Berkeley UNIX 4.3BSD. *IEEE Trans. Softw. Eng.* **1989**, *15*, 847–853. [CrossRef]
24. Elson, J.; Girod, L.; Estrin, D. Fine-grained network time synchronization using reference broadcasts. *ACM SIGOPS Oper. Syst. Rev.* **2002**, *36*, 147–163. [CrossRef]
25. Maróti, M.; Kusy, B.; Simon, G.; Ledeczi, A. The Flooding Time Synchronization Protocol. 2004; pp. 39–49. Available online: https://dl.acm.org/doi/abs/10.1145/1031495.1031501 (accessed on 28 May 2020).
26. Wang, S.; Shi, M.; Li, D.; Du, T. A Survey of Time Synchronization Algorithms for Wireless Sensor Networks. In Proceedings of the 2019 Chinese Control Conference (CCC), Guangzhou, China, 27–30 July 2019; pp. 6392–6397.
27. AT03155: Real-Time-Clock Calibration and Compensation. Available online: http://ww1.microchip.com/downloads/en/appnotes/atmel-42251-rtc-calibration-and-compensation_ap-note_at03155.pdf (accessed on 23 March 2020).
28. Abracon 32.768 kHz Low Profile Crystal. Available online: http://abracon.com/Resonators/ABS07.pdf (accessed on 28 November 2019).
29. Blazinsek, I.; Chowdhury, A. Enhancing the accuracy of standard embedded RTC module with random synchronization events and dynamic calibration. *Przeglad Elektrotechniczny* **2016**, *92*, 248–251. [CrossRef]
30. ISL12022 RTC Accuracy Optimization Calibration Procedure—Application Note. Available online: https://www.renesas.com/us/en/www/doc/application-note/an1400.pdf (accessed on 28 November 2019).
31. Underwood, S. Implementing a Temperature Compensated RTC—Application Note. Available online: http://www.ti.com/lit/ml/slap107/slap107.pdf (accessed on 28 November 2019).
32. Munoz Diaz, E.; Heirich, O.; Khider, M.; Robertson, P. Optimal sampling frequency and bias error modeling for foot-mounted IMUs. In Proceedings of the International Conference on Indoor Positioning and Indoor Navigation, Montbeliard-Belfort, France, 28–31 October 2013; pp. 1–9.
33. Provot, T.; Chiementin, X.; Oudin, E.; Bolaers, F.; Murer, S. Validation of a High Sampling Rate Inertial Measurement Unit for Acceleration During Running. *Sensors* **2017**, *17*, 1958. [CrossRef] [PubMed]
34. TDK MPU-9250 Datasheet. Available online: https://invensense.tdk.com/wp-content/uploads/2015/02/PS-MPU-9250A-01-v1.1.pdf (accessed on 28 November 2019).

12

Castration-Resistant Prostate Cancer Outcome Prediction Using Phased Long Short-Term Memory with Irregularly Sampled Serial Data

Jihwan Park [1,2], Mi Jung Rho [2], Hyong Woo Moon [3] and Ji Youl Lee [3,*]

1 Department of Biomedicine & Health Sciences, College of Medicine, The Catholic University of Korea, Seoul 06591, Korea; bosoagalaxy@gmail.com
2 Catholic Cancer Research Institute, College of Medicine, The Catholic University of Korea, Seoul 06591, Korea; romy1018@naver.com
3 Department of Urology, Seoul St. Mary's Hospital, College of Medicine, the Catholic University of Korea, Seoul 06591, Korea; aspasias@catholic.ac.kr
* Correspondence: uroljy@catholic.ac.kr

Abstract: It is particularly desirable to predict castration-resistant prostate cancer (CRPC) in prostate cancer (PCa) patients, and this study aims to predict patients' likely outcomes to support physicians' decision-making. Serial data is collected from 1592 PCa patients, and a phased long short-term memory (phased-LSTM) model with a special module called a "time-gate" is used to process the irregularly sampled data sets. A synthetic minority oversampling technique is used to overcome the data imbalance between two patient groups: those with and without CRPC treatment. The phased-LSTM model is able to predict the CRPC outcome with an accuracy of 88.6% (precision-recall: 91.6%) using 120 days of data or 94.8% (precision-recall: 96.9%) using 360 days of data. The validation loss converged slowly with 120 days of data and quickly with 360 days of data. In both cases, the prediction model takes four epochs to build. The overall CPRC outcome prediction model using irregularly sampled serial medical data is accurate and can be used to support physicians' decision-making, which saves time compared to cumbersome serial data reviews. This study can be extended to realize clinically meaningful prediction models.

Keywords: prostate cancer; castration-resistant prostate cancer; deep learning; phased long short-term memory

1. Introduction

Prostate cancer (PCa) is one of the most common male cancers. There are more than 3.3 million men suffering from PCa in the USA [1], and its incidence is increasing in Korea [2]. Recently, a national project in Korea has been developing artificial intelligence medical software for several diseases including PCa [3].

Androgen deprivation therapy (ADT) is commonly used to treat PCa patients. However, this fails patients that are classified as having castration-resistant prostate cancer (CRPC). According to the National Cancer Institute (NCI) of the National Institute of Health (NIH), CRPC is a "prostate cancer that keeps growing even when the amount of testosterone in the body is reduced to very low levels. Many early-stage prostate cancers need normal levels of testosterone to grow, but castration-resistant prostate cancers do not." It is important to administer appropriate treatments at the right time. When a patient has appropriate treatment, it will reduce the time and pain from the treatment such as chemotherapy. However, it is a complicated problem to make a treatment decision from cumbersome medical data, which has many irregularly sampled features. To overcome this situation, a CRPC prediction model can support physicians' decision-making and will help to identify appropriate treatments for PCa patients.

At present, PCa outcomes are usually predicted using nomograms [4–7]. Recently, researchers have begun to explore the use of deep learning methods, which show some promise [8–11], but the majority of these techniques rely on image segmentation and classification [12,13]. Data from longitudinal electronic health records (EHRs) that are irregularly sampled, such as PCa data, does not fit well with deep learning prediction models. Therefore, in this study, we adopt a phased long short-term memory (phased-LTSM) method with the aim of developing a model that can predict the outcome of PCa patients from asynchronously sampled data for various variables using deep learning [14]. In particular, we will develop a model that can identify CPRC patients.

2. Materials and Methods

2.1. Materials

Data from 1592 patients who had undergone prostatectomy were used to predict the use of CRPC medication. The data consisted of clinical stage information, laboratory data, and treatment events. In total, 8 patients received CRPC medication and 1584 patients did not. We used the receipt of CPRC medication as the binary classification condition. These medications included docetaxel, cabazitaxel, abiraterone, enzalutamide, and radium-223 (see Table 1).

Table 1. Demographics of prostate cancer patients.

Category	Non-Castration-Resistant Prostate Cancer (CRPC) Medication	CRPC Medication	p-Value (chi-Squared Test)
Number of cases (n = 1592 cases)	1584	8	
Age at diagnosis (%)			0.253
<40	1 (0.1)	0 (0.0)	
40–44	3 (0.2)	0 (0.0)	
45–49	16 (1.0)	0 (0.0)	
50–54	54 (3.4)	0 (0.0)	
55–59	165 (10.4)	2 (25.0)	
60–64	303 (19.1)	1 (12.5)	
65–69	461 (29.1)	0 (0.0)	
70–74	429 (27.1)	2 (25.0)	
75–80	146 (9.2)	3 (37.5)	
80–84	6 (0.4)	0 (0.0)	
Mean	63.64	66.5	
T-stage (%)			0.008
T1	1 (0.1)	0 (0.0)	
T1a	7 (0.4)	0 (0.0)	
T1c	3 (0.2)	0 (0.0)	
T2	100 (6.3)	0 (0.0)	
T2a	141 (8.9)	0 (0.0)	
T2b	56 (3.5)	0 (0.0)	
T2c	746 (47.1)	0 (0.0)	
T3	4 (0.3)	0 (0.0)	
T3a	312 (19.7)	3 (37.5)	
T3b	195 (12.3)	4 (50.0)	
T3c	1 (0.1)	0 (0.0)	
T4	14 (0.9)	1 (12.5)	
Tx	4 (0.3)	0 (0.0)	
N-stage (%)			0.305
N0	379 (23.9)	3 (37.5)	
N1	68 (4.3)	1 (12.5)	
Nx	1137 (71.8)	4 (50.0)	
M-stage (%)			0.422
M0	304 (19.2)	3 (37.5)	
M1	3 (0.2)	0 (0.0)	
Mx	1277 (80.6)	5 (62.5)	

CRPC patients are treated with specific treatments including chemotherapy, such as docetaxel [15], cabazitaxel [16], abiraterone [17], enzalutamide [18], and radium-223 [19]. These CRPC treatments are delivered in many different combinations alongside ADT medications such as leuprorelin, bicalutamide, goserelin, and degarelix.

We preprocessed the serial data into three-dimensional (3D) vectors to use as the input for the deep learning model. Seven features were used: two laboratory data, prostate specific antigen (PSA) and PSA doubling time (DT), the use of radiation therapy (RT), and four ADT medications—leuprorelin, bicalutamide, goserelin, and degarelix. The timesteps were the days when the features were observed. However, not all of the features are observed at every interval and each observation has irregularly sampled follow-up data (see Figure 1). Because PSA is commonly examined lab data through all of the patient's follow up periods, PSA is the most important factor. PSADT shows the characteristic of PSA kinetics.

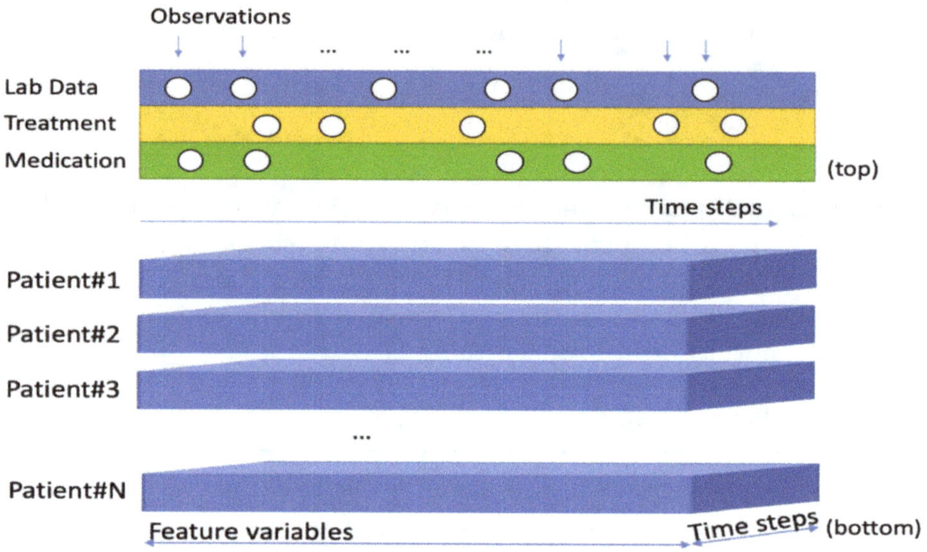

Figure 1. Irregularly collected events observations (top) 3D format input for serial data model (bottom).

2.2. *Ethics*

This study procedures were carried out in accordance with the Declaration of Helsinki and were approved by the Institutional Review Board of the Catholic University (IRB number: KC18SNDI0512). Identifying information was removed from the electronic health record (EHR) data, which was then formatted. Unless locally managed mapping information was exposed, specific patients could not be identified.

2.3. *Methods*

We used a 3D fixed time format to input serial data into the model. For the serial data modeling, a recurrent neural network (RNN) managed the data using a circular network model. Simple RNNs have a vanishing gradient problem, which cannot generate proper gradient values from repeated activation functions. The gradient value is an operator that directs the RNN's learning. The activation function calculates the gradient value for each iteration and will produce a value close to 0 after circular network executions. In contrast, long short-term memory (LSTM) uses a gating method to adjust the signal, which eliminates the vanishing gradient problem (see Figure 2). The input vector adjusts the value based on the tanh activation function. The forget vector adjust part of the previous input value to the current input. The output vector adjusts the output values using the previous input and current adjusted input. After all of these gating methods, the final output is used as the next input for the tanh and sigmoid layers.

Typically, the clinical event observations were not collected regularly. This irregular sampling meant that the intervals between consecutive events were not evenly spaced. LSTM cannot learn effectively from such data.

Phased-LSTM selectively updates the status to account for irregular sampling times through an additional time gate [14]. At each time step, the time gate switches on and off to update the state and the hidden output state. These updates only happen for the open phase. Otherwise, the previous values will be used. The time gate addresses the LSTM problems caused by irregularly sampled data (see Figure 3).

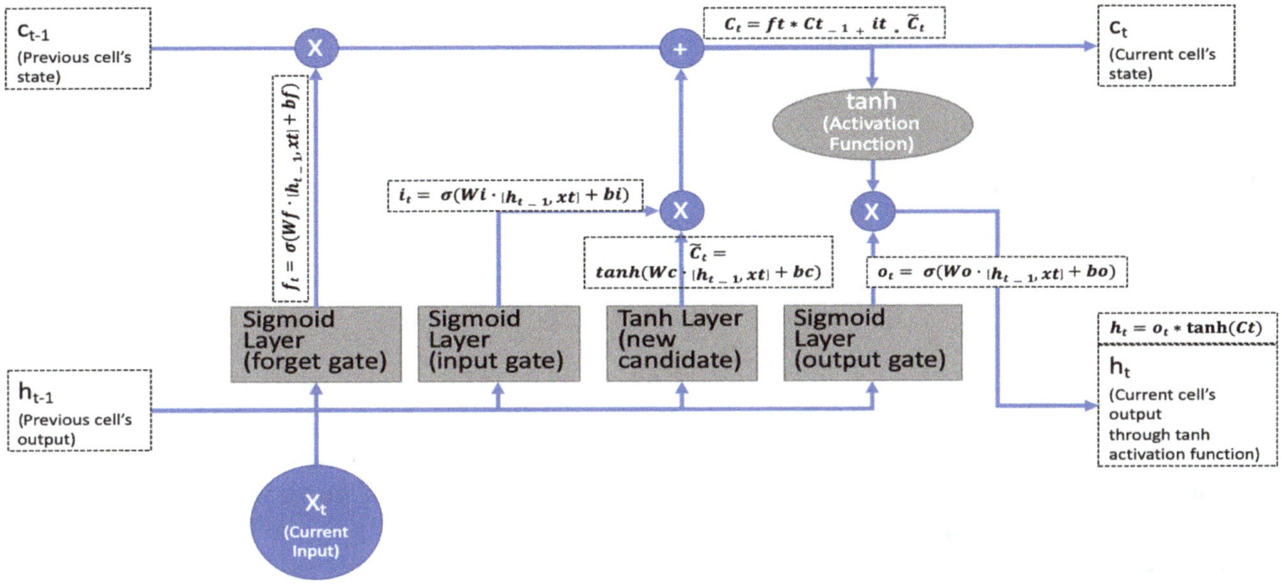

Figure 2. Standard long short-term memory (LSTM) using three gates (forget, input, and output) to eliminate the vanishing gradient problem.

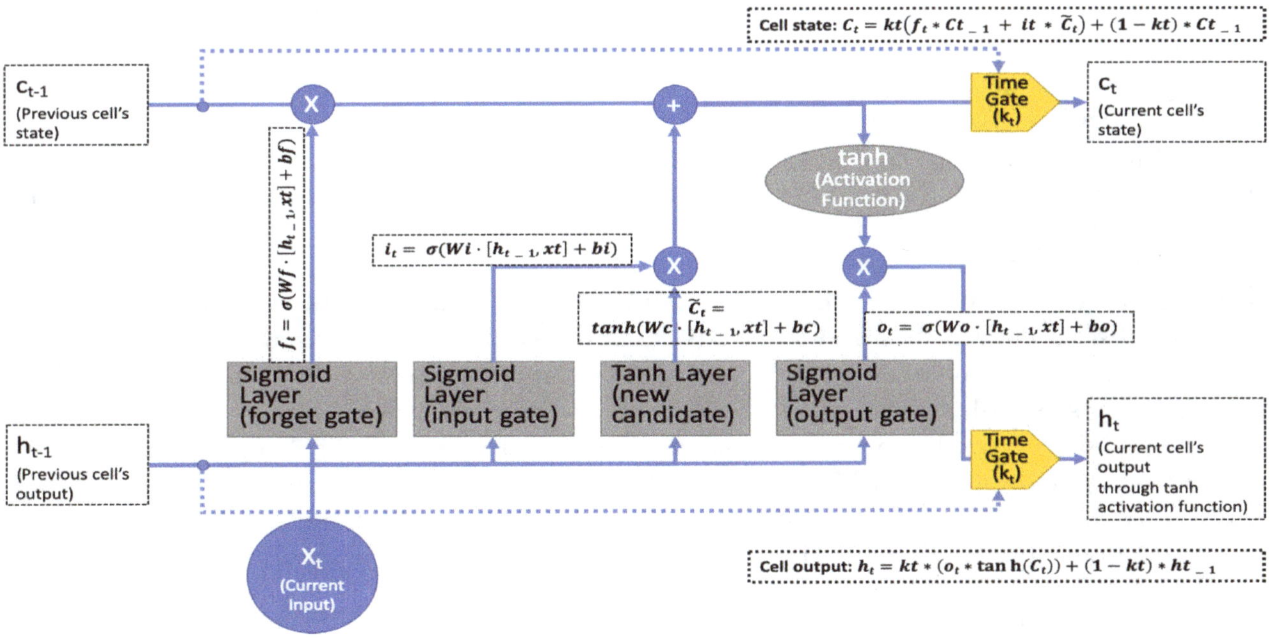

Figure 3. Phased LSTM using rectified linear units as the time-gate kt that propagates the gradient well.

There are two patterns of serial medical data: in the first, more than two features are sampled simultaneously and, in the second, some parts of the features are missing and others are not. To manage both patterns, missing imputation must be applied. The phased-LSTM's time gate addresses these patterns based on three phases (see Figure 4).

The time gate of phased-LSTM k_t has three phases: phase 1, "openness-rise" 0 to 1, phase 2, "openness-drop" 1 to 0, and phase 3, "closed" a leak at a rate α [14].

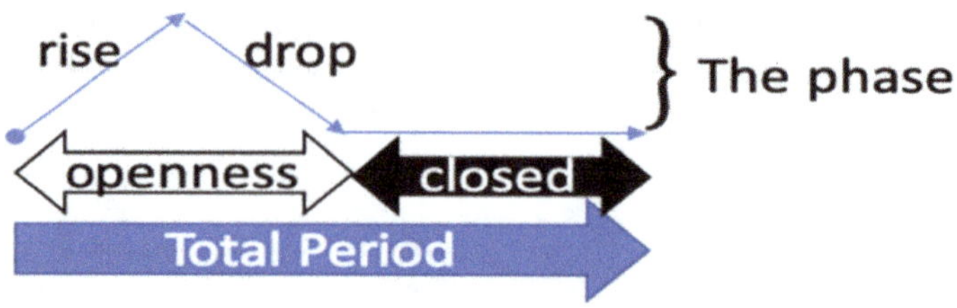

Figure 4. Phased LSTM time gate: phase visualization [14].

The time gate k_t is described by

$$\phi_t = \frac{(t-s) mod\ \tau}{\tau} \tag{1}$$

and

$$k_t \begin{cases} \frac{2\phi_t}{r_{on}}, & if\ \phi_t < \frac{1}{2} r_{on} \\ 2 - \frac{2\phi_t}{r_{on}}, & if\ \frac{1}{2} r_{on} < \phi_t < r_{on} \\ \alpha\phi_t, & otherwise \end{cases} \tag{2}$$

In this case, ϕ_t is an auxiliary variable that represents the phase of the cycle (Equation (1)), t is the time point, s is the phase shift, τ is the period that controls the real-time period, and r_{on} is the ratio of the open period to the total period τ [14].

Phased-LSTM's time gate k_t is a kind of rectified linear unit that can propagate gradient information effectively [14] (Equation (2)). Thus, k_t has three parameters: τ, s, and r_{on}. These parameters were used during the phased-LSTM model learning. During the open-phase, the rise or drop period in Figure 4 known as propagates new cell states or α-weighted gradient information. Ultimately, k_t is able to propagate irregularly sampled data selectively. In other words, it deals with complicated time series medical data effectively. Neil et al. presented this algorithm, which outperforms previous LSTM algorithms [14].

We used a chi-squared test to find the characteristic of patients' data. The chi-squared result showed the information of group differences, which represent how each of the groups performed in the study [20].

Due to the imbalance in the ratio of CRPC and non-CRPC patients, we used the synthetic minority oversampling technique (SMOTE) algorithm [21]. The SMOTE generates sample data that is similar to a prior set. This method is frequently used for imbalanced data analysis [22–25]. Based on the SMOTE oversampling algorithm, we generated a 50:50 ratio of CRPC data using the prior data.

We used k-fold cross validation to verify that the result of model training was not overfitted. The k-fold cross validation splits the data set into a k number of sets and validates the model with shuffled different sets [26]. We used 10-folds to verify the model.

The phased-LSTM prediction model was built using TensorFlow [27]. The model consists of a a phased-LSTM layer and used a SoftMax [28] dense layer to generate a binary result: CRPC or non-CRPC treated. It also used the Adam [29] optimizer and sparse_categorical_crossentropy loss function [12].

We used linear interpolation to build serial input data for the phased-LSTM model with an appropriate shape. Linear interpolation is one of the most common algorithms used to build connected serial data from data that has been irregularly recorded.

3. Results

The majority of age distribution resided between 55 and 80 years. The mean of age is 63.64 and 66.5 years for each Non-CRPC medication and CRPC medication group. The majority of T-stage data distribution resided between T2 and T3. Most of N-stage and M-stage data resided at a 0 or X stage, which means the absence of metastasis. Though it is highly imbalanced, the data distribution showed a similar shape from two groups.

Figure 5 shows the prior data shape, oversampling result, and scaling result for 120 and 360 days of serial data. We used SMOTE to generate CRPC-treated data similar to the prior CRPC cases. Lastly, we obtained balanced data (1575:1576, CRPC: non-CRPC treated) compared to the prior data that was highly imbalanced (8:1584, CRPC: non-CRPC treated).

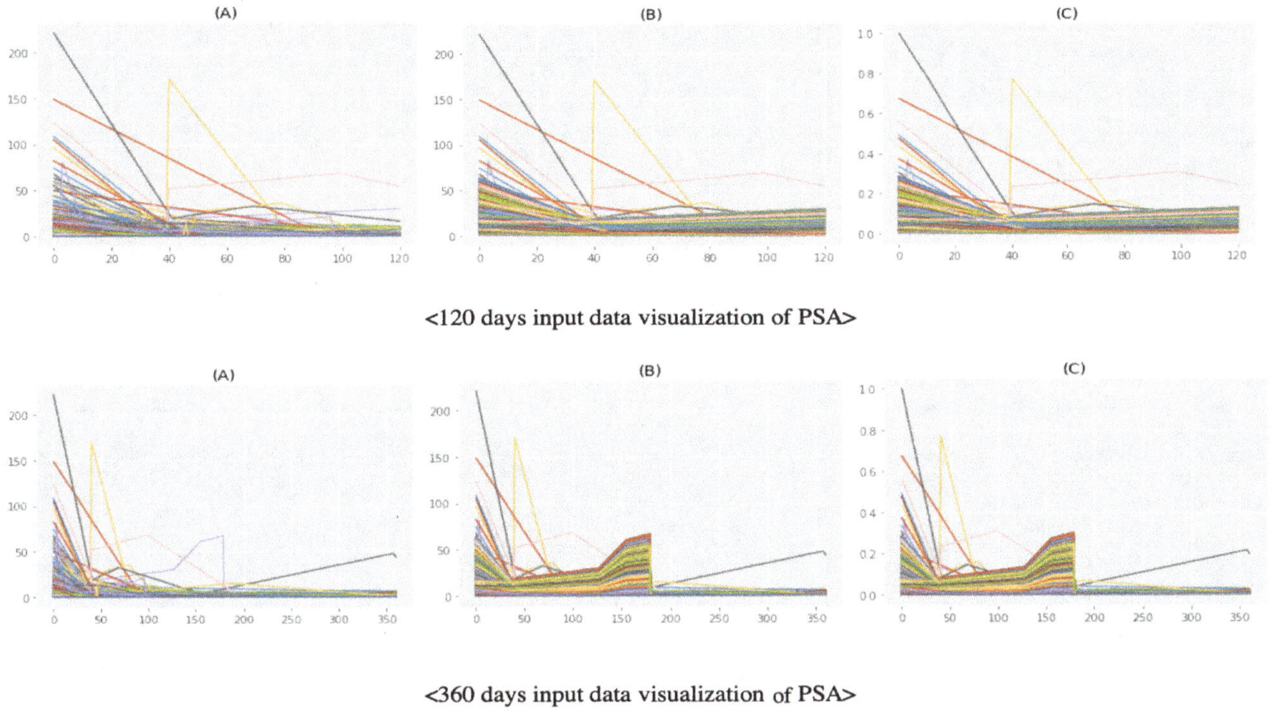

Figure 5. Shape of the input data for prostate specific antigens: (**A**) prior data, (**B**) oversampling result from prior data, and (**C**) scaling result from oversampling data.

We used two sets of serial data: 120 days and 360 days. Each set had a plus-one timestep. For instance, in the 120-day case, there were 121 (120 + 1) time steps including the start time point. The 120-day set contained 3152 cases, 121 timesteps, and seven features. The 360-day set contained 3152 cases, 361 timesteps, and seven features. The model parameter number for the model was 70,016, which was trained by the deep learning model.

Both sets used four epochs (blue lines), which is the number of training iterations. To prevent building the overfitted model, we manually determined four epochs by testing 10 epochs (see Table 2). Although the training time was short, the 120-day set has a recall precision of 91.6% and the 360-day set had a recall precision of 96.9%. The validation loss (red lines) of the 120-day set converged slowly, while that of the 360-day set converged quickly (see Figure 6). Ultimately, the Receiver Operating Characteristic/Area Under the Curve (ROCAUC) accuracy result of the 120-day model is 88.6% and the 360-day model is 94.8% (see Figure 7).

Because the loss of the model continued decreasing and the accuracy of the model continued increasing after four epochs, we did 10-fold cross-validation to verify 10 epochs' training results did not overfit (see Table 3). We have 97.81% and 97.68% average accuracy of the model's evaluations every 120 days and 360 days.

Table 2. Determining epochs to build model.

Running Result: 10 Epochs to Determine Early Stop				Running Result: Determine 4 Epochs for Preventing Overfitting			
Category	**Epoch (10)**	**Loss**	**Accuracy**	**Category**	**Epoch (4)**	**Loss**	**Accuracy**
120-day model	1	0.6892	0.5743	120-day model	1	0.6889	0.5168
	2	0.6722	0.5549		2	0.6705	0.6954
	3	0.5841	0.7257		3	0.5720	0.7756
	4	0.4445	0.8073		4	0.3924	0.8391
	5	0.2879	0.8957				
	6	0.1943	0.9379				
	7	0.1496	0.9560				
	8	0.1428	0.9615				
	9	0.1341	0.9637				
	10	0.1140	0.9701				
360-day model	1	0.6848	0.5698	360-day model	1	0.6882	0.4932
	2	0.5190	0.7969		2	0.5423	0.8196
	3	0.2708	0.9021		3	0.3228	0.8930
	4	0.2302	0.9180		4	0.2388	0.9288
	5	0.1519	0.9569				
	6	0.1065	0.9719				
	7	0.1060	0.9742				
	8	0.0861	0.9764				
	9	0.0749	0.9837				
	10	0.0942	0.9782				

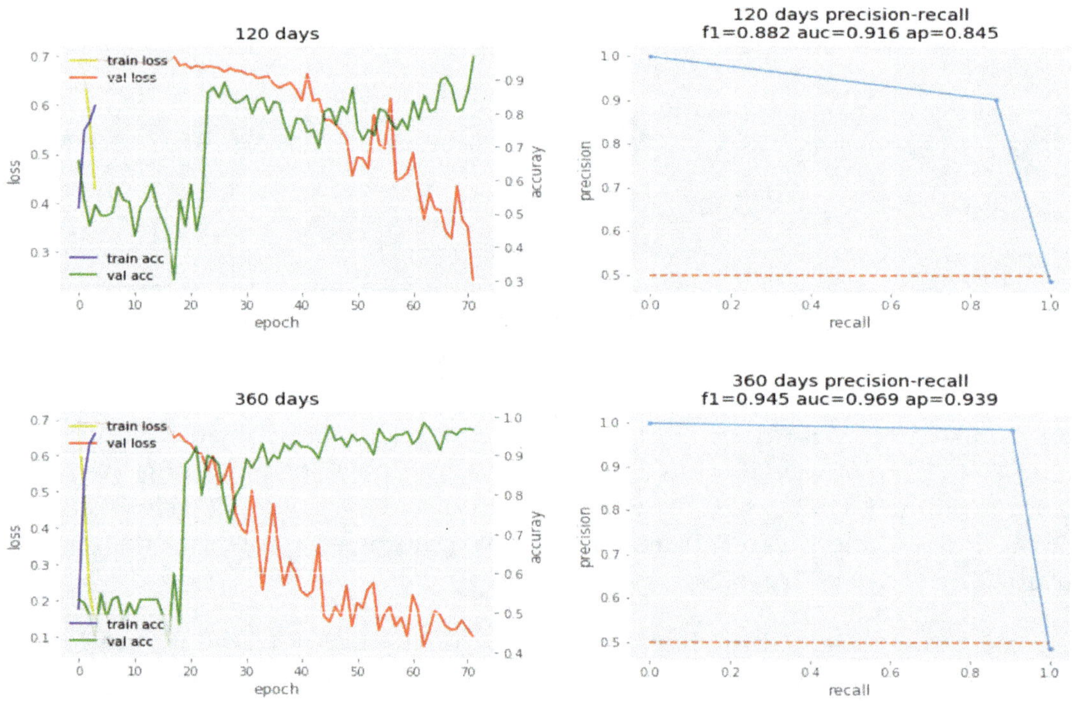

Figure 6. Phased LSTM training/validation (left) and precision-recall plots (right).

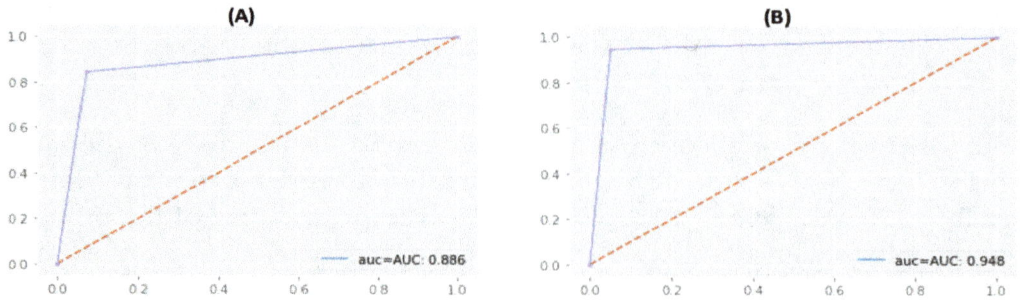

Figure 7. Accuracy Result (ROCAUC): (**A**) 120-day model's accuracy is 88.6%, (**B**) 360-day model's accuracy is 94.8%.

Table 3. 10-fold cross validation of the model.

10-Fold Cross Validation	120-Day Model		360-Day Model	
	Loss	Accuracy	Loss	Accuracy
1	0.1067	0.9778	0.2015	0.9937
2	0.0596	0.9810	0.0548	0.9873
3	0.0750	0.9778	0.1027	0.9714
4	0.1263	0.9587	0.1008	0.9778
5	0.2235	0.9841	0.0897	0.9746
6	0.1063	0.9714	0.1090	0.9746
7	0.1342	0.9905	0.0859	0.9683
8	0.2189	0.9937	0.0930	0.9746
9	0.0863	0.9810	0.1290	0.9651
10	0.1190	0.9651	0.0744	0.9810
Average	0.1256	0.9781	0.1041	0.9768

4. Discussion

In this study, we built a model to predict CPRC-treated patients. From this, we were able to draw the following conclusions.

Serial medical data is an important factor in predicting the likely outcome of patients with PCa. For example, predicting the likelihood of CRPC helps medical professionals to make appropriate decisions at the right time. Some previous studies have predicted time or variables related to CRPC. For example, Elishmereni et al. used a mathematical algorithm to predict the time until biochemical failure of ADT using data from 83 hormone sensitive prostate cancer patients [30]. Although this study only used data from 83 patients, it had a prediction accuracy of 90%. In this study, we used data from 1592 patients to predict CRPC, which is a large number of patients for building a prediction model. Another study by Humphreys et al. tried to find a relationship between age at diagnosis and CRPC. They found that those aged between 55 and 75 years have the shortest survival time [31]. We did not use age as an input variable since there was no significant difference (chi-squared test p-value of 0.253) between the groups with and without CRPC treatment (see Table 1). In another study, Angulo et al. used DNA hypermethylation profiles to predict CRPC. They found 61 genes related to CRPC [32]. However, DNA sequencing is not commonly used for PCa patients and it incurs extra expenses for the patient. We used typical follow-up data from PCa patients. A model based on commonly collected data make it more applicable in real out-patient scenarios.

We built a CRPC prediction model, which can support physicians' decision making and allows them to review more patients in a short period of time. When medical staff do not have enough time to track the status of each patient in need of significant interventions, human errors are more likely to occur and opportunities for treatment may be missed until the condition becomes serious. If prediction support is available, such as the likelihood of a PCa patient developing CPRC, patients in need of treatment can be identified quickly. Therefore, patients will receive the right treatment at the right time.

We used the state-of-the-art deep learning method to handle serial medical data. Because it is difficult to predict a patient's outcome with serial data that is collected irregularly, including medications, treatments, and laboratory test results such as blood tests. Typical deep learning methods such as RNN and LSTM can be used to analyze serial data. However, they must be improved in order to handle irregularly-sampled serial datasets. To overcome this, we adopted recently developed deep learning technology. The phased-LSTM [14] deep learning method builds a fast and accurate prediction model using serial medical data. The predictions show high precision recall scores, which means that they are highly accurate.

The results of this study can be extended to other areas such as emergency room or intensive care units, which receive a significant amount of serial data from patients. In addition, follow-up data from many patient care organizations can be used with this method to make accurate predictions that support clinicians' decision-making.

Although we produced meaningful results, this study still has some limitations. We used data from 1592 patients taken from one hospital. Because we were not permitted to use data from other hospitals for this study, we only used one hospital's data for this study. Though the data was from only one hospital, 10 years of follow-up data of 1592 patients is a big enough number to build a prediction model. Because there were many missing values for other features such as family history, genotype, and lifestyle, we built a model without those features.

In addition, we used imbalanced PCa treatment data with only a small number of CRPC-treated patients. Extremely imbalanced data is not enough to verify the model. For instance, when validation data have only a few CRPC patients out of hundreds of PCa patients, it does not make sense to verify the model's accuracy. Chawla et al. proposed SMOTE and presented results with imbalanced data sets, which has 10923 examples in the majority class and 260 examples in the minority class originally [21]. We used the SMOTE method to build oversampling data. Lastly, we got well balanced data, which has a similar shape to the prior data based on SMOTE.

In future studies, we will obtain more CRPC-treated cases in order to improve the model. However, our study is an example of how irregularly sampled serial medical data can be used to build a decision support prediction model.

Ultimately, this study shows how the state-of-the-art phased-LSTM deep learning method can be used to make meaningful prediction models based on serial medical data. This can help clinicians who want to know their patients' likely outcomes from irregularly sampled follow up data.

Author Contributions: J.P. wrote the article and helped to develop the CRPC prediction model. M.J.R. supported in writing the article and in developing the CRPC prediction model. H.W.M. gave medical advice for the development of the CRPC prediction model. J.Y.L. supervised the research and tested the CRPC prediction model. All four authors substantially contributed their expertise. All authors have read and agreed to the published version of the manuscript.

References

1. Siegel, R.; Miller, K.; Jemal, A. Cancer statistics, 2018. *CA Cancer J. Clin.* **2018**, *68*, 7–30. [CrossRef]
2. Jung, K.-W.; Won, Y.-J.; Kong, H.-J.; Lee, E.S. Cancer statistics in korea: Incidence, mortality, survival, and prevalence in 2016. *Cancer Res. Treat.* **2019**, *51*, 417–430. [CrossRef] [PubMed]
3. Park, J.; Rho, M.J.; Park, Y.H.; Jung, C.K.; Chong, Y.; Kim, C.-S.; Go, H.; Jeon, S.S.; Kang, M.; Lee, H.J. Promise clip project: A retrospective, multicenter study for prostate cancer that integrates clinical, imaging and pathology data. *Appl. Sci.* **2019**, *9*, 2982. [CrossRef]
4. Koh, H.; Kattan, M.W.; Scardino, P.T.; Suyama, K.; Maru, N.; Slawin, K.; Wheeler, T.M.; Ohori, M. A nomogram to predict seminal vesicle invasion by the extent and location of cancer in systematic biopsy results. *J. Urol.* **2003**, *170*, 1203–1208. [CrossRef] [PubMed]
5. Omlin, A.; Pezaro, C.; Mukherji, D.; Cassidy, A.M.; Sandhu, S.; Bianchini, D.; Olmos, D.; Ferraldeschi, R.; Maier, G.; Thompson, E. Improved survival in a cohort of trial participants with metastatic castration-resistant prostate cancer demonstrates the need for updated prognostic nomograms. *Eur. Urol.* **2013**, *64*, 300–306. [CrossRef] [PubMed]
6. Hirasawa, Y.; Nakashima, J.; Sugihara, T.; Takizawa, I.; Gondo, T.; Nakagami, Y.; Horiguchi, Y.; Ohno, Y.; Namiki, K.; Ohori, M. Development of a nomogram for predicting severe neutropenia associated with docetaxel-based chemotherapy in patients with castration-resistant prostate cancer. *Clin. Genitourin. Cancer* **2017**, *15*, 176–181. [CrossRef]
7. Mun, S.; Park, J.; Dritschilo, A.; Collins, S.; Suy, S.; Choi, I.; Rho, M. The prostate clinical outlook (pco) classifier application for predicting biochemical recurrences in patients treated by stereotactic body radiation therapy (sbrt). *Appl. Sci.* **2018**, *8*, 1620. [CrossRef]

8. Fakoor, R.; Ladhak, F.; Nazi, A.; Huber, M. Using deep learning to enhance cancer diagnosis and classification. In Proceedings of the International Conference on Machine Learning, Atlanta, GA, USA, 17–19 June 2013.
9. Liu, S.; Zheng, H.; Feng, Y.; Li, W. Prostate cancer diagnosis using deep learning with 3d multiparametric MRI. *arXiv* **2017**, arXiv:1703.04078.
10. Litjens, G.; Sánchez, C.I.; Timofeeva, N.; Hermsen, M.; Nagtegaal, I.; Kovacs, I.; Hulsbergen-Van De Kaa, C.; Bult, P.; Van Ginneken, B.; Van Der Laak, J. Deep learning as a tool for increased accuracy and efficiency of histopathological diagnosis. *Sci. Rep.* **2016**, *6*, 26286. [CrossRef]
11. Wang, X.; Yang, W.; Weinreb, J.; Han, J.; Li, Q.; Kong, X.; Yan, Y.; Ke, Z.; Luo, B.; Liu, T. Searching for prostate cancer by fully automated magnetic resonance imaging classification: Deep learning versus non-deep learning. *Sci. Rep.* **2017**, *7*, 15415. [CrossRef]
12. He, B.; Xiao, D.; Hu, Q.; Jia, F. Automatic magnetic resonance image prostate segmentation based on adaptive feature learning probability boosting tree initialization and cnn-asm refinement. *IEEE Access* **2017**, *6*, 2005–2015. [CrossRef]
13. Bhattacharjee, S.; Park, H.-G.; Kim, C.-H.; Prakash, D.; Madusanka, N.; So, J.-H.; Cho, N.-H.; Choi, H.-K. Quantitative analysis of benign and malignant tumors in histopathology: Predicting prostate cancer grading using svm. *Appl. Sci.* **2019**, *9*, 2969. [CrossRef]
14. Neil, D.; Pfeiffer, M.; Liu, S.-C. Phased lstm: Accelerating recurrent network training for long or event-based sequences Advances in neural information processing systems. *arXiv* **2016**, arXiv:1610.09513.
15. Bianchini, D.; Lorente, D.; Rodriguez-Vida, A.; Omlin, A.; Pezaro, C.; Ferraldeschi, R.; Zivi, A.; Attard, G.; Chowdhury, S.; De Bono, J.S. Antitumour activity of enzalutamide (mdv3100) in patients with metastatic castration-resistant prostate cancer (crpc) pre-treated with docetaxel and abiraterone. *Eur. J. Cancer* **2014**, *50*, 78–84. [CrossRef]
16. Miyoshi, Y.; Sakamoto, S.; Kawahara, T.; Uemura, K.; Yokomizo, Y.; Uemura, H. Correlation between automated bone scan index change after cabazitaxel and survival among men with castration-resistant prostate cancer. *Urol. Int.* **2019**, *103*, 279–284. [CrossRef]
17. Attard, G.; Reid, A.H.; A'Hern, R.; Parker, C.; Oommen, N.B.; Folkerd, E.; Messiou, C.; Molife, L.R.; Maier, G.; Thompson, E. Selective inhibition of cyp17 with abiraterone acetate is highly active in the treatment of castration-resistant prostate cancer. *J. Clin. Oncol.* **2009**, *27*, 3742. [CrossRef]
18. Penson, D.F.; Armstrong, A.J.; Concepcion, R.; Agarwal, N.; Olsson, C.; Karsh, L.; Dunshee, C.; Wang, F.; Wu, K.; Krivoshik, A. Enzalutamide versus bicalutamide in castration-resistant prostate cancer: The strive trial. *J. Clin. Oncol.* **2016**, *34*, 2098–2106. [CrossRef]
19. Parker, C.; Heinrich, D.; OSullivan, J.; Fossa, S.; Chodacki, A.; Demkow, T.; Cross, A.; Bolstad, B.; Garcia-Vargas, J.; Sartor, O. Overall survival benefit of radium-223 chloride (alpharadin) in the treatment of patients with symptomatic bone metastases in castration-resistant prostate cancer (crpc): A phase iii randomized trial (alsympca). *Eur. J. Cancer* **2011**, *47*, 3. [CrossRef]
20. McHugh, M.L. The chi-square test of independence. *Biochem. Med. Biochem. Med.* **2013**, *23*, 143–149. [CrossRef]
21. Chawla, N.V.; Bowyer, K.W.; Hall, L.O.; Kegelmeyer, W.P. Smote: Synthetic minority over-sampling technique. *J. Artif. Intell. Res.* **2002**, *16*, 321–357. [CrossRef]
22. Wang, J.; Xu, M.; Wang, H.; Zhang, J. Classification of imbalanced data by using the smote algorithm and locally linear embedding. In Proceedings of the 2006 8th international Conference on Signal Processing, Guilin, China, 16–20 November 2006.
23. Jeatrakul, P.; Wong, K.W.; Fung, C.C. Classification of imbalanced data by combining the complementary neural network and smote algorithm. In Proceedings of the International Conference on Neural Information Processing, Sydney, Australia, 22–25 November 2010; pp. 152–159.
24. Ditzler, G.; Polikar, R.; Chawla, N. An incremental learning algorithm for non-stationary environments and class imbalance. In Proceedings of the 2010 20th International Conference on Pattern Recognition, Istanbul, Turkey, 23–26 August 2010; pp. 2997–3000.
25. Torgo, L.; Ribeiro, R.P.; Pfahringer, B.; Branco, P. Smote for regression. In Proceedings of the Portuguese Conference on Artificial Intelligence, Azores, Portugal, 9–12 September 2013; pp. 378–389.
26. Boyce, M.S.; Vernier, P.R.; Nielsen, S.E.; Schmiegelow, F.K. Evaluating resource selection functions. *Ecol. Model.* **2002**, *157*, 281–300. [CrossRef]

27. Jia, Y.; Martín, A.; Ashish, A.; Paul, B.; Eugene, B.; Zhifeng, C.; Craig, C.; Greg, S.C.; Andy, D.; Jeffrey, D.; et al. Tensorflow: Large-Scale Machine Learning on Heterogeneous Systems. 2015. Available online: http://tensorflow.org/ (accessed on 1 October 2019).
28. Goodfellow, I.; Bengio, Y.; Courville, A. *Deep Learning*; MIT Press: Cambridge, MA, USA, 2016.
29. Kingma, D.P.; Ba, J. Adam: A method for stochastic optimization. *arXiv* **2014**, arXiv:1412.6980.
30. Elishmereni, M.; Kheifetz, Y.; Shukrun, I.; Bevan, G.H.; Nandy, D.; McKenzie, K.M.; Kohli, M.; Agur, Z. Predicting time to castration resistance in hormone sensitive prostate cancer by a personalization algorithm based on a mechanistic model integrating patient data. *Prostate* **2016**, *76*, 48–57. [CrossRef] [PubMed]
31. Humphreys, M.R.; Fernandes, K.A.; Sridhar, S.S. Impact of age at diagnosis on outcomes in men with castrate-resistant prostate cancer (crpc). *J. Cancer* **2013**, *4*, 304. [CrossRef]
32. Angulo, J.C.; Andrés, G.; Ashour, N.; Sánchez-Chapado, M.; López, J.I.; Ropero, S. Development of castration resistant prostate cancer can be predicted by a DNA hypermethylation profile. *J. Urol.* **2016**, *195*, 619–626. [CrossRef]

13

Blended Multi-Modal Deep ConvNet Features for Diabetic Retinopathy Severity Prediction

Jyostna Devi Bodapati [1], Veeranjaneyulu Naralasetti [2], Shaik Nagur Shareef [1], Saqib Hakak [3], Muhammad Bilal [4], Praveen Kumar Reddy Maddikunta [5] and Ohyun Jo [6,*]

[1] Department of CSE, Vignan's Foundation for Science Technology and Research, Guntur 522213, India; jyostna.bodapati82@gmail.com (J.D.B.); shaiknagurshareef6@gmail.com (S.N.S.)

[2] Department of IT, Vignan's Foundation for Science Technology and Research, Guntur 522213, India; veeru2006n@gmail.com

[3] Faculty of Computer Science, University of Northern British Columbia, Prince George, BC V2N 4Z9, Canada; saqib.hakak@unbc.ca

[4] Department of Computer and Electronics Systems Engineering, Hankuk University of Foreign Studies, Yongin-si 17035, Korea; m.bilal@ieee.org

[5] School of Information Technology and Engineering, The Vellore Institute of Technology (VIT), Vellore 632014, India; praveenkumarreddy@vit.ac.in

[6] Department of Computer Science, College of Electrical and Computer Engineering, Chungbuk National University, Cheongju 28644, Korea

* Correspondence: ohyunjo@chungbuk.ac.kr

Abstract: Diabetic Retinopathy (DR) is one of the major causes of visual impairment and blindness across the world. It is usually found in patients who suffer from diabetes for a long period. The major focus of this work is to derive optimal representation of retinal images that further helps to improve the performance of DR recognition models. To extract optimal representation, features extracted from multiple pre-trained ConvNet models are blended using proposed multi-modal fusion module. These final representations are used to train a Deep Neural Network (DNN) used for DR identification and severity level prediction. As each ConvNet extracts different features, fusing them using 1D pooling and cross pooling leads to better representation than using features extracted from a single ConvNet. Experimental studies on benchmark Kaggle APTOS 2019 contest dataset reveals that the model trained on proposed blended feature representations is superior to the existing methods. In addition, we notice that cross average pooling based fusion of features from Xception and VGG16 is the most appropriate for DR recognition. With the proposed model, we achieve an accuracy of 97.41%, and a kappa statistic of 94.82 for DR identification and an accuracy of 81.7% and a kappa statistic of 71.1% for severity level prediction. Another interesting observation is that DNN with dropout at input layer converges more quickly when trained using blended features, compared to the same model trained using uni-modal deep features.

Keywords: diabetic retinopathy (DR); pre-trained deep ConvNet; uni-modal deep features; multi-modal deep features; transfer learning; 1D pooling; cross pooling

---

1. Introduction

Diabetic Retinopathy (DR) is an adverse effect of Diabetes Mellitus (DM) [1] that leads to permanent blindness in humans. It is usually caused by the damage to blood vessels that provide nourishment to light-sensitive tissue called the retina. As per statistics [2], DR is the fifth leading cause for blindness across the globe. According to the World Health Organization (WHO), in 2013, around 382 million people were suffering from DR, and this number may rise to 592 million by 2025. It is possible to save many people from going blind if DR is identified in the early stages. Small lesions are formed in the eyes of DR-affected people and the type of lesions formed decides the level of severity of DR. Figure 1a shows types of lesions that include Micro Aneurysms (MA), exudates, hemorrhages, cotton wool spots, and improperly grown blood vessels on the retina.

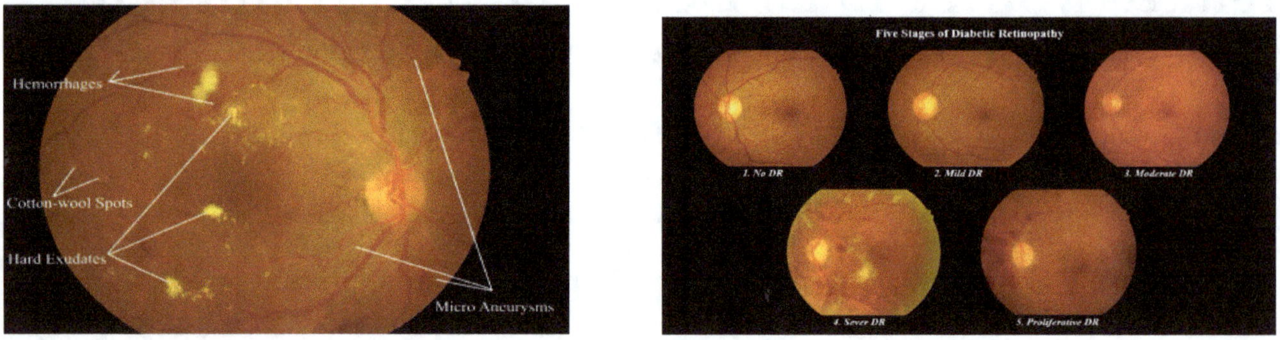

(**a**) (**b**)

Figure 1. Samples of DR-affected fundus images: (**a**) types of lesions formed; and (**b**) levels of severity.

DR can be categorized into five different stages [3]: no DR (Class 0), mild DR (Class 1), moderate DR (Class 2), severe DR (Class 3), and proliferative DR (Class 4). Sample retinal images with different severity levels of DR are shown in Figure 1b. Mild DR is the early stage during which the formation of Micro Aneurysms (MA) can be observed. As the disease progresses to moderate stage, swelling of blood vessels can be found, which leads to blurred vision. During the later non-proliferative DR (NPDR) stage, abnormal growth of blood vessels can be noticed. This stage is severe due to the blockage of a large number of blood vessels. Proliferative DR (PDR) is the advanced stage of DR; during this stage, retinal detachment along with large retinal break can be observed that leads to complete vision loss [4].

In traditional DR diagnosis approaches, manual grading of the retinal scan is required to identify the presence or absence of retinopathy. If DR is confirmed as positive, further diagnosis is recommended to identify severity level of the disease. This kind of diagnosis is quite expensive and time consuming as it demands human expertise. If DR identification is automated, then diagnosis of the disease becomes affordable to many people. In the recent past, several machine learning tools have been introduced to address this problem.

Early approaches to DR identification, where the presence or absence of DR is revealed, focuses on spotting the Hard Exudates (HEs). A dynamic threshold based Support Vector Machine (SVM) is used to segment HE in the retinal images [5]. Fuzzy C-means is used to detect HE and SVM is used to identify severity level of the disease to make the system more sophisticated [6]. SVM-based classifiers are adapted to find cotton wool spots in the retinal images.

With the introduction of deep learning, the focus of researchers has shifted from spotting HEs to MAs. A two-step CNN has been introduced to segment MAs in the given retinal scans [7]. Another CNN architecture that is trained using selective sampling approach is proposed to detect hemorrhages [8]. A max-out activation is introduced to improve the performance of a DNN model, for which DR is used as an application to find MA [9]. Recently, a bounding box based approach has been introduced to identify the region of interest in the retinal images [10]. Although many methods are available in the literature, they are either sub-optimal or complex. Hence, there is a need for a solution that is simple and robust.

The objective of this work is to design a simple and robust deep learning-based approach to recognize DR from the given retinal images. The major focus of this work is to obtain a better feature representation of the retinal images, which ultimately leads to a better model. To accomplish this, we propose uni- and multi-modal approaches. Initially, for the given retinal images, deep features are extracted from different pre-trained ConvNets such as VGG16, NASNet, Xception, and Inception ResNetV2. In the uni-modal approach, features extracted from a single pre-trained ConvNet gives the final feature representation. In the multi-modal approach, our idea is to blend the deep features extracted from multiple ConvNets to get the final feature representation. We propose different pooling-based approaches to blend multiple deep features. To check the efficiency of our feature representation, a Deep Neural Network (DNN) architecture is proposed for identification of DR (Task 1) and to recognize severity level of DR (Task 2). We observe that, in the multi-modal approach, blending deep features from Xception and Inception ResNet V2 outperforms others in both tasks. Another interesting observation is that there is a drop in the number of false positives, which is most desirable. Experimental studies on the benchmark APTOS 2019 dataset revealed that our blended feature representations trained using DNN model give superior performance compared to the existing methods.

The following are the major contributions of the proposed work:

- Effectiveness of the uni-modal feature representation is verified.
- A blended multi-modal feature representation approach is introduced
- Different pool-based approaches are proposed to blend deep features.
- A DNN architecture with dropout at the input layer is proposed to test the efficiency of the proposed uni-modal and blended multi-modal feature representations.
- APTOS 2019 benchmark dataset was used to compare the performance of the proposed approach with existing models.

2. Related Work

Recently, machine learning models are very popular to solve various problems such as image classification [11], text processing [12], real-time fault diagnosis [13], and healthcare tasks [14,15]. It is very common to use ML algorithms to address disease prediction [16–18].

In this section, we report various conventional models available in the literature for the task of DR recognition. In [19], an easy to remember scientific approach is introduced for DR severity identification. In [20], the authors presented a hybrid classifier by using both GMM and SVM as an ensemble model to improve the accuracy of the model. The same approach has been modified by augmenting the feature set with shape, intensity, and statistics of the affected region [21]. A random forest-based approach is proposed in [22,23] and segmentation-based approaches are proposed in [24]. In [25], a genetic algorithm-based feature extraction method is introduced. Different shallow classifiers such as GMM, KNN, SVM, and AdaBoost have been analyzed [26] to differentiate lesions from non-lesions. A hybrid feature extraction based approach is used in [27].

In the next few lines, deep learning models available in the literature for the task of DR severity identification are introduced. A large dataset consisting of 1,28,175 retinal images is used and trained using deep CNN. In [28], data augmentation method is used to generate the data on CNN architecture. Fuzzy models are used in [29]; a hybrid model that is designed based on fuzzy logic, Hough Transform, and numerous extraction methods are implemented as part of their system. A combination of fuzzy C-means and deep CNN architectures are used in [30]. A Siamese convolutional neural network is used in [31] to detect diabetic retinopathy.

With the introduction of deep learning models, focus has shifted to deep feature-based models. In [32], used features extracted from different layers of pre-trained ConvNets such as VGG19 and further applied PCA and SVD on those features for dimension reduction [33] to avoid overfitting. In the case of former models, the model is not robust, and, in the latter case, the models are robust, but large datasets are needed to train them. A PCA based fire-fly model [34] along with deep neural network is used for DR detection in [35], and the UCI repository is used for the experiments.

The performance of any ML algorithm is subject to the features extracted from the given data. Conventional ML models need a separate algorithm (GIST, HOG, and SIFT) for feature learning and give a global or local representation of the images and the features. Features extracted in this process are known as handcrafted features. Until the entry of deep learning models, these handcrafted features were dominant and being widely used for feature extraction.

Deep ConvNets for Feature Extraction and Transfer Learning

Deep learning models [36–38] learn the essential characteristics of the input images. This exceptional capability of the deep models make them representation models, as they can represent the data efficiently and reduce the use of the additional feature extraction phase where features are handcrafted. Deeper layers of the CNN models can represent the entire given input more efficiently than the early layers.

The downside of the deep learning models is that they need enormous amounts of data for training, which is usually scarce for most real-time applications. This problem can be addressed by the introduction of transfer learning, where the knowledge gained by a deep learning model can be transferred to other models. To achieve this, deep pre-trained CNN models such as VGG16 and ResNet152 are available for transfer learning. Pre-trained models are the models that are trained on large amounts of data, and the weights updated during the training of the complex model can be applied to similar kinds of tasks.

There are different types of pre-trained models which are trained on large scale datasets, such as ImageNet that consists of more than a million images. Popular pre-trained deep CNN models such as VGG16, VGG19, ResNet152, InceptionV3, Xception, NASNet, Inception ResNet V2 and DarkNet are briefly described below:

- **Visual Geometric Group (VGG 16):** VGG16 is a deep ConvNet trained on 14 million images belonging to 1000 different classes and topped the leader board in ILSVR (ImageNet) challenge. In this architecture, 2×2 filters are used with stride 1 for convolution operation, and 2×2 filters with stride two and the same padding are used for max-pooling operation across the network. At the end of architecture, two fully connected dense layers of 4096 neurons are connected followed by soft-max layer.
- **Neural Architecture Search Network (NASNet):** This is a special kind of deep CNN which searches for a better architectural building block on small datasets such as CIFAR10 and transfers it to larger datasets such as ImageNet. It has a better regularization mechanism called scheduled drop path, which significantly improves generalization.
- **Xception:** Xception is another deep ConvNet architecture that supports depth-wise separable convolution operations and outperformed ResNet and InceptionV3 in the ILSVR challenge.
- **Inception ResNetV2:** This is popularly known as InceptionV4, as it combines two different architectures: InceptionV3 and ResNet152. It has both inception and residual connections, which boost the performance of the model.

Deep neural networks give excellent performance only when trained with extensive data. If the data used to train are not sufficient, then the DNN models tend to overfit. Deep, convolutional neural networks are introduced in [39] for the task of scalable image recognition. Xception, a deep CNN, is developed using depth-wise separable convolutions to improve the performance [40]. A flexible architecture is defined in [41], which can search for a better convolutional cell with better regularization mechanism. All these models are trained on ImageNet Dataset for ILSVR challenge.

Our objective is to create a robust and efficient model to recognize DR with limited datasets and with limited computational resources. To achieve our objective of creating a robust model with small datasets, we seek the help of transfer learning and use various pre-trained ConvNets to extract deep features. We use the knowledge of these models to extract the most prominent features of color fundus images. A deep neural network with dropout introduced at early layers is trained to detect and classify the severity levels of diabetic retinopathy. As we introduced dropout at the input layer, deep neural network is immune to overfitting.

3. Proposed Methodology

In this work, our objective is to develop a robust and efficient model to automate DR diagnosis. We focus on the extraction of deep features that are most descriptive and discriminate, which ultimately improves the performance of DR recognition. To get an optimal representation, features are extracted from multiple pre-trained CNN architectures and are blended using pooling-based approaches. These final representations are used to train a deep neural network with a dropout at the input layer. The proposed model has three different modules: feature extraction, model training, and evaluation module.

3.1. Feature Extraction

Performance of any machine learning model is highly influenced by the feature representations and the same is applicable to models used for DR recognition. With this motivation, we propose two different approaches (uni-modal and multi-modal) to extract optimal features from the given retinal images.

In the proposed work, initial representations of the retinal images are obtained from the pre-trained VGG16, NASNet, Xception Net, and Inception ResNetV2. As each of the pre-trained models expects input images of varying sizes, the given retinal images are reshaped according to the input dimensions accepted by these models. For example, when VGG16 is used, images are reshaped to $224 \times 224 \times 3$. These reshaped retinal images are fed to the pre-trained models after removing the soft-max layer and freezing the rest of the layers. Activation outputs from the penultimate layers form the basis for the proposed feature extraction module. For each retinal image, deep features are extracted from the pre-trained ConvNets and the details are as follows:

- Each of the first (fc1) and second (fc2) fully connected layers of VGG16 produces a feature vector of 4096 dimensions.
- The final global average pooling layer of NASNet, Xception, and InceptionResNetV2 gives feature vectors of size 4032, 2048, and 1536, respectively.

Figure 2 gives the architectural details of the pre-trained VGG16, NASNet, Xception, and InceptionResNetV2 and pointers are marked at the feature extraction layers. These features form the input to the proposed uni-modal and blended multi-modal approaches to obtain the optimal feature representations of the retinal images.

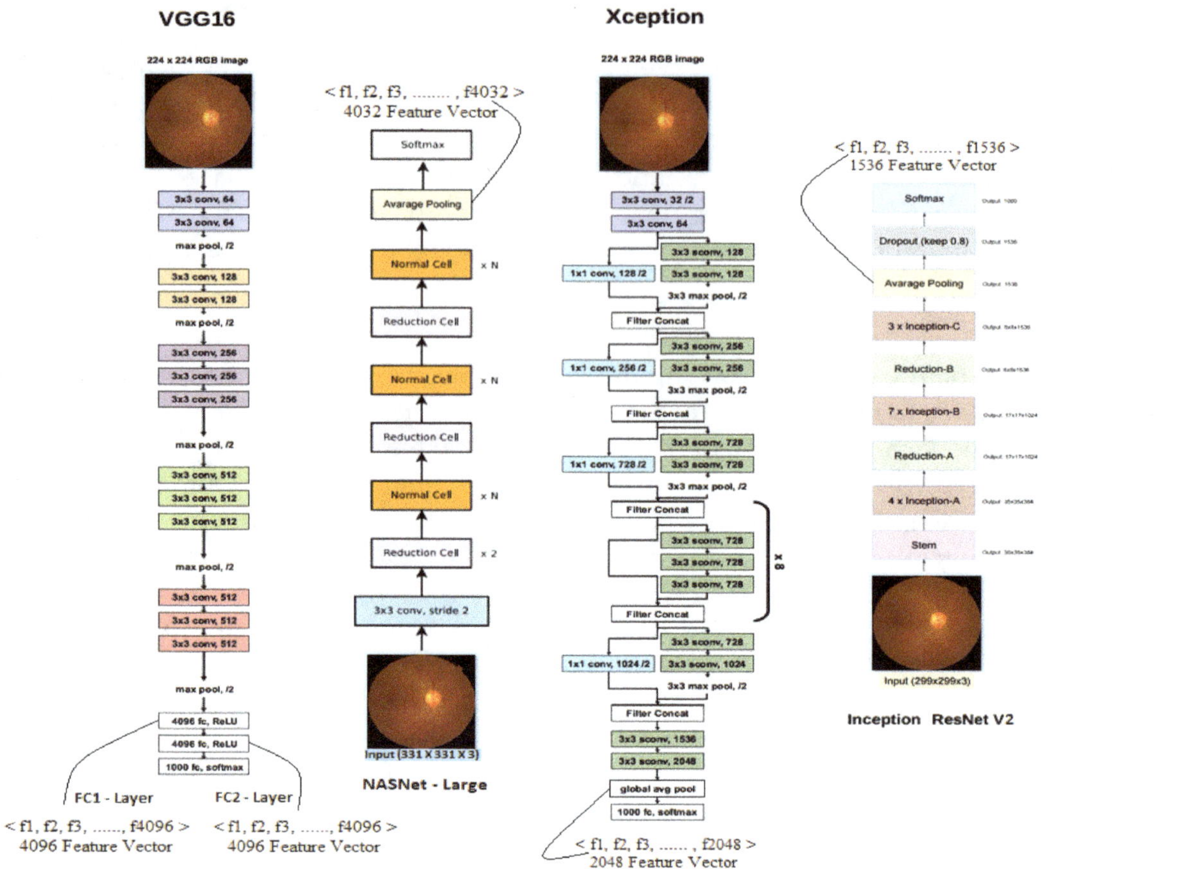

Figure 2. Architectures of various pre-trained models along with an indication of layers from which features are extracted.

3.2. Uni-Modal Deep Feature Extraction

In this approach, deep features are extracted from the final layers of one of the pre-trained ConvNets (VGG16, NASNet, Xception, or ResNet V2) to get the global representation of the retinal images. These deep features are fed to classification models for DR identification and recognition. We propose to use DNN architecture with a dropout at the input layer for DR identification and classification. Figure 3 gives the details of different stages involved in DR recognition process that uses uni-modal deep ConvNet features.

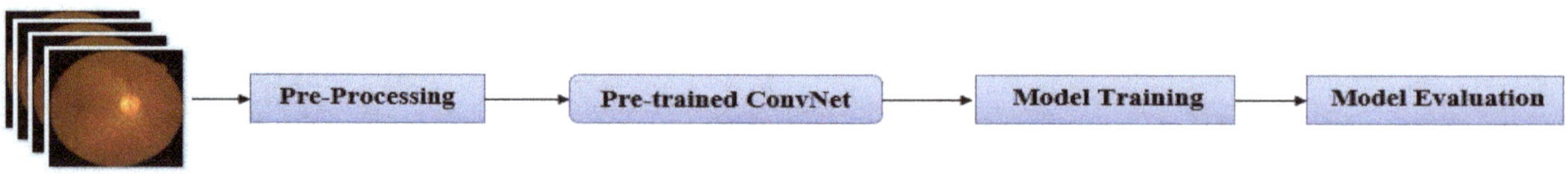

Figure 3. Stages involved in uni-modal deep feature based DR recognition.

3.3. Blended (Multi-Modal) Deep Feature Extraction

Unlike uni-modal approaches, multi-modal approaches use deep features extracted from multiple ConvNets and are blended using fusion techniques. The features obtained from different pre-trained models provide a different representation of the retinal images as they follow different architectures and are trained on different datasets. A stronger representation can be obtained by blending features from multiple ConvNets, as features of one ConvNet complement the features from other ConvNets involved in the process.

We propose various pooling approaches to fuse the deep features extracted from multiple pre-trained ConvNets. The final blended deep features provide better descriptive and discriminate representation of the retinal images. These blended features are fed to the classification models for DR identification or severity recognition. Figure 4 gives the details of different stages involved in DR recognition process that uses blended multi-modal deep ConvNet features. The proposed blended multi-modal feature extraction module uses features from both the fully connected layers of VGG16 (fc1 and fc2) and global average poling layer of Xception as input. The rationale behind choosing features of VGG16 and Xception over the others is two fold. In VGG16, each feature map of the final convolution block learns the presence of different lesions from the retinal images. Xception Net learns correlations across the 2D space; as a result, each feature map provides the comprehensive representation of the entire retinal scan. Figure 5 visualizes the feature maps obtained from the final convolution blocks of VGG16 and Xception models when a retinal image is passed to these models.

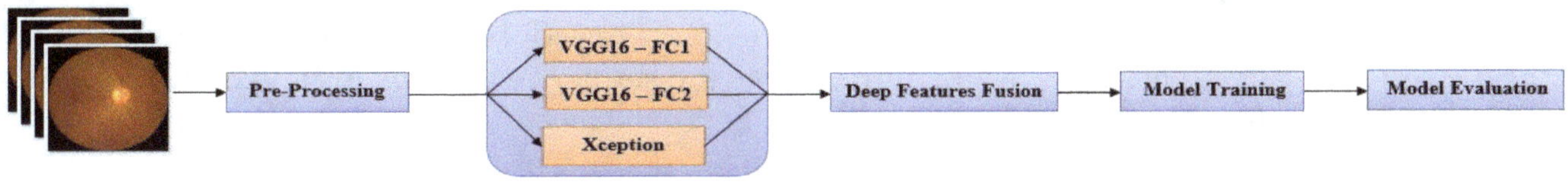

Figure 4. Stages involved in blended deep feature based DR recognition.

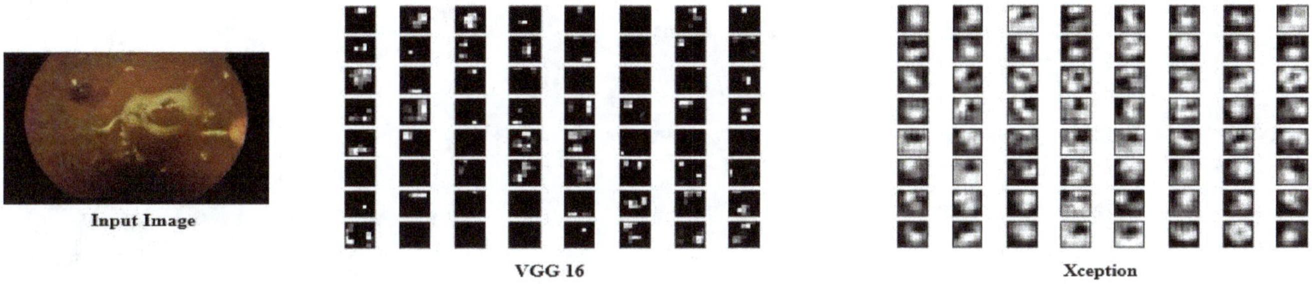

Figure 5. Visualization of the feature maps of the final convolution blocks of VGG16 and Xception models on passing retinal image as input.

Approaches to Blend Deep Features from Multiple ConvNets

In this work, two different pooling-based approaches (1D pooling and cross pooling) are proposed to fuse multi-modal deep features that are extracted from VGG16 (fc1 and fc2) and Xception. 1D pooling is used to select prominent local features from each region of VGG16, whereas cross pooling allows aggregating the prominent features obtained by 1D pooling with global representation of Xception.

1D pooling-based fusion takes one feature vector U as input and produces another feature vector $\hat{U}$, where $U \in R^{d1}$, $\hat{U} \in R^{d2}$, and $d_2 \leq d_1$. $\hat{U}$ is a reduced representation of U, where $U = \{u_1, u_2 ... u_{d1}\}$ and $\hat{U} = \{\hat{u}_1, \hat{u}_2 ... \hat{u}_{d2}\}$. Each feature element $\hat{u}_i$, of the output vector $\hat{U}$, is computed using one of the following three approaches:

$$\text{1D Max pooling:} \hat{u}_i = max(u_{i*2}, u_{i*2+1}) \; \forall i \in \{1, 2 ... d_2\} \tag{1}$$

$$\text{1D Min pooling: } \hat{u}_i = min(u_{i*2}, u_{i*2+1}); \; \forall i \in \{1, 2 ... d_2\} \tag{2}$$

$$\text{1D Average pooling: } \hat{u}_i = mean(u_{i*2}, u_{i*2+1}); \forall i \in \{1, 2 ... d_2\} \tag{3}$$

$$\text{1D Sum pooling:} \hat{u}_i = u_{i*2} + u_{i*2+1}; \forall i \in \{1, 2 ... d_2\} \tag{4}$$

In cross pooling-based feature fusion, two different feature vectors X and Y are passed as input and another feature vector Z is produced, where $X, Y, Z \in R^d$. Each feature element z_i, of the output vector Z, is computed using one of the following three approaches:

$$\text{Cross Max pooling: } z_i = max(x_i, y_i) \quad \forall i \in \{1, 2 ... d\} \tag{5}$$

$$\text{Cross Min pooling:} z_i = min(x_i, y_i) \quad \forall i \in \{1, 2...d\} \tag{6}$$

$$\text{Cross Average pooling:} z_i = mean(x_i, y_{i+1}) \forall i \in \{1, 2...d\} \tag{7}$$

$$\text{Cross Sum pooling:} \quad y_i = x_i + y_i \qquad \forall i \in \{1, 2...d\} \tag{8}$$

1D pooling is applied independently on features extracted from fc1 and fc2 layers of VGG16. Then, the cross pooling approach is applied on the resultant pooled features. This feature vector is merged with the features extracted from the Xception using cross pooling. Fusion module produces deep blended features, which are used to train the proposed DNN model. Figure 6 shows the proposed architecture of the deep feature fusion approach used to blend features from different ConvNets. As the final feature vector is a blended version of the local and global representations of the retinal images, it provides strong features. Algorithm 1 gives the sequence of steps involved in the blended multi-modal feature fusion-based DR recognition.

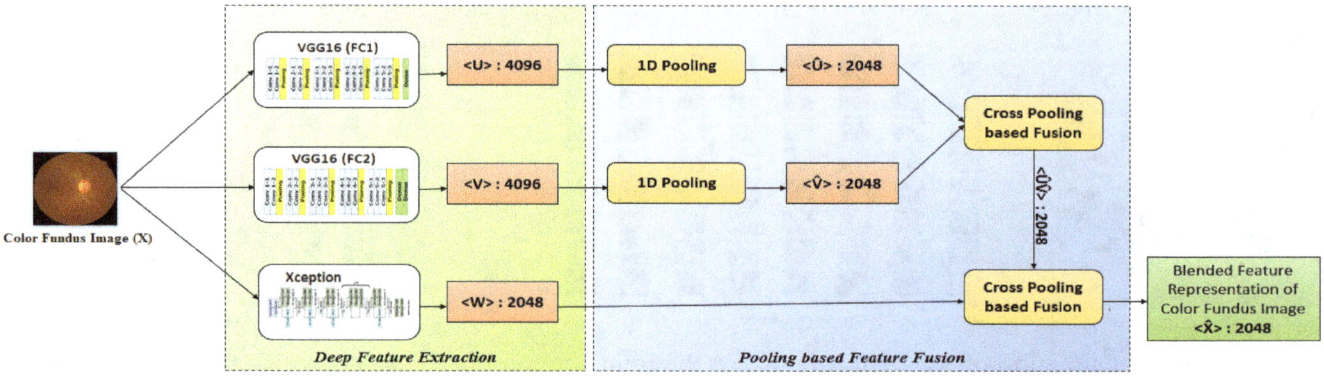

Figure 6. Approaches for fusion of features extracted from Deep ConvNets.

Algorithm 1: Blended multi-modal deep feature fusion based DR recognition task.

Input: Let D^{Tr} and D^{Tst} be the train and test datasets of fundus images, respectively, where $D^{Tr} = \{(x_i, y_i)_{i=1}^{N_{Tr}}\}$ and $D^{Tst} = \{(x_i)_{i=1}^{N_{Tst}}\}$. x_i represents ith color fundus image in the dataset and y_i is the severity level of DR associated with x_i. In the case of DR identification task, $y_i \in \{0, 1\}$, whereas, in the case of DR severity classification, task $y_i \in \{0, 1, 2, 3\}$.

Output: y_i for each $x_i \in D^{Tst}$

Step 1: Preprocess each image x_i in the dataset.

Step 2: Feature Extraction

For each preprocessed image x_i three different features (V_i, U_i, W_i) are extracted.

$V_i \leftarrow$ Features extracted from fc1 layer of VGG16

$U_i \leftarrow$ Features extracted from fc2 layer of VGG16

$W_i \leftarrow$ Features extracted from global avg pool layer of Xception

Where $V_i \in d1, U - i \in d2$ and $W_i \in d3$

Step 3: Deep feature fusion

Apply feature feature fusion on the deep features extracted from each image

$\hat{V}_i \leftarrow max(V_{i*2}, V_{i*2+1}); \quad \forall i \in \{1, 2...d_1\}$ (1D max pooling)

$\hat{U}_i \leftarrow max(U_{i*2}, U_{i*2+1}); \quad \forall i \in \{1, 2...d_2\}$ (1D max pooling)

$\hat{UV}_i \leftarrow \frac{(\hat{V}_i + \hat{U}_i)}{2}; \quad \forall i \in \{1, 2...d_2\}$ (Average Cross pooling)

$\hat{x}_i \leftarrow \frac{(\hat{UV}_i + W_i)}{2}; \quad \forall i \in \{1, 2...d_3\}$ (Average Cross pooling)

$\hat{x}_i$: blended feature vector corresponding to x_i

Step 4: Model Training

Training dataset is prepared using the blended features $D^{Tr} = \{(\hat{x}_i, y_i)\}_{i=1}^{N_{Tr}}$

Train a deep neural network (DNN) using D^{Tr}

Step 5: Model evaluation

Test dataset is prepared using the blended features $D^{Tst} = \{(\hat{x}_i)\}_{i=1}^{N_{Tst}}$

Evaluate the performance of D^{Tst}using the DNN trained in **Step 4**

3.4. Model Training and Evaluation

During this phase, we trained the ML model with deep blended pre-trained features. We preferred to use Deep Neural Network (DNN) model for training. For DR identification task, as it is a simple binary classification task, a DNN with two hidden layers with 256 and 128 units, respectively, with ReLU activation was used.

For DR severity classification task, a DNN with three hidden layers with 512, 256, and 128 units, respectively, using ReLU activation was used. For both the DNNs with the input layer, we applied 0.2 dropout to avoid the model from overfitting. This helped the model to become robust. Figure 7 represents the architecture of proposed approach for model training and evaluation.

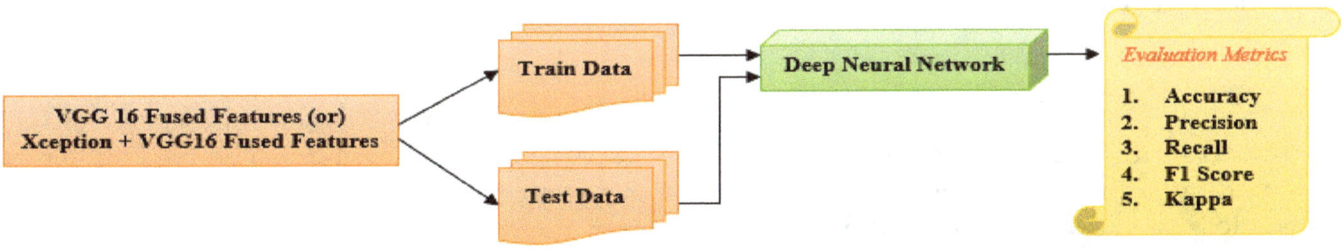

Figure 7. Training and Evaluation of DNN model for identification and recognition of DR.

4. Experimental Results

In this section, we provide details of experimental studies that were carried out to understand the efficiency of the proposed blended multi-modal deep features representation.

4.1. Dataset Summary

For the experimental studies, the APTOS 2019 kaggle benchmark dataset available as part of the blindness detection challenge was used [42]. This is a large dataset of retinal images taken using fundus photography under a variety of imaging conditions. The images are graded manually on a scale of 0 to 4 (0, no DR; 1, mild; 2, moderate; 3, severe; and 4, proliferative DR) to indicate different severity levels.

Table 1 gives the number of retinal images available in the dataset under each level of severity. We can observe that the dataset has an imbalance with more normal images and very few images in Class 3. In all experiments, 80% of the data were used for training and the remaining 20% were used for validation.

Table 1. Dataset summary of APTOS 2019 dataset.

Severity Level	# Samples
Class 0 (Normal)	1805
Class 1 (Mild Stage)	370
Class 2 (Moderate Stage)	999
Class 3 (Severe Stage)	193
Class 4 (Proliferative Stage)	295
Total	3662

4.2. Performance Measures

For the evaluation of the proposed model, we report different measures: accuracy, precision, recall, and F1 score. In addition, we used an additional metric called lappa statistic to compare an observed accuracy with an expected accuracy. Kappa Statistic is calculated as

$$\text{Kappa Score} = \frac{(\text{Observed Accuracy} - \text{Expected Accuracy})}{(1 - \text{Expected Accuracy})}$$

Observed accuracy is defined as the number of samples that are correctly classified. Expected accuracy is defined as the accuracy that a classifier would be expected to achieve, which is directly related to the number of examples of each class, along with the number of examples that the predicted value satisfied with the correct label.

4.3. DR Identification and Severity Level Prediction

The experiments carried out in this work were divided into two different tasks. In Task 1, presence or absence of DR was identified, whereas, in Task 2, the severity level was predicted for the given retinal image.

4.3.1. Task 1—DR Identification

In this task, given the DR image of a diabetic patient, we need to check whether the person is affected by retinopathy or not. DR identification is a binary classification task, thus binary cross entropy loss was used to measure the loss, and Adam optimizer was used to optimize the objective function. The dataset contains images belonging to five different classes, as shown in Table 1, and is not suitable for binary classification task. Merging all the DR-affected images into a single class gives 1857 positively labeled images and the remaining 1805 normal images are labeled as negative.

4.3.2. Task 2—Severity Level Prediction

The objective of Task 1 is to identify the presence or absence of DR, given a retinal image. While treating the DR-affected patients, mere identification of DR would not be sufficient and understanding the level of severity would be helpful for better treatment. Hence, we treat severity level identification as a separate task that categorizes the given retinal image into one of the five severity levels. Categorical cross entropy loss was used to represent loss and Adam optimizer was used to optimize the objective function.

4.4. Experimental Studies to Show the Representative Nature of Uni-Modal Features for Task 1

This experiment was carried out to understand how efficiently retinal images are represented using uni-modal features that are directly obtained from single pre-trained ConvNet. Models such as VGG16, Xception, NASNET, and ResNetV2 were considered to extract uni-modal features. For classification, models such as Naïve Bayes classifier, logistic regression, decision tree, k-Nearest Neighborhood (KNN) classifier, Multi Layered Perceptron (MLP), Support Vector Machine (SVM), and Deep Neural Network (DNN) were used.

Tables 2 and 3 show the performance of DR identification task using different ML models when the retinal images are represented with the features extracted from the first fully connected layer (fc2) of VGG16 and Xception, respectively. Based on these results, we concluded that DNN outperforms the rest of the ML models irrespective of the models. Hence, we decided to use DNN model alone in the rest of the experiments.

Table 2. Performance of ML algorithms on Task 1 using features from fc2 layer of VGG16.

Model	Accuracy	Precision	Recall	F1 Score	Kappa Statistic
Logistic Regression	97.13	97	97	97	94.27
KNN	95.36	96	95	95	90.73
Naive Bayes	77.08	82	77	76	54.45
Decision Tree	91.27	91	91	91	82.52
MLP	96.45	97	96	96	92.91
SVM (linear)	96.58	97	97	97	93.17
SVM (RBF)	96.86	97	97	97	93.73
DNN	97.32	98	98	98	94.63

Table 3. Performance of ML algorithms on Task 1 using features from Xception.

Model	Accuracy	Precision	Recall	F1 Score	Kappa Statistic
Logistic Regression	96.45	96	96	96	93
KNN	95.5	96	95	95	91
Naive Bayes	82.95	84	83	83	65.9
Decision Tree	87.59	88	88	88	75.17
MLP	96	96	96	96	91.89
SVM (linear)	96.18	96	96	96	92.36
SVM (RBF)	97.4	97	97	97	94.82
DNN	97.41	97	97	97	94.82

Table 4 shows the representative power of uni-modal features that are extracted from different pre-trained models. It is clear from the results that the performance of the DNN model varies depending on the uni-modal features used. This experiment gives a clue that each pre-trained model extracts a different set of features from retinal images. The features extracted from Xception yield better performance in terms of accuracy for the diabetic retinopathy identification task. A nominal difference in terms of accuracy and kappa score can be observed between the models trained using different uni-modal features.

Table 4. Task 1 performance using DNN trained on different uni-modal features.

Model	Accuracy	Precision	Recall	F1 Score	Kappa Statistic
VGG16-fc1	97.27	97	98	97	95.12
VGG16-fc2	97.32	98	98	98	94.63
NASNet	97.14	97	97	97	94.27
Xception	97.41	97	97	97	94.82
Inception ResNetV2	97.34	97	97	97	94.54

To better understand the representative nature of different uni-modal features, loss and number of epochs taken to converge by the DNN models are reported in Table 5. We can observe that the model trained using VGG16-Fc1 reaches minimum loss compared to the rest of the models. In terms of convergence, Xception takes only 16 epochs, whereas the Inception ResNetV2 outperforms the other models.

Table 5. Task 1: Comparison of DNN model (trained on uni-modal features) in terms of loss and number of epochs when trained on different uni-modal features.

Model	# Epochs	Loss	Accuracy
VGG16-fc1	65	0.0024	97.27
VGG16-fc2	67	0.0139	97.32
NASNet	37	0.0310	97.14
Xception	16	0.0213	97.41
Inception ResNet V2	19	0.0815	97.34

To summarize the experiments on DR identification task, features extracted from Xception, VGG16-fc2, and Inception ResnetV2 yields the same accuracy with nominal differences. However, models trained on the VGG16-fc1 features give better kappa scores compared to others. We can also observe that models trained on the VGG16-fc2 features give better performance in terms of precision, recall, and F1 scores. Regardless of the type of uni-modal features used, DNN consistently outperforms the rest of the models, especially in terms of kappa scores. The reason for the superior performance of the models trained using VGG16 and Xception features is that these models are good at extracting the lesion information that is useful to discriminate the DR-affected images from those that are not affected.

4.5. Experimental Studies to Show the Representative Nature of Uni-Modal Features for Task 2

We ran a set of experiments to understand the nature of uni-modal features for severity prediction of DR. Task 2 is more challenging compared to Task 1 as it involves multiple classes. DNN model with dropout at the input layer was used with different uni-modal features.

Based on the results reported in Table 6, we can observe the same trend that was observed in Task 1. The scores obtained for Task 2 show the complexity of severity prediction. The model trained on VGG-16+fc1 features shows superior performance to rest of the models. The same can be observed in terms of all the metrics.

Table 6. Task 2 performance using DNN trained on different uni-modal features.

Type of Uni-Modal Features	Accuracy	Precision	Recall	F1 Score	Kappa Statistic
VGG16-fc1	80.06	80	81	80	70.02
VGG16-fc2	79.81	79	80	79	68.88
NASNET	76.4	75	76	75	63.87
Xception	78.99	78	79	78	67.67
Inception ResNetV2	79.73	78	78	78	67.67

In Table 7, it is clear that, among all the pre-trained features, VGG16-fc1 yields superior performance with minimum loss. However, Xception converges in fewer epochs compared to other models.

Table 7. Task 2: Comparison of DNN model (trained on uni-modal features) in terms of loss and number of epochs when trained on different uni-modal features.

Model	# Epochs	Loss	Accuracy
VGG16-fc1	76	0.3623	80.06
VGG16-fc2	79	0.3986	79.81
NASNet	37	0.5612	76.39
Xception	23	0.4175	78.99
Inception ResNet V2	89	0.382	79.73

4.6. Performance Evaluation of the Proposed Blended Multi-Modal Features

A clue from the experiments on uni-modal features is that different uni-modal features extract different sets of features from the retinal images. If we can use multiple deep features extracted from different models, they complement each other and help to improve the scores. To benefit from more than one set of uni-modal features, we propose a blended multi-modal feature representation. This section is dedicated to show the representative power of the proposed feature representation with an application to DR identification and severity level prediction.

In addition, we applied the proposed pooling methods to blend the features from multiple pre-trained models. Initially, we blended features from the first and second fully connected layers of VGG16. Then, we extended this to the fusion of three different features from fc1 and fc2 layers of VGG16 and Xception.

4.6.1. Blended Multi-Modal Deep Features for Task 1

We experimented on the effect of blending deep features extracted from multiple pre-trained models on DR identification task. In addition, we verified the proposed maximum, sum, and average pooling approaches to blend multiple deep features.

In Table 8, we can observe that average pooling based fusion works better for DR Detection compared to other models. Using average fusion the models trained on multi-modal features leads to superior performance in terms of accuracy and kappa static. In addition, the model converges more quickly, in less than 50 epochs, and attains minimum loss. The accuracy obtained by model trained using multi-modal features is significantly better compared with to those trained on uni-modal features.

Table 8. DNN with blended multi-modal features with different fusions for Task 1.

Modalities	Pooling	Accuracy	Kappa Statistic	Epochs	Loss
VGG16-fc1 and VGG16-fc2	Max-pooling	96.12	91.89	68	0.0352
	Avg-pooling	97.39	94.61	51	0.0293
	Sum-pooling	95.5	91	64	0.0419
VGG16-fc1, VGG16-fc2 and Xception	Max-pooling	96.85	92.6	69	0.0314
	Avg-pooling	97.92	94.93	43	0.0201
	Sum-pooling	96.1	92.31	56	0.0396

4.6.2. Blended Multi-Modal Deep Features for Task 2

From the previous experiments, we understand that the models trained on multi-modal features give better performance compared to those trained on uni-modal features in the context of DR identification which is simple binary task. To understand that the proposed blended performs efficiently for more complex multi-class classification task, we applied the proposed feature representation for the severity prediction task shown in Table 9.

Table 9. DNN with blended multi-modal features with different fusions for Task 2.

Modalities	Pooling	Accuracy	Kappa Statistic	Epochs	Loss
VGG16-fc1 and VGG16-fc2	Maximum	78.06	66.87	72	0.4176
	Average	80.34	69.21	62	0.2987
	Sum	76.8	65.64	68	0.5693
VGG16-fc1, VGG16-fc2 and Xception	Maximum	79.25	67.29	74	0.3986
	Average	80.96	70.9	54	0.2619
	Sum	77.12	66.42	61	0.4782

In Table 10, we can see that average pooling based fusion of multiple deep features works better for diabetic severity prediction. Compared to the blended features from VGG16-fc1 and VGG16-fc2, the blended features from VGG16-fc1, VGG16-fc2, and Xception gives better representation. For severity prediction as well, the model that uses average pooling approach for fusion converges more quickly with better accuracy and kappa score when compared with the other approaches for fusion.

4.7. Comparison of Proposed Blended Feature Extraction with Existing Methods

In this experiment, we showed the effectiveness of the proposed DNN with dropout at the input layer trained using the proposed blended multi-modal deep feature representation and with the existing models in the literature for DR prediction. We compared the proposed model with the performances of the models used in [43,44]. In Table 10, we can see that the proposed method gives an accuracy of 80.96%, which is significantly better than existing models in the literature. When compared to the existing models, the proposed DNN model is simple with only three hidden layers with 512, 256 and 128 units each hidden layer. The confusion matrix in Figure 8 shows the mis-classifications produced by the proposed model when applied for DR severity prediction task. In the figure, we can see that most of the proliferate DR type images are predicted as moderate.

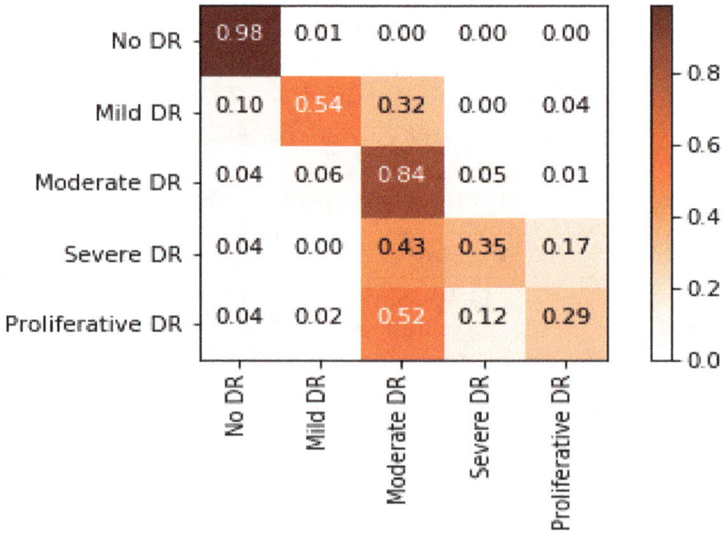

Figure 8. Confusion matrix for the severity prediction task.

As the final feature vector is a blended version of the local and global representations of the retinal images the final representation provides strong features. The reason for improvement in the performance of the proposed model is that each feature map of the final convolution block of VGG16 learns the presence of different lesions from the retinal images and Xception Net comprehensive representation of the entire retinal scan. When we combine the deep features from VGG16 and Xception gives a compact representation that gives the wholistic representation of DR images.

Table 10. Comparison of Proposed method using with existing methods.

Model	Accuracy
DR detection using Deep Learning [43]	57.2%
DR Classification Using Xception [44]	79.59
DR Classification Using InceptionV3 [44]	78.72
DR Classification Using MobileNet [44]	79.01
DR Classification Using ResNet50 [44]	74.64
Blended features + DNN (proposed)	80.96

5. Conclusions

The major objective of this work is to acquire a compact and comprehensive representation of retinal images as the feature representations extracted from retinal images significantly influence the performance of DR prediction. Initially, we extract features from deep pre-trained VGG16-fc1, CGG16-fc2 and Xception models. VGG16 model learns the lesions and Xception learns the global representation of the images. Then, the features from multiple ConvNets are blended to get final prominent representation of color fundus images. The final representation is obtained by pooling the representations from VGG16 and Xception features. A DNN model was trained using these blended features for the task of diabetic retinopathy severity level prediction. The proposed DNN model with dropout at the input avoids overfitting and converges more quickly. Our experiments on benchmark APTOS 2019 dataset showed the superiority of the proposed model when compared to the existing models. Among the proposed pooling approaches, average pooling used to fuse the features extracted from the penultimate layers of multiple pre-trained ConvNets gives better performance with minimum loss in fewer epochs compared to others.

Author Contributions: Conceptualization, J.D.B.; methodology, S.N.S.; software, S.H.; validation, M.B., P.K.R.M. and O.J.; formal analysis, O.J.; investigation, P.K.R.M.; resources, J.D.B.; writing—original draft preparation, J.D.B. and V.N.; writing—review and editing, V.N.; visualization, S.N.S.; supervision, M.B.; project administration, S.H.; funding acquisition, O.J. All authors have read and agreed to the published version of the manuscript.

References

1. Cheung, N.; Rogers, S.L.; Donaghue, K.C.; Jenkins, A.J.; Tikellis, G.; Wong, T.Y. Retinal arteriolar dilation predicts retinopathy in adolescents with type 1 diabetes. *Diabetes Care* **2008**, *31*, 1842–1846. [CrossRef] [PubMed]
2. Flaxman, S.; Bourne, R.; Resnikoff, S.; Ackland, P.; Braithwaite, T.; Cicinelli, M.; Das, A.; Jonas, J.; Keeffe, J.; Kempen, J.; et al. Global causes of blindness and distance vision impairment 1990-2020: A systematic review and meta-analysis. *Lancet Glob. Health* **2017**, *5*, e1221–e1234. [CrossRef]
3. Gulshan, V.; Peng, L.; Coram, M.; Stumpe, M.C.; Wu, D.; Narayanaswamy, A.; Venugopalan, S.; Widner, K.; Madams, T.; Cuadros, J.; et al. Development and validation of a deep learning algorithm for detection of diabetic retinopathy in retinal fundus photographs. *JAMA* **2016**, *316*, 2402–2410. [CrossRef] [PubMed]
4. Williams, R.; Airey, M.; Baxter, H.; Forrester, J.M.; Kennedy-Martin, T.; Girach, A. Epidemiology of diabetic retinopathy and macular oedema: A systematic review. *Eye* **2004**, *18*, 963–983. [CrossRef] [PubMed]
5. Long, S.; Huang, X.; Chen, Z.; Pardhan, S.; Zheng, D. Automatic detection of hard exudates in color retinal images using dynamic threshold and SVM classification: Algorithm development and evaluation. *BioMed Res. Int.* **2019**, *2019*, 3926930. [CrossRef]
6. Haloi, M.; Dandapat, S.; Sinha, R. A Gaussian scale space approach for exudates detection, classification and severity prediction. *arXiv* **2015**, arXiv:1505.00737.
7. Noushin, E.; Pourreza, M.; Masoudi, K.; Ghiasi Shirazi, E. Microaneurysm detection in fundus images using a two step convolution neural network. *Biomed. Eng. Online* **2019**, *18*, 67.

8. Grinsven, M.; Ginneken, B.; Hoyng, C.; Theelen, T.; Sanchez, C. Fast convolution neural network training using selective data sampling. *IEEE Trans. Med. Imaging* **2016**, *35*, 1273–1284. [CrossRef]
9. Haloi, M. Improved microaneurysm detection using deep neural networks. *arXiv* **2015**, arXiv:1505.04424.
10. Srivastava, R.; Duan, L.; Wong, D.W.; Liu, J.; Wong, T.Y. Detecting retinal microaneurysms and hemorrhages with robustness to the presence of blood vessels. *Comput. Methods Programs Biomed.* **2017**, *138*, 83–91. [CrossRef]
11. Bodapati, J.D.; Veeranjaneyulu, N. Feature Extraction and Classification Using Deep Convolutional Neural Networks. *J. Cyber Secur. Mobil.* **2019**, *8*, 261–276. [CrossRef]
12. Bodapati, J.D.; Veeranjaneyulu, N.; Shaik, S. Sentiment Analysis from Movie Reviews Using LSTMs. *Ingénierie des Systèmes d'Information* **2019**, *24*, 125–129. [CrossRef]
13. Zhuo, P.; Zhu, Y.; Wu, W.; Shu, J.; Xia, T. Real-Time Fault Diagnosis for Gas Turbine Blade Based on Output-Hidden Feedback Elman Neural Network. *J. Shanghai Jiaotong Univ. (Sci.)* **2018**, *23*, 95–102. [CrossRef]
14. Xia, T.; Song, Y.; Zheng, Y.; Pan, E.; Xi, L. An ensemble framework based on convolutional bi-directional LSTM with multiple time windows for remaining useful life estimation. *Comput. Ind.* **2020**, *115*, 103182. [CrossRef]
15. Moreira, M.W.; Rodrigues, J.J.; Korotaev, V.; Al-Muhtadi, J.; Kumar, N. A comprehensive review on smart decision support systems for health care. *IEEE Syst. J.* **2019**, *13*, 3536–3545. [CrossRef]
16. Gadekallu, T.R.; Khare, N.; Bhattacharya, S.; Singh, S.; Maddikunta, P.K.R.; Srivastava, G. Deep neural networks to predict diabetic retinopathy. *J. Ambient Intell. Humaniz. Comput.* **2020**. [CrossRef]
17. Patel, H.; Singh Rajput, D.; Thippa Reddy, G.; Iwendi, C.; Kashif Bashir, A.; Jo, O. A review on classification of imbalanced data for wireless sensor networks. *Int. J. Distrib. Sens. Netw.* **2020**, *16*, 1550147720916404. [CrossRef]
18. Reddy, G.T.; Reddy, M.P.K.; Lakshmanna, K.; Rajput, D.S.; Kaluri, R.; Srivastava, G. Hybrid genetic algorithm and a fuzzy logic classifier for heart disease diagnosis. *Evol. Intell.* **2019**, *13*, 185–196. [CrossRef]
19. Wu, L.; Fernandez-Loaiza, P.; Sauma, J.; Hernandez-Bogantes, E.; Masis, M. Classification of diabetic retinopathy and diabetic macular edema. *World J. Diabetes* **2013**, *4*, 290. [CrossRef]
20. Akram, M.U.; Khalid, S.; Khan, S.A. Identification and classification of microaneurysms for early detection of diabetic retinopathy. *Pattern Recognit.* **2013**, *46*, 107–116. [CrossRef]
21. Akram, M.U.; Khalid, S.; Tariq, A.; Khan, S.A.; Azam, F. Detection and classification of retinal lesions for grading of diabetic retinopathy. *Comput. Biol. Med.* **2014**, *45*, 161–171. [CrossRef] [PubMed]
22. Casanova, R.; Saldana, S.; Chew, E.Y.; Danis, R.P.; Greven, C.M.; Ambrosius, W.T. Application of random forests methods to diabetic retinopathy classification analyses. *PLoS ONE* **2014**, *9*, e98587. [CrossRef] [PubMed]
23. Verma, K.; Deep, P.; Ramakrishnan, A. Detection and classification of diabetic retinopathy using retinal images. In Proceedings of the 2011 Annual IEEE India Conference, Hyderabad, India, 16–18 December 2011; pp. 1–6.
24. Welikala, R.; Dehmeshki, J.; Hoppe, A.; Tah, V.; Mann, S.; Williamson, T.H.; Barman, S. Automated detection of proliferative diabetic retinopathy using a modified line operator and dual classification. *Comput. Methods Programs Biomed.* **2014**, *114*, 247–261. [CrossRef] [PubMed]
25. Welikala, R.A.; Fraz, M.M.; Dehmeshki, J.; Hoppe, A.; Tah, V.; Mann, S.; Williamson, T.H.; Barman, S.A. Genetic algorithm based feature selection combined with dual classification for the automated detection of proliferative diabetic retinopathy. *Comput. Med. Imaging Graph.* **2015**, *43*, 64–77. [CrossRef]
26. Roychowdhury, S.; Koozekanani, D.D.; Parhi, K.K. DREAM: Diabetic retinopathy analysis using machine learning. *IEEE J. Biomed. Health Inform.* **2013**, *18*, 1717–1728. [CrossRef]
27. Mookiah, M.R.K.; Acharya, U.R.; Martis, R.J.; Chua, C.K.; Lim, C.M.; Ng, E.; Laude, A. Evolutionary algorithm based classifier parameter tuning for automatic diabetic retinopathy grading: A hybrid feature extraction approach. *Knowl. Based Syst.* **2013**, *39*, 9–22. [CrossRef]
28. Porter, L.F.; Saptarshi, N.; Fang, Y.; Rathi, S.; Den Hollander, A.I.; De Jong, E.K.; Clark, S.J.; Bishop, P.N.; Olsen, T.W.; Liloglou, T.; et al. Whole-genome methylation profiling of the retinal pigment epithelium of individuals with age-related macular degeneration reveals differential methylation of the SKI, GTF2H4, and TNXB genes. *Clin. Epigenet.* **2019**, *11*, 6. [CrossRef]
29. Rahim, S.S.; Jayne, C.; Palade, V.; Shuttleworth, J. Automatic detection of microaneurysms in colour fundus images for diabetic retinopathy screening. *Neural Comput. Appl.* **2016**, *27*, 1149–1164. [CrossRef]

30. Dutta, S.; Manideep, B.; Basha, S.M.; Caytiles, R.D.; Iyengar, N. Classification of diabetic retinopathy images by using deep learning models. *Int. J. Grid Distrib. Comput.* **2018**, *11*, 89–106. [CrossRef]
31. Zeng, X.; Chen, H.; Luo, Y.; Ye, W. Automated diabetic retinopathy detection based on binocular Siamese-like convolutional neural network. *IEEE Access* **2019**, *7*, 30744–30753. [CrossRef]
32. Mateen, M.; Wen, J.; Song, S.; Huang, Z. Fundus image classification using VGG-19 architecture with PCA and SVD. *Symmetry* **2019**, *11*, 1. [CrossRef]
33. Reddy, G.T.; Reddy, M.P.K.; Lakshmanna, K.; Kaluri, R.; Rajput, D.S.; Srivastava, G.; Baker, T. Analysis of Dimensionality Reduction Techniques on Big Data. *IEEE Access* **2020**, *8*, 54776–54788. [CrossRef]
34. Bhattacharya, S.; Kaluri, R.; Singh, S.; Alazab, M.; Tariq, U. A Novel PCA-Firefly based XGBoost classification model for Intrusion Detection in Networks using GPU. *Electronics* **2020**, *9*, 219. [CrossRef]
35. Gadekallu, T.R.; Khare, N.; Bhattacharya, S.; Singh, S.; Reddy Maddikunta, P.K.; Ra, I.H.; Alazab, M. Early Detection of Diabetic Retinopathy Using PCA-Firefly Based Deep Learning Model. *Electronics* **2020**, *9*, 274. [CrossRef]
36. Jindal, A.; Aujla, G.S.; Kumar, N.; Prodan, R.; Obaidat, M.S. DRUMS: Demand response management in a smart city using deep learning and SVR. In Proceedings of the 2018 IEEE Global Communications Conference (GLOBECOM), Abu Dhabi, UAE, 9–13 December 2018; pp. 1–6.
37. Vinayakumar, R.; Alazab, M.; Srinivasan, S.; Pham, Q.V.; Padannayil, S.K.; Simran, K. A Visualized Botnet Detection System based Deep Learning for the Internet of Things Networks of Smart Cities. *IEEE Trans. Ind. Appl.* **2020**. [CrossRef]
38. Alazab, M.; Khan, S.; Krishnan, S.S.R.; Pham, Q.V.; Reddy, M.P.K.; Gadekallu, T.R. A Multidirectional LSTM Model for Predicting the Stability of a Smart Grid. *IEEE Access* **2020**, *8*, 85454–85463. [CrossRef]
39. Simonyan, K.; Zisserman, A. Very deep convolutional networks for large-scale image recognition. *arXiv* **2014**, arXiv:1409.1556.
40. Chollet, F. Xception: Deep learning with depthwise separable convolutions. In Proceedings of the 2017 IEEE Conference on Computer Vision and Pattern Recognition (CVPR), Honolulu, HI, USA, 21–26 July 2017; pp. 1251–1258.
41. Zoph, B.; Vasudevan, V.; Shlens, J.; Le, Q.V. Learning transferable architectures for scalable image recognition. In Proceedings of the 2018 IEEE/CVF Conference on Computer Vision and Pattern Recognition, Salt Lake City, UT, USA, 18–23 June 2018; pp. 8697–8710.
42. APTOS 2019. Available online: https://www.kaggle.com/c/aptos2019-blindness-detection (accessed on 30 December 2019).
43. Gargeya, R.; Leng, T. Automated identification of diabetic retinopathy using deep learning. *Ophthalmology* **2017**, *124*, 962–969. [CrossRef]
44. Kassani, S.H.; Kassani, P.H.; Khazaeinezhad, R.; Wesolowski, M.J.; Schneider, K.A.; Deters, R. Diabetic Retinopathy Classification Using a Modified Xception Architecture. In Proceedings of the 2019 IEEE International Symposium on Signal Processing and Information Technology (ISSPIT), Ajman, UAE, 10–12 December 2019; pp. 1–6.

Permissions

All chapters in this book were first published by MDPI; hereby published with permission under the Creative Commons Attribution License or equivalent. Every chapter published in this book has been scrutinized by our experts. Their significance has been extensively debated. The topics covered herein carry significant findings which will fuel the growth of the discipline. They may even be implemented as practical applications or may be referred to as a beginning point for another development.

The contributors of this book come from diverse backgrounds, making this book a truly international effort. This book will bring forth new frontiers with its revolutionizing research information and detailed analysis of the nascent developments around the world.

We would like to thank all the contributing authors for lending their expertise to make the book truly unique. They have played a crucial role in the development of this book. Without their invaluable contributions this book wouldn't have been possible. They have made vital efforts to compile up to date information on the varied aspects of this subject to make this book a valuable addition to the collection of many professionals and students.

This book was conceptualized with the vision of imparting up-to-date information and advanced data in this field. To ensure the same, a matchless editorial board was set up. Every individual on the board went through rigorous rounds of assessment to prove their worth. After which they invested a large part of their time researching and compiling the most relevant data for our readers.

The editorial board has been involved in producing this book since its inception. They have spent rigorous hours researching and exploring the diverse topics which have resulted in the successful publishing of this book. They have passed on their knowledge of decades through this book. To expedite this challenging task, the publisher supported the team at every step. A small team of assistant editors was also appointed to further simplify the editing procedure and attain best results for the readers.

Apart from the editorial board, the designing team has also invested a significant amount of their time in understanding the subject and creating the most relevant covers. They scrutinized every image to scout for the most suitable representation of the subject and create an appropriate cover for the book.

The publishing team has been an ardent support to the editorial, designing and production team. Their endless efforts to recruit the best for this project, has resulted in the accomplishment of this book. They are a veteran in the field of academics and their pool of knowledge is as vast as their experience in printing. Their expertise and guidance has proved useful at every step. Their uncompromising quality standards have made this book an exceptional effort. Their encouragement from time to time has been an inspiration for everyone.

The publisher and the editorial board hope that this book will prove to be a valuable piece of knowledge for researchers, students, practitioners and scholars across the globe.

List of Contributors

Jeongbae Jeon
Spatial Information Research Institute, Korea Land and Geospatial Informatix Corporation, Jeonju 54870, Korea

Solhee Kim
Interdisciplinary Program in Agricultural and Forest Meteorology, College of Agriculture and Life Sciences, Seoul National University, Seoul 08826, Korea

Gu Hyun Kang
Department of Emergency Medicine, KangNam Medical Center, College of Medicine, Hallym University, Seoul 07441, Korea

Kyo Suh
Graduate School of International Agricultural Technology, Institute of Green Bio Science Technology, Seoul National University, Pyeongchang 25354, Korea

Elias Moons, Abbas Akkasi and Marie-Francine Moens
Department of Computer Science, KU Leuven, 3000 Leuven, Belgium

Aditya Khanna
Department of Computer Science, KU Leuven, 3000 Leuven, Belgium
Department of Electrical Engineering, IIT Bombay, Maharashtra 400076, India

Junsheng Yu, Xiangqing Wang and Jinglin Guo
School of Electronic Engineering, Beijing University of Posts and Telecommunications, Beijing 100876, China

Xiaodong Chen
Queen Mary University of London, London E1 4NS, UK

Daniel Clavel, Cristian Mahulea and Manuel Silva
Department of Computer Science and Systems Engineering, University of Zaragoza, 50018 Zaragoza, Spain

Jorge Albareda
"Lozano Blesa" Hospital of Zaragoza, 50009 Zaragoza, Spain

Sarah A. Ebiaredoh-Mienye, Ebenezer Esenogho and Theo G. Swart
Center for Telecommunication, Department of Electrical and Electronic Engineering Science, University of Johannesburg, Johannesburg 2006, South Africa

Joaquín Rodríguez
Vibot ERL Laboratory, Université de Bourgogne Franche-Comté, IUT Le Creusot, 12 rue de la Fonderie, 71200 Le Creusot, France

Gilberto Ochoa-Ruiz
Tecnologico de Monterrey, School of Engineering and Sciences, Ave. Eugenio Garza Sada 2501, Monterrey, N.L., México 64849, Mexico

Christian Mata
Centre for Technological Risk Studies, Universitat Politècnica de Catalunya, 08034 Barcelona, Spain

Vytautas Abromavičius, Darius Plonis, Deividas Tarasevičius and Artūras Serackis
Department of Electronic Systems, Vilnius Gediminas Technical University, Naugarduko str. 41, 03227 Vilnius, Lithuania

Martín Hernández-Ordoñez and Guillermo Efren Ovando-Chacon
Department of Metal-Mechanics, México National Technological/I.T. Campus, Veracruz 91860, Mexico

Marco Aurelio Nuño-Maganda, Carlos Adrián Calles-Arriaga and José Margarito Canseco-Cortinas
Intelligent Systems Department, Polytechnic University of Victoria, Tamaulipas 87138, Mexico

Abelardo Rodríguez-León
Department of Systems and Computing, México National Technological/I.T. Campus, Veracruz 91860, Mexico

Rolando Salazar-Hernández
Facultad de Comercio, Administración y Ciencias Sociales, Universidad Autónoma de Tamaulipas, Tamaulipas 87000, Mexico

Omar Montaño-Rivas
Academy of Information Technologies, Polytechnic University of San Luis Potosí, San Luis 78369, Mexico

Muhammad Ijaz, Gang Li, Yussif Moro Awelisah and Ling Lin
State Key Laboratory of Precision Measurement Technology and Instrument, Tianjin University, Tianjin 300072, China
China and Tianjin Key Laboratory of Biomedical Detecting Techniques and Instruments, Tianjin University, Tianjin 300072, China

Huiquan Wang
School of life sciences, Tiangong University, Tianjin 300387, China

Ahmed M. El-Sherbeeny
Industrial Engineering Department, College of Engineering, King Saud University, Riyadh 11421, Saudi Arabia

Anis Koubaa
Robotics and Internet-of-Things Lab, Prince Sultan University, Riyadh 11586, Saudi Arabia
CISTER, INESC-TEC, ISEP, Polytechnic Institute of Porto, 4249-015 Porto, Portugal

Alam Noor
Robotics and Internet-of-Things Lab, Prince Sultan University, Riyadh 11586, Saudi Arabia

Zhengdong Lei, Laura Fasanella and Luc Mongeau
Department of Mechanical Engineering, McGill University, Montreal, QC H3A 0C3, Canada

Lisa Martignetti and Nicole Yee-Key Li-Jessen
School of Communication Sciences and Disorders, McGill University, Montreal, QC H3A 1G1, Canada

Giuseppe Coviello, Gianfranco Avitabile and Antonello Florio
Department of Electrical and Information Engineering, Polytechnic University of Bari, 70126 Bari, Italy

Jihwan Park
Department of Biomedicine & Health Sciences, College of Medicine, The Catholic University of Korea, Seoul 06591, Korea
Catholic Cancer Research Institute, College of Medicine, The Catholic University of Korea, Seoul 06591, Korea

Mi Jung Rho
Catholic Cancer Research Institute, College of Medicine, The Catholic University of Korea, Seoul 06591, Korea

Hyong Woo Moon and Ji Youl Lee
Department of Urology, Seoul St. Mary's Hospital, College of Medicine, the Catholic University of Korea, Seoul 06591, Korea

Jyostna Devi Bodapati and Shaik Nagur Shareef
Department of CSE, Vignan's Foundation for Science Technology and Research, Guntur 522213, India

Veeranjaneyulu Naralasetti
Department of IT, Vignan's Foundation for Science Technology and Research, Guntur 522213, India

Saqib Hakak
Faculty of Computer Science, University of Northern British Columbia, Prince George, BC V2N 4Z9, Canada

Muhammad Bilal
Department of Computer and Electronics Systems Engineering, Hankuk University of Foreign Studies, Yongin-si 17035, Korea

Praveen Kumar Reddy Maddikunta
School of Information Technology and Engineering, The Vellore Institute of Technology (VIT), Vellore 632014, India

Ohyun Jo
Department of Computer Science, College of Electrical and Computer Engineering, Chungbuk National University, Cheongju 28644, Korea

Index

www.ingramcontent.com/pod-product-compliance
Lightning Source LLC
LaVergne TN
LVHW081028210926
848485LV00004B/969